Neurosurgery Research Progress

Medicine & Health
New York

Neurosurgery Research Progress

Advances in Neurosurgery Research
Amit Agrawal, MD, Pradeep Chouksey, MD, Adesh Shrivastava, MD, Sumit Raj, MD and Rakesh Mishra, MD (Editors)
2022. ISBN: 978-1-68507-859-1 (Hardcover)
2022. ISBN: 979-8-88697-061-6 (eBook)

Neurosurgery Research: An Update
Amit Agrawal, MD (Editor)
Pradeep Chouksey, MD (Editor)
Adesh Shrivastava, MD (Editor)
Sumit Raj, MD (Editor)
Rakesh Mishra, MD (Editor)
2022. ISBN: 978-1-68507-837-9 (Hardcover)
2022. ISBN: 979-8-88697-076-0 (eBook)

The Handbook of Neuromodulation (2 Volume Set)
Albert J. Fenoy, MD, Georgios Matis, MD, PhD, Pritam Majumdar, PhD, Sait Ozturk, MD (Editors)
2022. ISBN: 978-1-68507-617-7 (Hardcover)
2022. ISBN: 978-1-68507-789-1 (eBook)

Neuroendoscopic Procedures and Challenges
Soner Duru, MD (Editor)
2021. ISBN: 978-1-68507-092-2 (Softcover)
2021. ISBN: 978-1-68507-155-4 (eBook)

More information about this series can be found at
https://novapublishers.com/product-category/series/neurosurgery-research-progress/

Irina Savvina
Editor

Aneurysmal Subarachnoid Hemorrhage

From Diagnosis to Treatment

nova
Medicine & Health
New York

DOI: https://doi.org/10.52305/DNGF4073

Library of Congress Cataloging-in-Publication Data

ISBN: 979-8-88697-251-1

Published by Nova Science Publishers, Inc. † New York

Contents

Foreword

I have the privilege of accepting an invitation from the editor and publisher of the manuscript Aneurysmal Subarachnoid Hemorrhage: From Diagnosis to Treatment to write this foreword.

As a neurosurgeon, I think it is of great importance to discuss the problem of emergency neurosurgery due to cerebral aneurysm rupture in a combination of diagnostic and therapeutic approaches based on the latest knowledge in the field of fundamental medicine.

The manuscript Aneurysmal Subarachnoid Hemorrhage: From Diagnosis to Treatment reviews the pathophysiology, morphology, clinical presentation, diagnosis, and management of patients with nontraumatic SAH due to the rupture of cerebral aneurysms. This type of hemorrhagic stroke is a neurosurgical emergency with still high morbidity and mortality.

Over the past decades, the incidence of SAH has remained the same; however, hospital mortality has decreased significantly. We believe that this is because of our deeper understanding of the pathophysiological mechanisms of this type of stroke, admission of patients to high-volume centers under the management of specialized teams with a multidisciplinary approach involving neuroradilogists, neurosurgeons, anesthesiologists and neurointensivists; rapid identification and cure the source of bleeding.

For forty years, we have been moving towards more minimally invasive surgical procedures to secure the aneurysm. In the book, international experts highlight that endovascular treatment with coil embolization, stents and flow diverters has now become the first line option for most patients. Nevertheless, microsurgical clipping and timely decompression of the brain remain extremely important options in the treatment of patients with aneurysmal SAH.

"I am as big as anesthesiology allows me to be", the great American heart surgeon Michael DeBakey said. We should never forget about the contribution of anesthetic factors to the success of cerebral aneurysm surgery, which is the subject of the relevant chapter of this manuscript.

Specialized neurocritical care units with close monitoring for delayed cerebral ischemia, blood pressure control, enteral nimodipine and induced hypertension have considerably improved the survival of patients with aneurysmal SAH.

Treatment of SAH in pregnancy and in pediatric practice has some features that are discussed in the relevant chapters.

Despite a decline in the above-mentioned discharge mortality, SAH remains a condition with severe morbidity. Survivors often have a permanent neurological disability and cognitive deficits. As a result, they suffer a decrease in their health-related quality of life. Symptomatic cerebral vasospasm or delayed cerebral ischemia remains a major cause of poor outcomes. The need for improved treatment modalities is apparent. This is stated in the last chapter on Future Direction of Aneurysmal Subarachnoid Hemorrhage Management.

New times bring new challenges. Whether SARS-CoV-2 infection affects the aneurysm formation and the incidence of SAH requires further research, as the author from Greece postulates.

The international team's manuscript highlights new insights into aneurysmal SAH and provides updates in both diagnostics and treatment approaches.

Prof. Alexey Krivoshapkin, MD, PhD, FRCS (England)
Correspondent Member of RAS
Head of the Department of Neurology and Neurosurgery,
RUDN University, Moscow, Russia

Preface

The rupture of a cerebral aneurysm and its accompanying SAH is a dramatic scenario, the ending of which for the patient can be difficult to predict.

Therefore, the clear actions of a multidisciplinary team at all stages of care, fast and timely diagnosis, neurosurgical tactics and pathogenetically substantiated intensive care will undoubtedly determine the outcomes of treatment for such a severe category of patients.

The title Aneurysmal Subarachnoid Hemorrhage: From Diagnosis to Treatment represents a knowledge-based book that includes questions of the etiology and morphogenesis of cerebral aneurysms, pathophysiological and pathomorphological aspects of subarachnoid hemorrhage and cerebral vasospasm, the relationship between constitution and developmental risk of subarachnoid hemorrhage, hemostasiological disorders in patients with aneurysmal subarachnoid and intracranial hemorrhage, peculiarities of diagnosis and methods of conservative and neurosurgical treatment in different types of patients with subarachnoid hemorrhage – adults, pregnant women and children. Anesthetic management of cerebral aneurysm surgery is an important topic of discussion. A special chapter is devoted to the analysis of the COVID-19 pandemic's influence on the dynamic of subarachnoid hemorrhage incidence as a neurovascular emergency. Finally, it's a very interesting chapter regarding concerns, developments, and future direction of aneurysmal subarachnoid hemorrhage management.

This book was written by neurologists, neuroradiologists, neurosurgeons, anesthesiologists and intensive care specialists, pathologists, laboratory diagnosticians and hemostasiologists - 23 authors from 4 countries, whose daily work is to manage and treat emergency vascular neurosurgical patients.

"Work hard and love will follow", - wrote the most famous Estonian writer Anton Hansen-Tammsaare. We sincerely hope that this manuscript by an international team of authors will be useful to readers in solving clinical problems of daily practice.

Saint Petersburg, Russia-Toronto, Canada Irina A. Savvina

Acknowledgments

I thank the departments of neurosurgery, anesthesiology, intensive care, neuroradiology, laboratory diagnostics and pathomorphology, each of which has provided opportunities for colleagues to contribute to the writing of the book using their knowledge and clinical experience.

Special thanks are also due to Alexey L. Krivoshapkin for the Foreword.

I would like to acknowledge the publisher, editors, and support staff at Nova Science Publishers, they were very helpful in the various stages of developing and producing the volume.

And especially thanks to the contributing authors from different countries whose expertise has been particularly important in making this manuscript edition possible.

I express my heartfelt gratitude to my family for patience and faith.

"Viam supervadet vadens".

Irina A. Savvina, Dr. Sc. Med.

Chapter 1

Aneurysmal Subarachnoid Hemorrhage in the Pandemic Era

Andreas Theofanopoulos*, MD
and Constantine Constantoyannis, MD, PhD
Neurosurgery Department, University Hospital of Patras, Patras, Greece

Abstract

Aneurysmal subarachnoid hemorrhage (SAH) is a neurovascular emergency with an often-malignant clinical course, requiring highly specialized treatment to maximize favorable outcomes. Since the outbreak of the COVID-19 pandemic in early 2020, there have been numerous reports from various fields of clinical medicine noting variations in the incidence of several clinical entities during the pandemic period in comparison with the baseline figures. Acute coronary syndromes are reportedly on the decline, as well as neurological emergencies in the form of acute stroke. The situation when it comes to aneurysmal SAH is more obscure, as several studies have been published with often conflicting results. Early reports noted a decline in SAH incidence, while several others claimed no significant variation or even a significant increase. A review of the available literature is presented in an attempt to draw insights into the impact of the pandemic on aneurysmal SAH. Conclusions are bound to facilitate rational healthcare resource reallocation, to effectively deal with COVID-19 while not neglecting patients suffering from threatening classical diseases.

*Corresponding Author's Email: andreastheofano@gmail.com.

In: Aneurysmal Subarachnoid Hemorrhage
Editor: Irina Savvina
ISBN: 979-8-88697-251-1

Keywords: Coronavirus disease 19 (COVID-19); SARS-CoV2; pandemic; subarachnoid hemorrhage (SAH); admission rate; aneurysm

Introduction

Acute subarachnoid hemorrhage (SAH) due to aneurysmal rupture is a devastating vascular disease associated with severe morbidity and mortality and accounting for approximately 5% of strokes (Grasso, Alafaci, and Macdonald 2017). Approximately one-third of patients eventually succumb, and one-third face long-term neurological sequelae while the rest return to normal activity (Etminanet al., 2019; Kundra et al., 2014). The incidence of acute SAH is estimated at 10 cases per 100000 persons per year. Patients'age distribution peaks around 40-60 years (Petridis et al., 2017). Aneurysmal rupture has been associated with smoking, uncontrolled hypertension, familial history of aneurysms, and connective tissue diseases (Petridis et al., 2017). Females and slightly more often affected, especially in older age groups. SAH also varies significantly with geographic region, as rates are higher in Japan and Finland and lower in Central and South America (de Rooij et al., 2007).

The global pandemic of COVID-19 has interestingly had an impact on the incidence of several seemingly unrelated diseases. Since the official pandemic outbreak in March 2020, there have been studies in the fields of cardiology and neurology presenting a decline in acute coronary syndromes and neurological emergencies respectively (Padmanabhan et al., 2021; Garcia et al., 2020; de Rosa et al., 2020). Early series reported similar downward trends in aneurysmal SAH admissions (Diestro et al., 2020; A. L. Bernat et al., 2020; A.-L. Bernat et al., 2020). A marked decline in the overall emergency neurosurgical admissions between early 2020 compared to the same period in 2019 was noted in other studies, which however pointed out the fact that the admissions of SAH remained unchanged during the early COVID-19 era (Hecht et al., 2020; Luostarinen et al., 2020). On the contrary, other studies demonstrated an increased frequency of aneurysmal SAH during the early stages of the pandemic (Theofanopoulos et al., 2021). In this chapter, we attempt to elucidate the intricate relationship between this important neurovascular emergency and the novel healthcare and socioeconomic milieu imposed by the pandemic. Conclusions drawn are bound to be valuable in shaping resilient healthcare systems with sufficient resource reserves to ensure adequate treatment for victims of neurosurgical emergencies at the dawn of the pandemic era (The Lancet Planetary Health 2021).

Literature Review

The outbreak of the global pandemic of COVID-19 at the dawn of the year 2020 has had profound effects on the function of health systems worldwide, with resource allocation inevitably gravitating toward dealing with the acute, unprecedented crisis. This situation raised concerns within the medical community about adequate continuity of treatment of the so-called 'classic' diseases outside the COVID-19 spectrum, the incidence of which should theoretically remain the same. However, some seemingly paradoxical observations about alterations in the actual incidence of several diseases during the pandemic period, which were unaccounted for by factors other than the pandemic itself, led to multiple investigations worldwide attempting to verify and quantify this effect and propose possible explanations.

The first relevant reports arrived from the field of interventional cardiology. A large study of the case volume of 9 high-volume (>100 PPCIs/year) cardiac catheterization laboratories in the United States from January 1, 2019, to March 31, 2020, showed a 38% reduction in the cardiac catheterization laboratory STEMI (ST-elevation myocardial infarction) activations in the period after COVID-19, defined as the period after March 1, 2020 (Garcia et al., 2020). The authors had expected an increase in STEMIs due to both heightened environmental and psychosocial stress and a higher load of STEMIs induced by COVID-19 infection. Tentative explanations offered for the surprising results were possible avoidance of hospital-based medical care by the general public out of fear of exposure to COVID-19, STEMI misdiagnosis, or predilection for medical instead of interventional management, possibly as a result of overloading of the health system.

Almost simultaneously, similar results were published by a collaboration of Italian investigators who conducted a multicentre observational study of admissions in cardiac care units (CCUs) of 54 Italian hospitals (de Rosa et al., 2020). By comparing admissions during a week within the pandemic (March 2020) to the equivalent week of 2019, the authors reported a marked decrease of about 50% in acute myocardial infarction (AMI) admissions during the pandemic. Interestingly, they also reported a substantially higher case fatality rate (13.7% compared to 4.1%) during the pandemic, an effect which remained similar even after excluding AMI patients positive for SARS-CoV-2, who had even higher care fatality rates of up to 28.6%. The explanation attempted is generally in line with that of the US group.

Shortly thereafter, Spanish investigators published a similar trend of approximately a 40% reduction in urgent revascularization procedures

(Negreira Caamaño, Piqueras Flores, and Mateo Gómez 2020). Therefore, this trend of reduction in presentation of acute ischemic myocardial disease during the pandemic seems to be well documented, albeit its explanation remains elusive.

Another major ischemic disease whose incidence diminished during the pandemic was ischemic stroke. Royal Stoke University Hospital in the United Kingdom reported a 39.5% decrease in stroke or transient ischemic attack (TIA) admissions during the first month of COVID-19, with a simultaneous increase in stroke severity measured according to the NIHSS (Padmanabhan et al., 2021). Corresponding downward trends in stroke admissions were also reported by several other studies (Hoyer et al., 2020; Rudilosso et al., 2020). Similar were the results of a survey consisting of data derived from the Big Data Observatory Platform for Stroke of China consisting of 280 hospitals across China, which showed a 40% decrease in hospital admissions for stroke (Zhao et al., 2020). Most of the above studies cited patient reluctance to present to hospitals due to fear of COVID-19 infection as a major possible contributing factor to the observed changes.

However, also reported in the aforementioned Chinese study (Zhao et al., 2020) is a marked reduction in the aggressive medical treatment and neurointerventional procedures for acute ischemic stroke, i.e., thrombolysis and thrombectomy, with a reduction of 26.7% and 25.3% respectively. These findings are corroborated by the reports from stroke centers in France with a 21% reduction in mechanical thrombectomy (Kerleroux et al., 2020) as well as a combined study from centers in France, Portugal, Italy, Switzerland, Spain, Germany, Canada, and the United States (Hajdu et al., 2020) with approximate 30% reduction. The latest two studies, as well as numerous others -indicative are a US-based (Schirmer et al., 2020) and an Italian (Frisullo et al., 2020)- concurrently demonstrate a notable increase both in the mean time between disease onset to hospital presentation (time since last-known-well) and between presentation and intervention (door-to-groin time). These observations are once again attributed to a reluctance of the public to seek medical care, however delays in the time since last-known-well and door-to-groin hint at inadequacies of the healthcare system to cope with the stress imposed on it by the pandemic.

The effect of the pandemic on aneurysmal subarachnoid hemorrhage (SAH) is, however, far more obscure. Early reports hinted at a downward trend, not unlike the cardiovascular and ischemic stroke emergencies already discussed. Diestroet al., 2020 in Toronto, Canada, found a striking decrease in ruptured aneurysms ranging from 64% to 75% during the early COVID-19 period (March – April 2020) (Diestro et al., 2020). Bernat et al., 2020 also report a steep decline in aneurysmal SAH admissions in Neurosurgical units throughout Paris during the last two weeks of March 2020 (A. L. Bernat et al., 2020; A.-L. Bernat et al., 2020). Here, speculation over possible reasons for the phenomenon is once again centered on the hesitation of patients to seek medical attention when experiencing relatively mild symptoms, due to either fear of COVID-19 infection or unwillingness to contribute to healthcare system overload. Ever present is also the suspicion of misdiagnosis as a result of extreme pressure on the healthcare system -especially for patients presenting with headache as the sole symptom, conceivably mimicking early SARS-CoV-2 infections. However, there is also a novel explanation proposed by the authors, who posit that containment measures imposed by the government and the resultant decrease in the usual daily stressful activities may have led to a decrease in aneurysm rupture via reducing stress levels.

At about the same time, others reported no significant variation in the rates of aneurysmal SAH. Hecht et al., 2020 in Berlin, Germany, found similar rates of SAH in early 2020 (February to April) compared to 2019, albeit with a decrease in other neurovascular emergencies (Hecht et al., 2020). Luostarinen et al., 2020 in Helsinki, Finland, came to similar conclusions over observations during a similar period (January to May – the initiation of containment measures in the country starting mid-March) (Luostarinen et al., 2020). In both studies, authors admit that their respective countries' healthcare systems were relatively less overloaded -even if still considerably affected- by the pandemic and better capable of continuing to provide for neurosurgical emergencies than countries hit more severely. This is cited as a possible factor contributing to consistency in SAH admissions.

On the contrary, a marked increase in aneurysmal SAH during the pandemic was found in a study from Greece (Theofanopoulos et al., 2021). This is probably the study spanning the widest timeline during the COVID-19 period (February to June 2020). SAH admissions were analyzed as cases per week and the test period was compared with the corresponding period in the previous year as well as with the rest of the previous year, to account for possible seasonal variance. The authors report a statistically significant surprising increase in aneurysmal SAH, with admissions being 1.5-fold higher during the COVID period. No statistically significant difference was found in mortality, length of hospital stay, geographical origin, and gender distribution, however, the mean age of patients was remarkably lower (54 compared to 62 years of age), with similar standard deviations (SD).

Such results come in contrast with the previous reports and warrant careful evaluation. The study is a retrospective, observational, single-center one. Nevertheless, the reporting University Hospital of Patras is the sole referral center for neurovascular emergencies requiring neurosurgical and neurointerventional coverage in the whole Wcstern Greece area, with an estimated population of about 2 million inhabitants, therefore serving a well-defined catchment area and somewhat mitigating the single-center design limitation. Taking into consideration the fact that this study spans a broader period than previously discussed reports, it may well represent a real upward trend in aneurysmal SAH cases during the pandemic.

Attempting to delve into possible explanations for the contrast of this study's findings with previous reports, we should notice that during the first wave of the COVID-19 pandemic, Greece implemented early, very strict, and synchronously applied confinement measures. Statistics showed that this led to fewer infected patients, intubated cases, and deaths due to the COVID-19 virus even when compared to countries with similar populations. Consequently, pressure on the Greek healthcare system was not excessive compared to other European countries, possibly aiding in avoiding misdiagnosis, especially for SAH patients. This may have avoided falsely low numbers of SAH due to failure of such cases to be detected.

While management of elective surgical cases was significantly decreased in all Greek hospitals during the COVID-19 period, it is reported that referral of emergency cases such as ruptured aneurysms was not modified. Given the concurrent strict travel ban, it is considered unlikely that tourism has influenced the demographics in the author's area. The aforementioned factors are therefore unlikely to have contributed to the observed increase in SAH cases. It is however speculated that socioeconomic repercussions of the pandemic may have contributed to temporary population relocations and a possible increase in patient input in the specific hospital's healthcare geographical region.

The authors consider the sudden increase in the average civilian's stress level during the pandemic as a possible cause for the notable increase in the number of patients with aneurysmal rupture. Unprecedented alterations in social interactions and forced social isolation, compounded by lockdown-driven economic recession and the resultant financial strain, as well as job insecurity may have placed undue psychological burdens on people's minds. The aforementioned psychological factors' physical manifestations could trigger chronic and acute elevation of both systolic and mean arterial pressure, while also activating inflammatory cascades, both events potentially increasing the chance of aneurysmal rupture and SAH (Texakalidis et al., 2019; Signorelli et al., 2018).

The question of whether SARS-CoV-2 infection has any causal effect on aneurysmal formation or rupture has not been adequately researched. A case series from five high-volume cerebrovascular centers in the United States comprised of 10 patients with ruptured aneurysms who were also concurrently positive for COVID-19 reported a possibly distinct pattern compared with the common SAH patients (Dodd et al., 2021). The authors report a lower-than-expected median and mean patient age and a higher-than-expected frequency of small aneurysms and dissecting aneurysms. Still, indications that COVID-19 significantly impacts the pathophysiology of aneurysmal SAH remain scarce.

Discussion

Before 2019, the word pandemic in most people's minds evoked images of long-forgotten times. Very few heeded the warnings from numerous infectious disease experts about the real possibility of large-scale epidemics in the globalized world. Most chose to believe that modern societies were sheltered from that sort of danger; extreme examples being anti-vaxxer movements emerging in most western developed countries during the last decades. The COVID-19 pandemic dispelled such delusions and proved beyond any reasonable doubt the vulnerability of the 21st-century interconnected, globalized social environment that relies on rapid transport of goods and people to the rapid spread of contagious infections. Current strategies that focus on containment, tracing, and travel restrictions following disease detection seem insufficient to limit the spread of highly contagious, rapidly evolving pathogens, while being largely economically inefficient. The cost of the SARS-CoV-2 pandemic in loss of life is in the millions, with the economic cost in loss of production and wider damages estimates in the trillions of US dollars. Experts claim that the emergence of pandemics will possibly accelerate in the following years, owing to various interacting factors such as ecological disruption, climate change, and shifting wildlife species distribution (The Lancet Planetary Health 2021). We seem therefore to be entering a "Pandemic Era," where phenomena such as the recent COVID-19 outbreak will no longer appear as a once-in-a-century event.

The recent pandemic imposed a heavy burden on healthcare systems around the world. The different results in fatality rates demonstrate varying degrees of ability to cope with the added stress, accordingly to each country's system's available reserves. Nevertheless, drastic changes in resource allocation were a common phenomenon in all healthcare systems, as none is designed to absorb massive waves of critically ill patients in short time periods. Therefore, the universal need to shift resources and personnel to tracking, diagnosis, and treatment of COVID-19 infections may have resulted in suboptimal or delayed treatment of other common medical conditions.

Conclusion

The studies reviewed above indicate that aneurysmal subarachnoid hemorrhage, a neurological emergency with a highly malignant course, remains a threat in the face of the pandemic. The severity of SAH as a disease entity, combined with its high morbidity and mortality burden and the highly specialized care required to obtain favorable outcomes, necessitate access to intensive care and trained and experienced personnel. It is evident that the need for diagnosis and treatment of neurosurgical emergencies is consistent even during pandemic scenarios and should neither be underestimated. Patients who do present with such pathology generally require neurosurgical treatment, indicating that neurosurgery should be prioritized in the allocation of available resources in periods of systemic stress. The current COVID-19 pandemic could serve as an example of the effect of similar epidemics on the incidence of emergencies such as aneurysmal subarachnoid hemorrhage. Through it, insights can be drawn guiding the design of resilient healthcare systems, better able to afford continued high-caliber care for patients in times of extreme spikes in work- and caseload.

References

A.-L. Bernat, T. Gaberel, L. Giammattei, F. Rault, C. Gakuba, E. Magro, C. Peltier, T. Graillon, B. Baussart, K. Premat, F. Clarençon, A. Nouet, V. Civelli, S. Froelich. 2020. "Intracranial Hemorrhage Related to Brain Vascular Disease and COVID-19 Containment: Where Are the Patients?" *Neurochirurgie* 66(5):400–401. https://doi.org/10.1016/j.neuchi.2020.06.127.

Anne L. Bernat, Lorenzo Giammattei, Rosaria Abbritti, and Sebastien Froelich. 2020. "Impact of COVID-19 Pandemic on Subarachnoid Hemorrhage." *Journal of Neurosurgical Sciences* 64(4). https://doi.org/10.23736/S0390-5616.20.04963-2.

Diestro, Jose Danilo Bengzon, Yang Mei Li, Carmen Parra-Fariñas, Dipanka Sarma, Aditya Bharatha, Thomas R. Marotta, and Julian Spears. 2020. "Letter to the Editor 'AneurysmalSubarachnoidHemorrhage:Collateral Damage of COVID?'" *World Neurosurgery* 139 (July). https://doi.org/10.1016/j.wneu.2020.05.206.

Dodd, William S., Pascal M. Jabbour, Ahmad Sweid, Stavropoula Tjoumakaris, Michael R. Gooch, Fadi al Saiegh, David M. Hasan, Robert M. Starke, Peter T. Kan, Adam J. Polifka, Dimitri Laurent, Katharina M. Busl, Ritam Ghosh, Brian L. Hoh, Nohra Chalouhi, 2021. "Aneurysmal Subarachnoid Hemorrhage in Patients with Coronavirus Disease 2019 (COVID-19): A Case Series." *World Neurosurgery* 153 (September): e259–64. https://doi.org/10.1016/j.wneu.2021.06.092.

Etminan, Nima, Han-Sol Chang, Katharina Hackenberg, Nicolien K. de Rooij, Mervyn D. I. Vergouwen, Gabriel J. E. Rinkel, and Ale Algra. 2019. "Worldwide Incidence of AneurysmalSubarachnoidHemorrhageAccording to Region, Time Period, Blood Pressure, and Smoking Prevalence in the Population." *JAMA Neurology* 76(5):588. https://doi.org/10.1001/jamaneurol.2019.0006.

Frisullo, Giovanni, Valerio Brunetti, Riccardo di Iorio, Aldobrando Broccolini, Pietro Caliandro, Mauro Monforte, Roberta Morosetti, Carla Piano, Fabio Pilato, Paolo Calabresi, Giacomo Della Marca, 2020. "Effect of Lockdown on the Management of Ischemic Stroke: An Italian Experience from a COVID Hospital." *Neurological Sciences* 41 (9): 2309–13. https://doi.org/10.1007/s10072-020-04545-9.

Garcia, Santiago, Mazen S. Albaghdadi, Perwaiz M. Meraj, Christian Schmidt, Ross Garberich, Farouc A. Jaffer, Simon Dixon, 2020. "Reduction in ST-Segment ElevationCardiacCatheterizationLaboratory Activations in the United States During COVID-19 Pandemic." *Journal of the American College of Cardiology* 75 (22): 2871–72. https://doi.org/10.1016/j.jacc.2020.04.011.

Grasso, Giovanni, Concetta Alafaci, and RLoch Macdonald. 2017. "Management of Aneurysmal Subarachnoid Hemorrhage: State of the Art and Future Perspectives." *Surgical Neurology International* 8(1):11. https://doi.org/10.4103/2152-7806.198738.

Hajdu, Steven D., ValeriePittet, Francesco Puccinelli, Wagih ben Hassen, Malek ben Maacha, Raphaël Blanc, Sandra Bracco, Gabriel Broocks, Bruno Bartolini, Tommaso Casseri, Frederic Clarençon, Olivier Naggara, François Eugène, Jean-Christophe Ferré, Alexis Guédon, Emmanuel Houdart, Timo Krings, Pierre Lehmann, Nicola Limbucci, Paolo Machi, Juan Macho, Nicolo Mandruzzato, Sergio Nappini, Marie Teresa Nawka, Patrick Nicholson, João Pedro Marto, Vitor Pereira, Manuel A Correia, Teresa Pinho-E-Melo, João Nuno Ramos, Eytan Raz, Patrícia Ferreira, João Reis, Maksim Shapiro, Eimad Shotar, Noel van Horn, Michel Piotin, Guillaume Saliou, 2020. "Acute Stroke Management During the COVID-19 Pandemic." *Stroke* 51(8):2593–96. https://doi.org/10.1161/STROKEAHA.120.030794.

Hecht, Nils, Lars Wessels, Finn-Ove Werft, Ulf C. Schneider, Marcus Czabanka, and Peter Vajkoczy. 2020. "Need for Ensuring Care for Neuro-Emergencies—Lessons Learned from the COVID-19 Pandemic." *Acta Neurochirurgica* 162 (8):1795–1801. https://doi.org/10.1007/s00701-020-04437-z.

Hoyer, Carolin, Anne Ebert, Hagen B. Huttner, Volker Puetz, Bernd Kallmünzer, Kristian Barlinn, Christian Haverkamp, Andreas Harloff, Jochen Brich, Michael Platten, Kristina Szabo, 2020. "Acute Stroke in Times of the COVID-19 Pandemic." *Stroke* 51 (7): 2224–27. https://doi.org/10.1161/STROKEAHA.120.030395.

Kerleroux, Basile, Thibaut Fabacher, Nicolas Bricout, Martin Moïse, Benoit Testud, Sivadji Vingadassalom, Héloïse Ifergan, Janot, K., Consolli, A., Ben Hassen, W., Shotar, E., Ognard, J., Charbonnier, G., L'allinec, V., Guedon, A., Bolognini, F., Marnat, G., Forestier, G., Rouchaud, A., ... Boulouis, G. 2020. "Mechanical Thrombectomy for Acute Ischemic Stroke Amid the COVID-19 Outbreak." *Stroke* 51(7):2012–17. https://doi.org/10.1161/STROKEAHA.120.030373.

Kundra, Sandeep, Vidhi Mahendru, Vishnu Gupta, and Ashwani Kumar Choudhary. 2014. "Principles of Neuroanesthesia in Aneurysmal Subarachnoid Hemorrhage." *Journal of Anaesthesiology Clinical Pharmacology* 30(3):328. https://doi.org/10.4103/0970-9185.137261.

Luostarinen, Teemu, Jyri Virta, Jarno Satopää, Minna Bäcklund, Riku Kivisaari, Miikka Korja, and Rahul Raj. 2020. "Intensive Care of Traumatic Brain Injury and Aneurysmal Subarachnoid Hemorrhage in Helsinki during the Covid-19 Pandemic." *Acta Neurochirurgica* 162(11):2715–24. https://doi.org/10.1007/s00701-020-04583-4.

Negreira Caamaño, Martín, Jesús Piqueras Flores, and Cristina Mateo Gómez. 2020. "Impacto de La Pandemia COVID-19 Sobre Los Ingresos Hospitalarios En Cardiología." *Medicina Clínica* 155(4): 179–80. https://doi.org/10.1016/j.medcli.2020.05.013.

Padmanabhan, Nishita, Indira Natarajan, Rachel Gunston, Marko Raseta, and Christine Roffe. 2021. "Impact of COVID-19 on Stroke Admissions, Treatments, and Outcomes at a Comprehensive Stroke Centre in the United Kingdom." *Neurological Sciences* 42 (1):15–20. https://doi.org/10.1007/s10072-020-04775-x.

Petridis, Athanasios K., Marcel A. Kamp, Jan F. Cornelius, Thomas Beez, Kerim Beseoglu, Bernd Turowski, and Hans-Jakob Steiger. 2017. "Aneurysmal Subarachnoid Hemorrhage." *Deutsches Aerzteblatt Online*, [*German Medical Journal Online*] March. https://doi.org/10.3238/arztebl.2017.0226.

Rooij, N K de, F H H Linn, J A van der Plas, A Algra, and G J E Rinkel. 2007. "Incidence of Subarachnoid Haemorrhage: A Systematic Review with Emphasis on Region, Age, Gender and Time Trends." *Journal of Neurology, Neurosurgery&Psychiatry* 78(12):1365–72. https://doi.org/10.1136/jnnp.2007.117655.

deRosa, Salvatore, Carmen Spaccarotella, Cristina Basso, Maria Pia Calabrò, Antonio Curcio, Pasquale Perrone Filardi, Massimo Mancone, Giuseppe Mercuro, Saverio Muscoli, Savina Nodari, Roberto Pedrinelli, Gianfranco Sinagra, Ciro Indolfi, 2020. "Reduction of Hospitalizations for Myocardial Infarction in Italy in the COVID-19 Era." *European Heart Journal* 41(22):2083–88. https://doi.org/10.1093/eurheartj/ehaa409.

Rudilosso, Salvatore, Carlos Laredo, Víctor Vera, Martha Vargas, Arturo Renú, Laura Llull, Víctor Obach, Sergio Amaro, Xabier Urra, Ferrán Torres, Francesc Xavier Jiménez-Fàbrega, Ángel Chamorro, 2020. "Acute Stroke Care Is at Risk in the Era of COVID-19." *Stroke* 51(7):1991–95. https://doi.org/10.1161/STROKEAHA.120.030329.

Schirmer, Clemens M, Andrew J Ringer, Adam S Arthur, Mandy J Binning, W Christopher Fox, Robert F James, Michael R Levitt, Rabih G Tawk, ErolVeznedaroglu, Melanie Walker, Alejandro M Spiotta, 2020. "Delayed Presentation of Acute Ischemic Strokes during the COVID-19 Crisis." *Journal of Neuro Interventional Surgery* 12 (7): 639–42. https://doi.org/10.1136/neurintsurg-2020-016299.

Signorelli, Francesco, Sapir Sela, Loreto Gesualdo, Sophie Chevrel, Félix Tollet, Cyril Pailler-Mattei, LeonelloTacconi, Francis Turjman, Angelo Vacca, and David B. Schul. 2018. "Hemodynamic Stress, Inflammation, and Intracranial Aneurysm Development and Rupture: A Systematic Review." *World Neurosurgery* 115 (July): 234–44. https://doi.org/10.1016/j.wneu.2018.04.143.

Texakalidis Pavlos, Ahmad Sweid, Nikolaos Mouchtouris, Eric C. Peterson, Chrissa Sioka, Leonardo Rangel-Castilla, John Reavey-Cantwell, and Pascal Jabbour. 2019. "Aneurysm Formation, Growth, and Rupture: The Biology and Physics of Cerebral Aneurysms." *World Neurosurgery* 130(October):277–84. https://doi.org/10.1016/j.wneu.2019.07.093.

The Lancet Planetary Health. 2021. "A Pandemic Era." *The Lancet Planetary Health* 5 (1):e1. https://doi.org/10.1016/S2542-5196(20)30305-3.

Theofanopoulos Andreas, Dionysia Fermeli, Spyros Boulieris, George Kalantzis, Zinovia Kefalopoulou, Vasilios Panagiotopoulos, Dimitrios Papadakos, and Constantine Constantoyannis. 2021. "Effects of COVID-19 on the Admissions of AneurysmalSubarachnoidHemorrhage: The West Greece Experience." Neurological Sciences: *Official Journal of the Italian Neurological Society and of the Italian Society of Clinical Neurophysiology* 42(6). https://doi.org/10.1007/s10072-021-05190-6.

Zhao Jing, Hang Li, David Kung, Marc Fisher, Ying Shen, and Renyu Liu. 2020. "Impact of the COVID-19 Epidemic on Stroke Care and Potential Solutions." *Stroke* 51(7):1996–2001. https://doi.org/10.1161/STROKEAHA.120.030225.

Chapter 2

Subarachnoid Hemorrhage and Vasospasm: Understanding the Pathophysiology

Yusuf Mehkri[1], William Dodd[1], Alec Clark[2], Coulter Small[1], Abeer Dagra[1], Eric Williams[1] and Brandon Lucke-Wold[1,*]

[1]Department of Neurosurgery, University of Florida, Gainesville, USA
[2]University of Central Florida, College of Medicine, Orlando, USA

Abstract

Symptomatic vasospasm is deleterious following subarachnoid hemorrhage and limited treatment options currently exist. Blood pressure augmentation and/or endovascular management with balloon angioplasty and intra-arterial calcium channel blockers are commonly employed with varying degrees of success. The subsequent delayed cerebral ischemia that can develop after vasospasm can lead to devastating consequences for patients. In order to improve treatment options, understanding the pathophysiology of vasospasm development is critical. In this chapter, we highlight several key mechanisms that are currently being investigated regarding their role in vasospasm development. The compiled summary will serve as a springboard for further investigation and inspire inquiry into effective multimodality treatment approaches.

Keywords: subarachnoid hemorrhage, vasospasm, secondary mechanisms, novel targets

---

*Corresponding Author's Email: Brandon.Lucke-Wold@neurosurgery.ufl.edu.

In: Aneurysmal Subarachnoid Hemorrhage
Editor: Irina Savvina
ISBN: 979-8-88697-251-1

Introduction

Cerebral vasospasm for aneurysmal subarachnoid hemorrhage (SAH) continues to be a severe and debilitating problem. It is well known that 30-40% of SAH patients have symptomatic vasospasm during admission. Understanding of the pathophysiology is limited thereby limiting current interventions. Frequently, blood pressure is driven up to allow permissive hypertension. Furthermore, patients are often taken to the endovascular suite for balloon angioplasty, stent assisted dilation, or intra-arterial verapamil injection. Recent clinical and pre-clinical data has shed light on some emerging pathways of interest. The below sections highlight some of these pathways. As our understanding improves, better treatment options may be developed that offer more sustainable clinical utility.

IL-6 Pathway

The role of IL-6, a pleiotropic cytokine, has long been established in both the formation and eventual rupture of aneurysms (Chalouhi and Ali 2012, 1259). Elevated levels of cytokines such as IL-6 have been detected in aneurysm tissue and aneurysm growth has been shown to be reduced using anti-inflammatory inhibitors via a signaling pathway involving IL-6 (Ikedo and Minami 2017, 6). IL-6 has also been implicated in aneurysm rupture. IL-6 receptor inhibition in estrogen-deficient mice was shown to suppress cerebral aneurysm rupture (Wajima and Hourani 2020, 86), and the use of a peroxisome proliferator-activated receptor-γ (PPARγ) agonist, pioglitazone, reduced the incidence of rupture primarily by reducing M1 macrophage infiltration and levels of inflammatory cytokines including IL-6 (Shimada and Furukawa 2015, 46). Although the underlying molecular pathways involved in the pathophysiology of cerebral aneurysms are largely unknown, neuroinflammatory signaling including IL-6 appears to play a large role.

The involvement of IL-6 in the development of vasospasm and subsequent delayed cerebral ischemia (DCI) following SAH is also currently under investigation. Serum and CSF analysis have been used to assess the role that IL-6 may play in disease progression following SAH.

Muroi and colleagues (Muroi and Bellut 2011, 18), compared daily serum IL-6 levels in the acute phase and found significantly higher levels in patients with SAH and vasospasm when compared to patients experiencing non-aneurysmal SAH (naSAH). They found no difference in serum levels between patients with aSAH without vasospasm and those with naSAH. Although not proving that systemic inflammation has a direct impact on the development of vasospasm, it may be involved. Other groups have either supported (Tang and Lu 2015, 8; Chaudhry and Stoffel-Wagner 2017, 18; Wang and Gao 2018, 15), or contradicted these results (Chou and Feske 2012, 60; Rasmussen and Bache 2019, 128).

McMahon and colleagues (McMahon and Hopkins 2013, 5), evaluated the systemic inflammatory response following SAH with DCI as the primary outcome of interest. They found no association between initial, average, peak or final serum IL-6 levels with the development of DCI. They did, however, find rate of change in IL-6 levels to be predictive of impending DCI, with IL-6 levels declining significantly slower. This likely demonstrates an acute, delayed inflammatory event associated with DCI that can be detected in serum analyses. These findings have both been replicated (Tang and Lu 2015, 8), and contradicted (Rasmussen and Bache 2019, 128; Chamling and Gross 2017, 104; Wennebergand and Hergès 2021, 143) by other groups.

Muroi and colleagues (Muroi and Hugelshofer 2013, 72), further assessed the time course of systemic inflammatory markers with the development of DCI and associated neurological deficits. Unlike C-reactive protein (CRP), leukocyte count and procalcitonin levels, serum IL-6 was found to be predictive of DCI with elevated levels between days 5 and 10. IL-6 also showed a biphasic pattern, with peaks on day 3 and 10. The second peak, although likely DCI related, was not significantly associated with DCI diagnosis. This was also shown by Chaudhry and colleagues (Chaudhry and Stoffel-Wagner 2017, 18), who found the strongest associations between IL-6 and DCI around days 3 and 9. The second peaks suggest a secondary inflammatory event that may not be systemic in nature.

Cerebral spinal fluid (CSF) analyses have shown strong associations with the development of vasospasm and DCI, and the literature is more definitive. Wu and colleagues (Wu and Guan 2016, 53) found significantly elevated CSF IL-6 levels, more-so than TNF-α, on day two of admission in patients with aSAH who developed vasospasm than those without. They further confirmed these findings with a meta-analysis including thirteen studies.The time course of CSF inflammatory markers with the development of vasospasm has also been investigated. Elevated CSF levels of IL-6 on admission (Kwon and Jeon 2001,16; Hendryk and Jarzab 2004, 25), days 1-2 (Hendryk and Jarzab 2004, 25), day 3 (Hendryk and Jarzab 2004, 25; Gaetani and Tartara 1998, 20; Ni and Gu 2011, 110) and days 4-5 (Schoch and Regel 2007; 60) were all associated with development of vasospasm. Similarly, DCI was associated with elevated IL-6 on days 0-3 (Hendryk and Jarzab 2004, 25), day 5 (Ridwan and Grote 2021, 11) and day 7 (Schoch and Regel 2007; 60).

Interestingly, studies on both serum and CSF levels of IL-6 have generally only found positive associations with CSF analyses. Ridwan and colleagues (Ridwan and Grote 2021, 11), not only found significantly higher levels of IL-6 in CSF, but also found stronger associations with DCI, and specifically DCI with infarctions. Lenski and colleagues (Lenski and Huge 2017, 99), similarly showed that the diagnostic potential of both serum and CSF levels combined was lower than that of CSF alone. They found an increased posttest probability for vasospasm in patients with CSF levels between 529 and 3081pg/mL.

Multiple conclusions can be drawn from this literature. CSF levels of IL-6 appear to be more reliable and specific for the development of vasospasm and DCI following SAH. This is especially true given that CSF levels are magnitudes higher than systemic levels and local changes in IL-6 may not be reflected in serum samples (Hopkins and McMahon 2012, 9; Mathiesen and Andersson 1993, 78). In addition, neuroinflammation is a key player in the vascular and ischemic changes following SAH. Although CSF IL-6 may not be a useful diagnostic marker, largely due to an unclear time course, it has potential as a therapeutic target.

Several preclinical studies have allowed us to gain a better understanding of the role IL-6 may play in the development of vasospasm and DCI. Croci and colleagues (Croci and Nevzati 2019, 63), investigated the relationship between IL-6 and endothelin-1 (ET-1) in a simple rabbit model. Rabbits with induced SAH were compared to both those given cisterna magna IL-6 injections and controls. The SAH group experienced more pronounced vasospasm and there was a significant association between CSF levels of IL-6 and ET-1. They found that IL-6 triggered vasospasm following SAH is ET-1 dependent. A similar study (Croci and Nevzati 2020, 29), investigated whether increases in CSF IL-6 may be due to sphingolipid pathways, which have been shown to be involved in cerebral vasoconstriction and ischemic stroke pathophysiology, in addition to inducing expression of IL-6 (Altura and Gebrewold 2002, 58; Li and Zhang 1999, 33; Perry and Newcomb 2014, 289). Although they recorded changes in levels of CSF IL-6, there were no changes in any CSF lipid profiles, suggesting no relationship.

Targeting IL-6 to reduce occurrence of vasospasm following SAH appears to be promising. Bowman and colleagues (Bowman and Dixit 2004, 54), have shown in a rat femoral artery model that administration of a polyclonal antibody against rat IL-6 was effective at reducing the degree of vasospasm in a dose-dependent manner. They showed similar results using a novel, broad spectrum, proinflammatory cytokine inhibitor (CNI-1493), including vasospasm reversal with their highest dose (Bowman and Bonneau 2006, 5). IL-6 receptor antagonists have also shown to be effective. Croci and colleagues (Croci and Wanderer 2021,12), administered Tocilizumab intravenously after SAH induction in a rabbit model. Compared to animals not given the antagonist and control animals, Tocilizumab-treated animals showed significantly reduced vasospasm and neuronal death.

IL-6 and its downstream effects can also be targeted indirectly. One mechanism is via mast cell (MC) activity modulation. MCs are the central nervous system's main proinflammatory effector cell involved in cytokine release (Parrella and Porrini 2019, 8) and are known to have increased expression in ruptured aneurysms (Hasan and Chalouhi 2012, 9). The use of LJ-529, a partial PPARγ agonist and adenosine A_3 receptor agonist, was shown to attenuate this mast cell mediated inflammation, reduce levels of IL-6 and subsequent post-SAH injury (Zhang and Huang 2021, 340). Another mechanism is via targeting endothelial dysfunction that is a direct result of inflammation mediated by factors such as IL-6 and can lead to vascular reactivity and cerebral ischemia (Frijns and Kasius 2006, 77). Lipoxin A4, an endogenous anti-inflammatory lipoxygenase-derived eicosanoid mediator, suppressed levels of pro-inflammatory IL-6 via modulation of the NF-κB pathway and significantly improved endothelial dysfunction when administered to rates with induced SAH (Liu and Zhang 2019, 408). A third mechanism is targeting the C-Jun N-terminal kinase (JNK) signaling pathway which contributes to the release of IL-6 and is a key driver of neuroinflammation (Zhang and Chen 2016, 3421060). Yatsushige and colleagues (Yatsushige and Yamaguchi 2005, 36), showed an increased expression of phosphorylated JNK mirroring an increase in IL-6 in dogs with induced SAH that later developed vasospasm. Administration of a JNK inhibitor, SP600125, attenuated the vasospasm in a dose-dependent manner. A final mechanism that requires further investigation involves soluble gp130 (sgp130), a signal transduction receptor and therefore regulator of IL-6 (Jostock and Müllberg 2001, 268). Nakura and colleagues (Nakura and Osuka 2011, 82), found decreasing concentrations of sgp130 five days post-SAH, coinciding with and likely contributing to vasospasm and DCI.

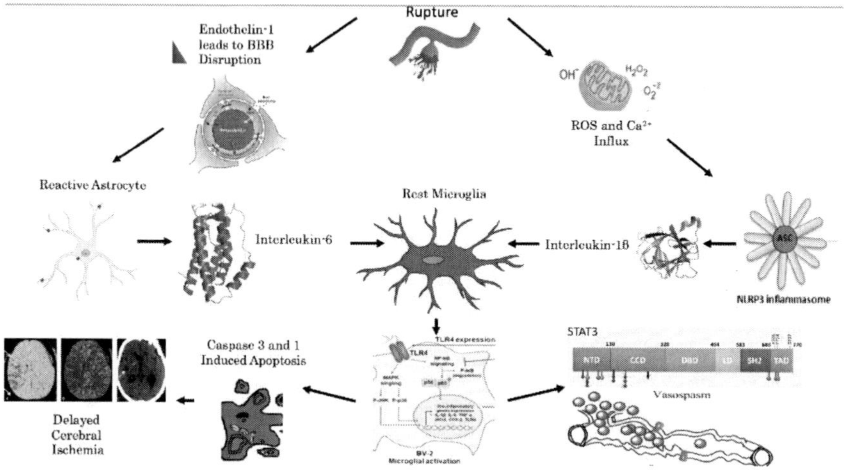

Figure 1. Shared pathway for Vasospasm.

Although much is still unknown regarding the role of IL-6 in the development of vasospasm and DCI, multiple pathways are involved, with neuroinflammation as the primary underlying mechanism (Figure 1). The nonspecific nature of IL-6, an acute phase reactant, limits its diagnostic potential. However, it's significant role has led to the discovery of multiple therapeutic targets that are currently under investigation.

NLRP3 Pathway

Inflammasomes are innate immune regulatory complexes which function to regulate the post-translational processing of pro-inflammatory factors, including IL-1β, IL-18, and GSDMD (Lupfer and Kanneganti 2013, 4). Inflammasomes are classified by their structural platform protein which serves to oligomerize and physically approximate the common elements of inflammasomes, ASC and caspase-1. Caspase-1 is the effector protein responsible for cleavage of pro-IL-1β into its active form as well as promotion of pyroptosis, a pro-inflammatory programmed cell death cascade (Lamkanfi and Dixit 2014, 157).

The NLRP3 inflammasome is uniquely pathogenic during SAH-induced neuroinflammation due to its distinct activation and expression profile (Swanson and Deng 2019, 19). After SAH, the characteristic damage-associated molecular patterns (DAMPs) are those associated with lysed RBCs, such as heme-containing proteins and ATP. TLR4 and P2X7, transmembrane receptors which activate the NLRP3 pathway, are known to bind and be activated by heme and ATP, respectively (Man and Kanneganti 2015, 265). Knockout of the either the TLR4 or P2X7 gene in mice is beneficial after subarachnoid hemorrhage, suggesting a common downstream element would be an ideal therapeutic target (Hanafy 2013, 83). NLRP3 also shares similar tissue expression patterns; it is expressed in TLR4+ and P2X7+ microglia, which are the central inflammatory cells of the CNS (Gustin and Kirchmeyer 2015, 10; Xiong and Liu 2016, 142). Overall, SAH is a uniquely powerful stimulus to the TLR4-NLRP3 and P2X7-NLRP3 pathways.

There is also direct evidence for the neuroprotective effect of NLRP3 inhibition after SAH. Multiple studies have documented decreased neuronal cell death after NLRP3 inhibition (Luo and Lu 2019, 146), including one that also reported NLRP3 inhibition ameliorated cerebral vasospasm (Dodd and Noda 2021, 18). One of the primary challenges in the translational study of this pathway is clearly delineating the mechanism of NLRP3-mediated vasospasm and DCI. It is not yet known which cell type is the primary source of NLRP3 activation after SAH or which is most involved in the development of vasospasm. One of the benefits of NLRP3 however is the availability of a specific small molecule inhibitor with well-defined mechanism of inhibition (Coll and Robertson 2015, 21). NLRP3 is a promising therapeutic target and future clinical trials will be vital to establishing safety and efficacy of any NLRP3 inhibitor in humans.

There is already some clinical evidence the NLRP3 pathway is activated after SAH in humans. IL-1β increases within the CSF after SAH and rise in IL-1β concentration during the second week post-SAH is most predictive of vasospasm and poor outcome (Coll and Hill 2019, 15). Further, caspase-1 enzymatic activity is elevated after SAH and predictive of poor outcome (Hendryk and Jarzab 2004, 25). Collectively, these data suggest that the, since IL-1β must be post-translationally activated by the inflammasome, the delayed activation of the NLRP3 pathway may be critical to development of vasospasm and DCI. In principle, the function of the NLRP3 pathway after SAH in humans seems to be similar to that in rodents, thus further supporting the basis for clinical trials of NLRP3 inhibitors for prevention of vasospasm and DCI.

Endothelial Injury

The blood-brain barrier (BBB) is a diffusion barrier that regulates the movement of compounds from the blood to the brain (Ballabh and Braun 2004, 16). The BBB is comprised of endothelial cells, the capillary basement membrane, pericytes enclosed within the capillary basement membrane, and astrocyte foot processes (Ballabh and Braun 2004, 16). As the central nervous system (CNS) is a sensitive organ, this barrier is highly selective, and this selectivity primarily results from the tight junctions—composed of transmembrane proteins including claudins, occludins, and junctional adhesion molecules (JAMs)—between the endothelial cells (Wolburg and Noell 2009, 335).In addition to their role in maintaining the BBB, endothelial cells regulate various aspects of vessel function, including thrombus formation, vascular tone, angiogenesis, and inflammation (Kumar and McBride 2019, 56; Sasaki and Kassell 1986, 19).

The inciting event in the pathogenesis of subarachnoid hemorrhage is the rupture of a cerebral aneurysm, which causes the release of blood under arterial pressure into the subarachnoid space where it mixes with the CSF (Kumar and McBride 2019, 56). Aneurysm rupture leads to aberrant blood flow dynamics, which subsequently cause endothelial cell damage (Kumar and McBride 2019, 56) through free radical generation (Fang and Chen 2009, 426346; Ayer and Zhang 2008, 104; Won and Lee 2011, 43), elevated intracellular calcium (Zhang and Weir 1996, 277), pro-inflammatory cytokines (Ansar and Larsen 2010, 1316; Guo and Sun 2010, 32; Zhou and Yamaguchi 2005, 25), and the direct cytotoxic effects of oxyhemoglobin (Meguro and Chen 2001, 77). Furthermore, following the Monro-Kellie doctrine, the contents within the cranium are restricted by the fixed space within the cranium including blood, CSF, and brain parenchyma existing in equilibrium (Rabelo and da Silva Brito 2021, 12). Therefore, an increase in one of these aforementioned components will result in an increase in intracranial pressure (ICP) (Rabelo and da Silva Brito 2021, 12). As cerebral perfusion pressure (CPP) is dependent upon the difference between mean arterial pressure (MAP) and ICP, a rise in ICP will cause a commensurate decrease in CPP (Armstead 2016, 465-77). This reduction in CPP causes a reduction in cerebral blood flow, which further contributes to endothelial cell injury following subarachnoid hemorrhage (Alkan and Tureyen 2001, 109; Clower and Yamamoto 1994, 240).

After the initial aneurysm rupture, endothelial cell dysfunction may result in impaired regulation of vascular tone and subsequent cerebral vasospasm

(Kumar and McBride 2019, 56; Iuliano and Pluta 2004, 100). Nitric oxide production is one of the principal vasodilators produced by endothelial cells, and impaired nitric oxide production is associated with cerebral vasospasm in primate models (Iuliano and Pluta 2004, 100). Notably, exogenous nitric oxide administration has shown efficacy in preventing cerebral vasospasm in rat models (Gabikian and Clatterbuck 2002, 33). As endothelial cells produce nitric oxide, endothelial cell dysfunction results in lower levels of nitric oxide (Iuliano and Pluta 2004, 100). In subarachnoid hemorrhage, this deficiency of nitric oxide is exacerbated by the presence of blood products in the subarachnoid space (Kumar and McBride 2019, 56). Evidence suggests that the autooxidation of oxyhemoglobin to methemoglobin produces free radicals that induce malfunction in the enzyme nitric oxide synthase (Kolias and Sen 2009, 87; Sabri and Ai2011, 31) and extracellular hemoglobin may act as a scavenger of available nitric oxide (Kumar and McBride 2019, 56). Furthermore, after subarachnoid hemorrhage, endothelial cells have demonstrated an up regulation of multiple vasoconstrictive proteins, including the endothelin B receptor, the serotonin (5HT1B) receptor, and the endothelin-1 molecule (Kumar and McBride 2019, 56).

Additionally, after subarachnoid hemorrhage, there is an inflammatory response caused by the activation of toll-like receptor 4 (TLR4) from downstream products of erythrocyte lysis (Kumar and McBride 2019, 56; Pradilla and Chaichana 2010, 21). Activation of TLR4 induces an inflammatory cascade—particularly through TNF-α production—that upregulates cell adhesion molecules, which in turn facilitates leukocyte adhesion and eventual extravasation, as well as causing endothelial cell damage (Zhou and Yamaguchi 2005, 25; Pradilla and Chaichana 2010, 21). However, due to alterations in the BBB, leukocytes that undergo extravasation may become trapped in the subarachnoid space and continue to release pro-inflammatory cytokines and reactive oxygen species, contributing to further endothelial cell dysfunction and inflammatory-induced vasoconstriction (Chaichana and Pradilla 2010, 73) (Figure 2).

Again, the BBB is comprised of endothelial cells, the capillary basement membrane, pericytes enclosed within the capillary basement membrane, and astrocyte foot processes (Ballabh and Braun 2004, 16). Endothelial cells are paramount in maintaining the function of the BBB; therefore, any mechanism causing aberrant function or destruction of endothelial cells ultimately leads to disruption of the BBB (Kumar and McBride 2019, 56). One mechanism of endothelial cell damage that was previously discussed is the generation of pro-inflammatory cytokines (Ansar and Larsen 2010, 1316; Guo and Sun 2010,

32; Zhou and Yamaguchi 2005, 25); however, it is worth noting that these pro-inflammatory cytokines have additional downstream effects, including the induction of matrix metalloproteinase 9 (MMP-9) (Guo and Sun 2010, 32; Rosenberg and Estrada 1995, 703). MMP-9 degrades the extracellular matrix and serves to further disrupt the BBB (Guo and Sun 2010, 32). A disrupted BBB has devastating consequences by causing red blood cell leakage, impaired transport, impaired vascular homeostasis, brain edema, and subsequent neuronal and glial cell injury; all of which contribute to delayed injury after the subsequent insult (Kumar and McBride 2019, 56).

Oxidative Stress Cascade

SAH is a neurologic emergency due to a ruptured aneurysm of the cerebral vasculature, leading to bleeding within the subarachnoid space. The incidence of SAH is between 1-7/2500 people (Rodriguez-Rodriguez and Egea-Guerrero 2014, 341). The prognosis of SAH patients is related to clinical status on admission (stratified according to metrics such as the Hunt-Hess scale or World Federation of Neurological Surgeon (WFNS)), magnitude of bleeding (quantified by the Fisher/modified Fischer scale) and the development of cerebral vasospasm (Hollig and Stoffel-Wagner 2017, 8). Cerebral vasospasm leading to delated ischemia is a devastating complication of SAH and is a major cause of morbidity and mortality after SAH and is estimated to be responsible for the deterioration or death of 15-20% of SAH patients (Longstreth and Nelson 1993, 43). SAH can trigger a vigorous immune response that is suspected to increase the risk of arteriolar vasospasm, contributing to the development of delayed cerebral ischemia. The role of inflammatory markers has been documented in recent years with a burgeoning body of evidence suggesting the increase in inflammatory markers in serum and CSF after subarachnoid hemorrhage is associated with subsequent brain injury. The clinical and prognostic value of these markers of inflammation however has remained uncertain (Etminan and Chang 2019, 76).

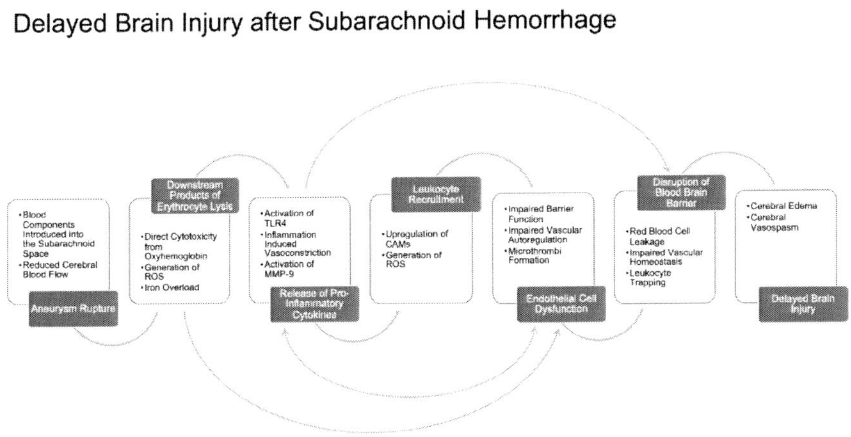

Figure 2. Role of endothelial cell dysfunction following SAH.

There are many biomarkers that have been associated with subarachnoid hemorrhage some with elevations in CSF while others are elevated in serum or both. Rodriguez et al. investigated the role of several biomarkers (Table 1). To date, these biomarkers have not been demonstrated to be a useful tool for predicting vasospasm or outcome after SAH due to their marginal specificity (Ascenzi and Bocedi 2005, 57). Höllig et al. conducted a study which examined the time course of inflammatory markers after SAH. This study discussed the time course of interleukin 6 (IL-6), leukemia inhibitory factor (LIF), C-reactive protein (CRP), matrix metalloproteinase 9 (MMP9), and intercellular adhesion molecule 1 (ICAM1), to determine a reliable prognostic indicator. Of note, they observed that using the WFNS scale score, IL-6 levels were found to be indicators for injury severity but the study notes that IL-6 is non-specific and ambiguous, rising during a variety of other stimuli. The time course of serum inflammatory markers related to occurrence of DCI showed no significant difference.

Chaichana et al. investigated the interaction between leukocyte-endothelial cell interactions in the pathogenesis of vasospasm after SAH. This study discussed how cell adhesion molecules (CAMs) are upregulated during SAH and may represent the root of chronic vasospasm, which is currently thought to be due to the second immune response/chronic inflammation characterized by lymphocytes and plasma cells (Filer and Pitzalis 2006, 6). Al-Kholy et al. also investigated the role of biomarkers. This study demonstrated a relationship between occurrence of inflammation with rising CRP level and development of vasospasm post-SAH. The noted CRP, total leukocyte count and IL-6 to be significantly higher in the patients who were to develop post SAH vasospasm and determined IL-6 and total leukocyte count may be strong predictors of vasospasm, which is congruent with previous studies by Mazlam and Hodgson identifying leukocyte action on the vasculature as a cause of a vasospasm and ischemia (Cahill and Calvert 2006, 26).

Table 1. Biomarkers of SAH

Biomarker	Activity	Situation in SAH	Research results	
Oxidative stress	NO·	Vasoconstrictor	↓0–24 h ↑>24 h	Administration of NO· donors improves recovery and reduces CVS incidence
	NOX	Produces ROS	↑	Inhibition of NOX prevents vasoconstriction and improves CBF in rat model
	SOD	Eliminates O_2	↓	Administration/overexpression SOD: –Rabbit model: ↓ CVS incidence –Dog model: no effect on preventing CVS –Mice model: ↓ CVS incidence
	GPx	Eliminates H_2O_2	↑ activity	Increased activity in SAH patients suffering CVS
	MDA	LPO	↑	Predicts neurological outcome
Inflammation	TNF-α	Pro-inflammatory	↑	Related to poor outcome. No association with CVS development
	IL-6	Stimulates mature B cell growth and promotes synthesis of acute phase proteins	↑ CSF (not serum)	Related to CVS development
	IL-1β	Pro-inflammatory	↑ in jugular vein	Slight increase promotes pathological processes
	IL-1ra	Inflammatory inhibitor	↑ CSF	Related to poor outcome
	IL-8	Neutrophil and monocyte chemotactic properties	↑ CSF (not serum)	No relation with CVS development

Biomarker	Activity	Situation in SAH	Research results	
Vascular pathology	ET-1	Vasoconstrictor	↑	Remains inconclusive whether ET-1 levels differ from SAH developing CVS or not
	Rho-kinase	Smooth muscle constriction	↑ activity	Administration of Rho-kinase inhibitors reduces the incidence of CVS development in animal models
	Neuropeptides	Control of vascular tone	↑/↓	Inconclusive results
Brain injury	S100B	[nM]: promotes neural growth [μM]: induces neural apoptosis	↑	Inconclusive whether related to poor outcome and CVS development or not.
	NSE	Glycolytic pathway. Mainly located in neurons	↑	Correlates with clinical deterioration and WFNS, but not with amount of blood or CVS development
	GFAP	Structural (astrocytes)	↑	Correlates with WFNS and poor clinical outcome
	KLK6	Remyelination	↓	As a consequence of cell death following SAH, KLK6 release decreases
	pNF-H	Neurofilament structure (white matter)	↑	Predicts poor outcome
	UCHL1	Gray matter structure	↑	Predicts poor outcome

Risk for cerebral vasospasm begins to take place around day 4 after subarachnoid hemorrhage and continues until the second week and is characterized by diffuse narrowing of arteries (O'Shea and Murray 2008, 28). The pathophysiology of the vasospasm is due thought to be a result of a vigorous inflammatory cascade. As the red blood cells within the subarachnoid space begin to breakdown, they release hemoglobin, which is toxic (Serhan and Savill 2005, 6). Some hemoglobin is neutralized by serum haptoglobin, a protein whose function is to clear free hemoglobin to avoid iron loss, but an immense primary immune response is triggered by the remaining hemoglobin, leading to the migration of macrophages and polymorphonuclear cells into the subarachnoid space with the help of cell adhesion molecules on the surface of endothelial cells (Serhan 2006, 341-64). The expression of CAMs is upregulated by the lysis of red blood cells (Gallia and Tamargo 2006, 28), which are phagocytized by the migrating leukocytes, that then die and degranulate with 2-4 days. Upon the death of these immune cells, which remained trapped in the subarachnoid space due to the absence of lymphatic vessels and impaired CSF flow due to SAH (Cahill and Calvert 2006, 26), endothelin's and free radicals are released. Endothelins are potent vasoconstrictors while free radicals within the subarachnoid space have been observed to cause smooth muscle constriction (via activation of protein kinase C and Rho kinase). Oxygen free radicals, also known as reactive oxygen species, cause lipid peroxidation, which contributes to delayed ischemic injury after SAH. These oxygen free radicals disrupt the blood brain barrier and induce pro-apoptotic enzymes (Miller and Turan 2014, 384342).

Corticosteroids are potent anti-inflammatories and been tested in human SAH trials. High dose methylprednisolone has been shown to improve neurological outcomes, reduce mortality and delayed cerebral ischemia (Pradilla and Chaichana 2010, 21). Intravenous hydrocortisone administration after SAH has more controversial results, with one large multicenter study showing improved mental status, speech and motor function at 1 month after treatment and another showing no improvement in neurological outcome. Nonsteroidal anti-inflammatory drugs (NSAIDs) have been shown to reduce vasospasm in animal models of SAH, however the mode of treatment (administration 30 minutes prior and 3 hours after SAH) makes replication for human trials difficult (Ryba and Grieb 1991, 22).

Immunosuppressants have also been tested with moderate success (White and Robertson 1983, 12). Clinical studies with cyclosporin showed no benefit in outcomes for patients with severe SAH but showed improved outcomes in patients with early clipping after SAH when combined with nimodipine. Monoclonal antibodies against CAMs, and drugs that decrease expression of CAMs have been shown to decrease vasospasm in experimental studies (Ryba and Grieb 1991, 22). Overall, therapies aimed at preventing inflammation may prevent or reverse vasospasm but outcomes for SAH patients depend on more than the development of vasospasm, as demonstrated by the varied success of anti-inflammatories. And although anti-inflammatories may improve the lives of patients, neuroinflammation has beneficial effects and may play a role in recovery (Chaichana and Pradilla 2010, 73).

Calcium Calmodulin Protein Kinase System

The calcium/calmodulin-dependent protein kinase (CaMK) family of proteins are important intracellular Ca+2 sensors and signaling proteins in a number of biological systems, with calcium/calmodulin-dependent protein kinase II (CaMKII) being prominently expressed in the brain, heart, and vasculature (Zhang and Connelly 2021, 12). Ca+2 action in the cytosol is crucial for smooth-muscle contractility modulation (Yamaura and Tani 1993, 79). Smooth-muscle contraction is controlled by Ca+2/CaM-regulated myosin light-chain kinase (MLCK) and myosin light-chain phosphatase (MLCP) dependent phosphorylation and dephosphorylation of myosin light chain (MLC). Increased intracellular Ca+2 forms a compound with calmodulin (CaM), which activates MLCK and causes smooth muscle contraction. The activity of MLCP reverses this contraction (Sato and Tani 1997, 87). Pathways that result in persistent activation of MLCK as a biproduct of elevated intracellular calcium and/or autophosphorylation of the kinase are thought to be involved in the delayed onset of vasospasm after SAH.

Increased Ca+2 sensitivity, persistent activation of CaMKII, and inhibition of myosin phosphatase (through phosphorylation at its myosin-binding subunit), are all factors that contribute to the development of Ca+2-dependent and Ca+2-independent vasospasm after SAH (Williams and Becker 1987, 235). Furthermore, it is well understood that an elevated sympathetic tone coupled with increased circulating catecholamine may occur after SAH, and increase endothelin activation, which is implicated in precipitating vasospasm (Chen and Li 2014, 858496). It has also been shown that shear stress on endothelial cells, as seen in vessel rupture resulting in SAH, causes increased exposure to histamine, thrombin, oxyhemoglobin, and other blood products, which leads to increased calcium release from intracellular stores and decreases NO availability (a vasodilator scavenged by oxyhemoglobin) (Johansson and Haase 2014, 29). Cerebral vasospasm is defined by an increase in intracellular Ca+2 levels and leading to greater sustained activation of MLC in vascular smooth-muscle cells, which might lead to subsequent ischemic damage in SAH patients.

SAH patients have a significant initial death rate (12%) before seeking treatment (Kolias and Sen 2009, 87). In roughly 40% of SAH patients, delayed cerebral ischemia and cerebral vasospasm develop after several days post SAH which leads to a decreased cerebral blood flow (CBF) (Vergouwen and Etminan 2011, 31). Many patients who survive SAH have long-term memory and cognitive problems, which have a negative influence on their quality of life (Al-Khindi and Macdonald 2010, 41). Interventions that target intracellular calcium and CaMKII availability to prevent vasospasm following SAH have been studied in several research investigations (Figure 3).

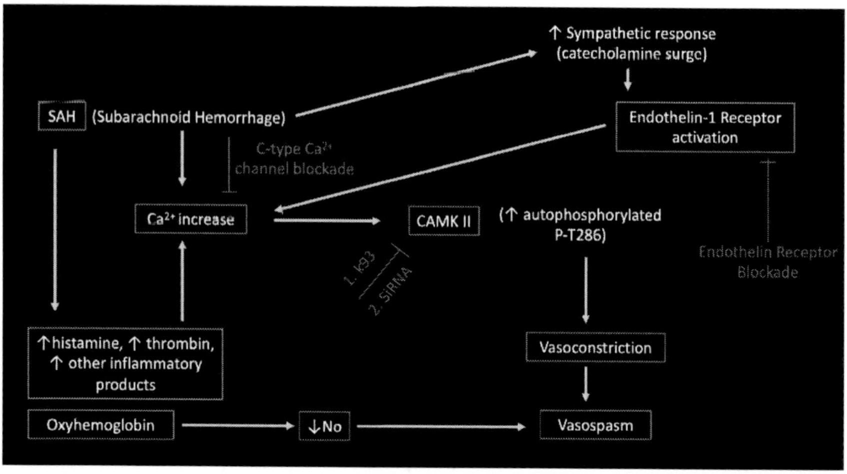

Figure 3. Ca/Calmodulin pathway contribution to vasospasm.

A meta-analysis of a large single-center study with 3361 patients across 16 trials (6 trials specifically for oral nimodipine (969 patients total)) found that oral nimodipine (L-type Ca+2 channel blocker) reduces the incidence of adverse outcomes and delays cerebral ischemia after SAH, possibly by reducing intracellular calcium and preventing vasospasms after SAH. Another study found that infusing high doses of nicardipine intravenously as soon as 24 hours after SAH has significant beneficial effect on the development of delayed cerebral ischemia, implying that pharmacological reduction of intracellular Ca2+ in the cerebral artery is an important measure to prevent the development of vasospasm (Pickard and Murray 1989, 298).

A study conducted by Parker et al. utilized quantitative mass spectrometry–based phosphoproteomic analysis in cerebral artery tissue lysates obtained from a rat model of SAH to examine early SAH-induced phosphorylation events at two different time points (0.5hr and 1hr after SAH respectively), finding sustained activation of CaMKII via phosphorylation at its autophosphorylation site T286 that could be blocked by treating the rat with KN93 prior to SAH hence reducing the delayed vasospastic and ischemic events (Dodd and Laurent 2021, 10). Another group utilizing siRNA that targets CaMKII (Edvinsson and Povlsen 2014, 11), confirmed the positive benefits of decreasing CaMKII activity for improved outcomes after SAH in animal models. Furthermore, CaMKII knockdown by siRNA injected intracerebroventricularly 48 hours before surgery improved neurobehavior and significantly reduced p-TAK1, p-JNK, and nucleotide-binding domain-like receptor protein 3 (NLRP3) inflammasome expression (Parker and Larsen 2013, 33), indicating a reduced inflammatory response that may be involved in reduced vasospasm, improved CBF, and prevention of secondary ischemia (Zhou and Enkhjargal 2018, 49).

Protein Kinase C Pathway

There are several known isoforms of protein kinase C (PKC) (Mellor and Parker 1998, 332; Kaleli and Ozer 2020, 9; Karhu and Ruskoaho 2021, 99). Among PKC isoforms, PKCα and PKCδ are the most widely implicated in vasospasm following subarachnoid hemorrhage (Nishizawa and Obara 2000, 98; Ansar and Edvinsson 2008, 39; Pyne-Geithman and Nair 2008, 13). Other studies have suggested that isoform PKCε may play a role as well (Takuwa and Matsui 1993, 13; Wickman and Lan 2003, 92), but this evidence is less substantial. Our understanding of the PKC isoforms involved in vasospasm post-subarachnoid hemorrhage comes mainly from canine studies. However, several of these studies, along with mechanisms of PKC described in other bodies of literature, shed light on the role that PKC may play in inducing vasospasm in the setting of subarachnoid hemorrhage.

PKC is a well-characterized class of serine/threonine kinases that are involved in numerous cell processes, including survival and proliferation, and are implicated in a wide variety of disease states, including cardiovascular disease (Griner and Kazanietz 2007, 7; Garg and Benedetti 2014, 33). Since first being described in literature over 30 years ago, several isoforms of PKC have been identified and categorized into three distinct groups: classical (isoforms PKCα, PKCβI, PKCβII, PKCγ), novel (isoforms PKCδ, PKCε, PKCη, PKCθ), and atypical (isoforms PKCζ, PKCι) (Garg and Benedetti 2014, 33). There are multiple endogenous substances that activate PKC isoforms, but diacylglycerol (DAG) is among the most discussed (Huang 1989, 425-32). Moreover, activation by DAG has been further stratified by PKC isoform subtype. Namely, only the classical and novel subtypes are activated by DAG (Newton 2018, 208-30). Thus, since the isoforms PKCα and PKCδ belong to the classical and novel subtypes, respectively, it follows then that processes involving an increase in DAG must be considered in the context of this discussion. Other potential mechanisms for the development of cerebral vasospasm following subarachnoid hemorrhage are also discussed below, including the role of calcium, nitric oxide (NO), and phosphorylation of the myosin regulatory light chains (MLC20).

One proposed mechanism of PKC activation leading to cerebral vasospasm involves the elevation of oxyhemoglobin levels in the setting of subarachnoid hemorrhage which stimulates vascular endothelial cells to produce endothelin-1 (Wu and Chen 2016, 121). Endothelin-1 then promotes the generation of DAG from breakdown of phosphatidylinositol bisphosphate (PIP2) (Lan and Das 2004, 286). DAG subsequently activates PKC, which potentiates calcium influx and causes smooth muscle cell contraction (Dietrich and Dacey 2000, 46). The role of PKC in further increasing calcium entry into vascular smooth muscle cells is well-characterized in the cardiac literature (Dietrich and Dacey 1994, 90), and these observations would likely translate to PKC-mediated cerebral vasospasm. Further, since the PKC isoforms PKCα and PKCδ thought to be involved in cerebral vasospasm following subarachnoid hemorrhage are activated by DAG, this mechanism appears to be plausible. Additionally, PKC has been shown to both monophosphorylate and biphosphorylate myosin light chain (MLC), contributing to the perpetuation of coronary artery vasospasm in porcine models (Kadokami and Shimokawa 1996, 94). A mechanism of cerebral vasospasm under the influence of PKC may be formulated from this framework, as there are phosphorylation sites on MLC20 that are specific to PKC. Upon phosphorylation by PKC, these sites can drastically slow cross bridge cycling, subsequently leading to calcium sensitization and contraction maintenance even in low calcium states (Shimokawa 2000, 1-12).

Endothelin-1 has also been shown to reduce NO production in vascular smooth muscle cells through activation of PKC (Ramzy and Rao 2006, 114). In fact, the two isoforms shown to have this effect are PKCα and PKCδ, the same isoforms thought to be involved in cerebral vasospasm following subarachnoid hemorrhage (Nishikawa and Yamamoto 1997, 73). Thus, in the setting of subarachnoid hemorrhage, where endothelin-1 levels are high, another mechanism by which PKC may cause cerebral vasospasm is through inhibition of the vasodilatory NO. As such, the presence of endothelin-1 has the potential to both initiate vasoconstriction through PKC-mediated calcium potentiation and reduce vasodilation through attenuation of NO production. Interestingly, the transient receptor potential vanilloid 1 (TRPV1) channel located on vascular smooth muscle cells, known to play an independent role in the pathogenesis of coronary vasospasm, have recently been discovered to be partially acted upon by PKC under the influence of endothelin-1 as well (Korishettar and Nishijima 2021, 178). These channels may also have an effect on cerebral vasospasm under the direct influence of PKC that is yet to be characterized. Bilirubin oxidation products may also play a role in the development of cerebral vasospasm, with peak production in cerebrospinal fluid between 3-8 days after the onset of subarachnoid hemorrhage, which closely mirrors the timeline for cerebral vasospasm development following subarachnoid hemorrhage (Weir and Grace 1978, 48). Bilirubin oxidation products have also been shown to activate PKC isoforms PKCα and PKCδ and may initiate subsequent cerebral vasospasm through this mechanism (Nishziawa 2011, 27-30). Some researchers have even shown evidence that PKCδ activation is initiated on approximately day 4 following the onset of subarachnoid hemorrhage and is mainly responsible for the initial development of cerebral vasospasm. On the other hand, it is postulated that PKCα activation is initiated on approximately day 8 following the onset of subarachnoid hemorrhage and is mainly responsible for maintaining cerebral vasospasm (Nishziawa 2011, 27-30). This has profound implications for the development of delayed cerebral ischemia, which is a primary concern in this setting. Delayed cerebral ischemia is a major predictor of morbidity in patients who sustain a subarachnoid hemorrhage (Dodd and Laurent 2021, 10). With evidence of multiple mechanisms that describe both the onset and maintenance of cerebral vasospasm due to PKC activation, it follows that PKC may be an important factor in the cascade of events leading to the development of delayed cerebral ischemia (Figure 4).

In summary, although the exact interplay of mechanisms is not known, it is clear that PKC may play a significant role in the development of cerebral vasospasm following subarachnoid hemorrhage and, thus, may play an important role in the development of delayed cerebral ischemia leading to significant patient morbidity and mortality. An overview of these proposed mechanisms has been highlighted in Figure 4. An understanding of the role that PKC plays in this setting is of particular importance, with the potential of guiding the development of future clinical interventions, such as those involving modulation or inhibition of PKC.

Conclusion

This chapter highlighted some emerging pathways that are at play in the pathophysiology of vasospasm following SAH. Ongoing work is needed to fully understand the time course of progression. Once the pathophysiology is more completely understood, targeted treatment approaches can be implemented. It will be important for the teams that investigate this important topic to be multidisciplinary and include both pre-clinical and clinical expertise. Substantial funding will be warranted to institute multi-institutional studies for discovery and validation.

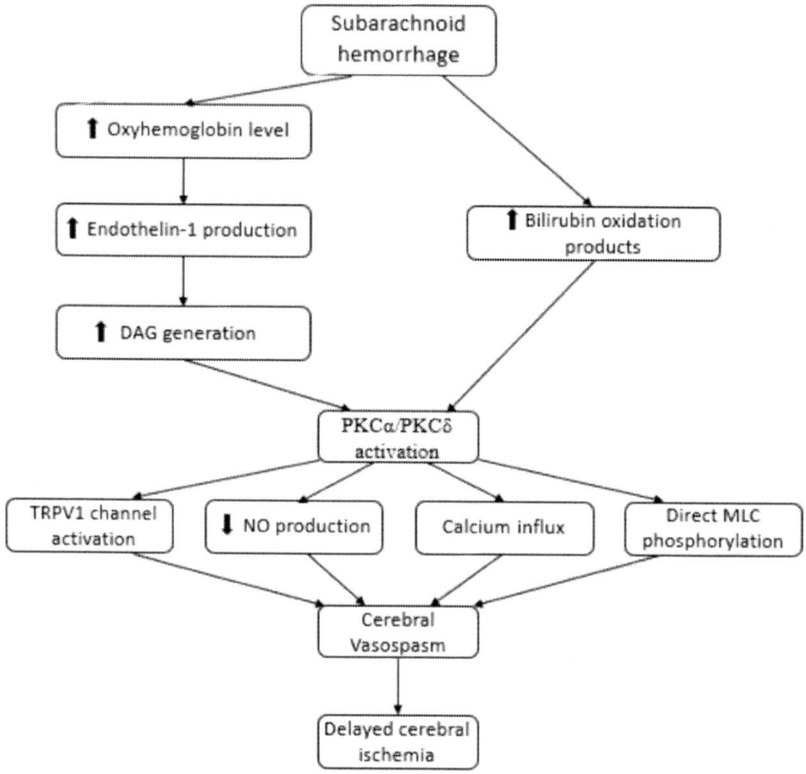

Figure 4. Protein Kinase C pathway.

References

Alkan T., Tureyen K., Ulutas M., Kahveci N., Goren B., Korfali E., et al. 2001. Acute and delayed vasoconstriction after subarachnoid hemorrhage: local cerebral blood flow, histopathology, and morphology in the rat basilar artery. *Arch Physiol Biochem.* 109(2):145-53.

Al-Khindi T., Macdonald R. L., Schweizer T. A. 2010. Cognitive and functional outcome after aneurysmal subarachnoid hemorrhage. *Stroke.* 41(8):e519-36.

Altura B. M., Gebrewold A., Zheng T., Altura, B. T. 2002. Sphingomyelinase and ceramide analogs induce vasoconstriction and leukocyte-endothelial interactions in cerebral venules in the intact rat brain: Insight into mechanisms and possible relation to brain injury and stroke. *Brain Res Bull*. 58(3):271-8.

Ansar S., Edvinsson L. 2008. Subtype activation and interaction of protein kinase C and mitogen-activated protein kinase controlling receptor expression in cerebral arteries and microvessels after subarachnoid hemorrhage. *Stroke*. 39(1):185-90.

Ansar S., Larsen C., Maddahi A., Edvinsson L. 2010. Subarachnoid hemorrhage induces enhanced expression of thromboxane A2 receptors in rat cerebral arteries. *Brain Res*. 1316:163-72.

Armstead W. M. 2016. Cerebral Blood Flow Autoregulation and Dysautoregulation. *Anesthesiol Clin*. 34(3):465-77.

Ascenzi P., Bocedi A., Visca P., Altruda F., Tolosano E., Beringhelli T., et al. 2005. Hemoglobin and heme scavenging. *IUBMB Life*. 57(11):749-59.

Ayer R. E., Zhang J. H. 2008. Oxidative stress in subarachnoid haemorrhage: significance in acute brain injury and vasospasm. *Acta Neurochir Suppl*. 104:33-41.

Ballabh P., Braun A., Nedergaard M. 2004. The blood-brain barrier: an overview: structure, regulation, and clinical implications. *Neurobiol Dis*. 16(1):1-13.

Bjerkne Wenneberg S., Odenstedt Hergès H., Svedin P., Mallard C., Karlsson T., Adiels M., et al. 2021. Association between inflammatory response and outcome after subarachnoid haemorrhage. *Acta Neurol Scand*. 143(2):195-205.

Bowman G., Dixit S., Bonneau R. H., Chinchilli V. M., Cockroft K. M. 2004. Neutralizing antibody against interleukin-6 attenuates posthemorrhagic vasospasm in the rat femoral artery model. *Neurosurgery*. 54(3):719-25, discussion 25-6.

Bowman G., Bonneau R. H., Chinchilli V. M., Tracey K. J., Cockroft K. M. 2006. A novel inhibitor of inflammatory cytokine production (CNI-1493) reduces rodent post-hemorrhagic vasospasm. *Neurocrit Care*. 5(3):222-9.

Cahill J., Calvert J. W., Zhang J. H. 2006. Mechanisms of early brain injury after subarachnoid hemorrhage. *J Cereb Blood Flow Metab*. 26(11):1341-53.

Chaichana K. L., Pradilla G., Huang J., Tamargo R. J. 2010. Role of inflammation (leukocyte-endothelial cell interactions) in vasospasm after subarachnoid hemorrhage. *World Neurosurg*. 73(1):22-41.

Chalouhi N., Ali M. S., Jabbour P. M., Tjoumakaris S. I., Gonzalez L. F., Rosenwasser R. H., et al. 2012. Biology of intracranial aneurysms: role of inflammation. *J Cereb Blood Flow Metab*. 32(9):1659-76.

Chamling B., Gross S., Stoffel-Wagner B., Schubert G. A., Clusmann H., Coburn M., et al. 2017. Early Diagnosis of Delayed Cerebral Ischemia: Possible Relevance for Inflammatory Biomarkers in Routine Clinical Practice? *World Neurosurg*. 104:152-7.

Chaudhry S. R., Stoffel-Wagner B., Kinfe T. M., Güresir E., Vatter H., Dietrich D., et al. 2017. Elevated Systemic IL-6 Levels in Patients with Aneurysmal Subarachnoid Hemorrhage Is an Unspecific Marker for Post-SAH Complications. *Int J Mol Sci*. 18(12).

Chen S., Li Q., Wu H., Krafft P. R., Wang Z., Zhang J. H. 2014. The harmful effects of subarachnoid hemorrhage on extracerebral organs. *Biomed Res Int*. 2014:858496.

Chou S. H., Feske S. K., Atherton J., Konigsberg R. G., DeJager P. L., Du R., et al. 2012. Early elevation of serum tumor necrosis factor-α is associated with poor outcome in subarachnoid hemorrhage. *J Investig Med*. 60(7):1054-8.

Clower B. R., Yamamoto Y., Cain L., Haines D. E., Smith R. R. 1994. Endothelial injury following experimental subarachnoid hemorrhage in rats: effects on brain blood flow. *Anat Rec*. 240(1):104-14.

Coll R. C., Robertson A. A., Chae J. J., Higgins, S. C., Munoz-Planillo R., Inserra M. C., et al. 2015. A small-molecule inhibitor of the NLRP3 inflammasome for the treatment of inflammatory diseases. *Nat Med*. 21(3):248-55.

Coll R. C., Hill J. R., Day C. J., Zamoshnikova A., Boucher D., Massey N. L., et al. 2019. MCC950 directly targets the NLRP3 ATP-hydrolysis motif for inflammasome inhibition. *Nat Chem Biol*. 15(6):556-9.

Croci D., Nevzati E., Danura H., Schöpf S., Fandino J., Marbacher S., et al. 2019. The relationship between IL-6, ET-1 and cerebral vasospasm, in experimental rabbit subarachnoid hemorrhage. *J Neurosurg Sci*. 63(3):245-50.

Croci D., Nevzati E., Muroi C., Schöpf S., Hornemann T., Widmer H. R., et al. 2020. Changes in the cerebrospinal fluid lipid profile following subarachnoid hemorrhage in a closed cranium model: Correlations to cerebral vasospasm, neuronal cell death and Interleukin-6 synthesis. A pilot study. *J Stroke Cerebrovasc Dis*. 29(9):105054.

Croci D. M., Wanderer S., Strange F., Grüter B. E., Sivanrupan S., Andereggen L., et al. 2021. Tocilizumab Reduces Vasospasms, Neuronal Cell Death, and Microclot Formation in a Rabbit Model of Subarachnoid Hemorrhage. *Transl Stroke Res*. 12(5):894-904.

Dietrich H. H., Dacey R. G. Jr. 2000. Molecular keys to the problems of cerebral vasospasm. *Neurosurgery*. 46(3):517-30.

Dodd W. S., Noda I., Martinez M., Hosaka K., Hoh B. L. 2021. NLRP3 inhibition attenuates early brain injury and delayed cerebral vasospasm after subarachnoid hemorrhage. *J Neuroinflammation*. 18(1):163.

Dodd W. S., Laurent D., Dumont A. S., Hasan D. M., Jabbour P. M., Starke R. M., et al. 2021. Pathophysiology of Delayed Cerebral Ischemia After Subarachnoid Hemorrhage: A Review. *J Am Heart Assoc*. 10(15):e021845.

Edvinsson L., Povlsen G. K., Ahnstedt H., Waldsee R. 2014. CaMKII inhibition with KN93 attenuates endothelin and serotonin receptor-mediated vasoconstriction and prevents subarachnoid hemorrhage-induced deficits in sensorimotor function. *J Neuroinflammation*. 11:207.

Etminan N., Chang H. S., Hackenberg K., deRooij N. K., Vergouwen M. D. I., Rinkel G. J. E., et al. 2019. Worldwide Incidence of Aneurysmal Subarachnoid Hemorrhage According to Region, Time Period, Blood Pressure, and Smoking Prevalence in the Population: A Systematic Review and Meta-analysis. *JAMA Neurol*. 76(5):588-97.

Fang Q., Chen G., Zhu W., Dong W., Wang Z. 2009. Influence of melatonin on cerebrovascular proinflammatory mediators expression and oxidative stress following subarachnoid hemorrhage in rabbits. *Mediators Inflamm*. 2009:426346.

Filer A., Pitzalis C., Buckley C. D. 2006. Targeting the stromal microenvironment in chronic inflammation. *Curr Opin Pharmacol*. 6(4):393-400.

Frijns C. J., Kasius K. M., Algra A., Fijnheer R., and Rinkel G. J. 2006. Endothelial cell activation markers and delayed cerebral ischaemia in patients with subarachnoid haemorrhage. *J NeurolNeurosurg Psychiatry*. 77(7):863-7.

Gabikian P., Clatterbuck R. E., Eberhart C. G., Tyler B. M., Tierney T. S., Tamargo R. J. 2002. Prevention of experimental cerebral vasospasm by intracranial delivery of a nitric oxide donor from a controlled-release polymer: toxicity and efficacy studies in rabbits and rats. *Stroke*. 33(11):2681-6.

Gaetani P., Tartara F., Pignatti P., Tancioni F., Rodriguez Y., Baena R., DeBenedetti F. 1998. Cisternal CSF levels of cytokines after subarachnoid hemorrhage. *Neurol Res*. 20(4):337-42.

Gallia G. L., Tamargo R. J. 2006. Leukocyte-endothelial cell interactions in chronic vasospasm after subarachnoid hemorrhage. *Neurol Res*. 28(7):750-8.

Garg R., Benedetti L. G., Abera M. B., Wang H., Abba M., Kazanietz M. G. 2014. Protein kinase C and cancer: what we know and what we do not. *Oncogene*. 33(45): 5225-37.

Griner E. M., Kazanietz M. G. 2007. Protein kinase C and other diacylglycerol effectors in cancer. *Nat Rev Cancer*. 7(4):281-94.

Guo Z., Sun X., He Z., Jiang Y., Zhang X., Zhang J. H. 2010. Matrix metalloproteinase-9 potentiates early brain injury after subarachnoid hemorrhage. *Neurol Res*. 32(7): 715-20.

Gustin A., Kirchmeyer M., Koncina E., Felten P., Losciuto S., Heurtaux T., et al. 2015. NLRP3 Inflammasome Is Expressed and Functional in Mouse Brain Microglia but Not in Astrocytes. *PLoS One*. 10(6): e0130624.

Hanafy K. A. 2013. The role of microglia and the TLR4 pathway in neuronal apoptosis and vasospasm after subarachnoid hemorrhage. *J Neuroinflammation*. 10:83.

Hasan D., Chalouhi N., Jabbour P., Hashimoto T. 2012. Macrophage imbalance (M1 vs. M2) and upregulation of mast cells in wall of ruptured human cerebral aneurysms: preliminary results. *J Neuroinflammation*. 9:222.

Hendryk S., Jarzab B., Josko J. 2004. Increase of the IL-1 beta and IL-6 levels in CSF in patients with vasospasm following aneurysmal SAH. *Neuro Endocrinol Lett*. 25(1-2):141-7.

Hollig A., Stoffel-Wagner B., Clusmann H., Veldeman M., Schubert G. A., Coburn M. 2017. Time Courses of Inflammatory Markers after Aneurysmal Subarachnoid Hemorrhage and Their Possible Relevance for Future Studies. *Front Neurol*. 8:694.

Hopkins S. J., McMahon C. J., Singh N., Galea J., Hoadley M., Scarth S., et al. 2012. Cerebrospinal fluid and plasma cytokines after subarachnoid haemorrhage: CSF interleukin-6 may be an early marker of infection. *J Neuroinflammation*. 9:255.

Huang K. P. 1989. The mechanism of protein kinase C activation. *Trends Neurosci*. 12(11):425-32.

Ikedo T., Minami M., Kataoka H., Hayashi K., Nagata M., Fujikawa R., et al. 2017. Dipeptidyl Peptidase-4 Inhibitor Anagliptin Prevents Intracranial Aneurysm Growth by Suppressing Macrophage Infiltration and Activation. *J Am Heart Assoc*. 6(6).

Ito A., Shimokawa H., Nakaike R., Fukai T., Sakata M., Takayanagi T., et al. 1994. Role of protein kinase C-mediated pathway in the pathogenesis of coronary artery spasm in a swine model. *Circulation*. 90(5):2425-31.

Iuliano B. A., Pluta R. M., Jung C., Oldfield E. H. 2004. Endothelial dysfunction in a primate model of cerebral vasospasm. *J Neurosurg*. 100(2):287-94.

Johansson P. I., Haase N., Perner A., Ostrowski S. R. 2014. Association between sympathoadrenal activation, fibrinolysis, and endothelial damage in septic patients: a prospective study. *J Crit Care*. 29(3):327-33.

Jostock T., Müllberg J., Ozbek S., Atreya R., Blinn G., Voltz N., et al. 2001. Soluble gp130 is the natural inhibitor of soluble interleukin-6 receptor transsignaling responses. *Eur J Biochem*. 268(1):160-7.

Kadokami T., Shimokawa H., Fukumoto Y., Ito A., Takayanagi T., Egashira K., et al. 1996. Coronary artery spasm does not depend on the intracellular calcium store but is substantially mediated by the protein kinase C-mediated pathway in a swine model with interleukin-1 beta *in vivo*. *Circulation*. 94(2):190-6.

Kaleli H. N., Ozer E., Kaya V. O., Kutlu O. 2020. Protein Kinase C Isozymes and Autophagy during Neurodegenerative Disease Progression. *Cells*. 9(3).

Karhu S. T., Ruskoaho H., Talman V. 2021. Distinct Regulation of Cardiac Fibroblast Proliferation and Transdifferentiation by Classical and Novel Protein Kinase C Isoforms: Possible Implications for New Antifibrotic Therapies. *Mol Pharmacol*. 99(2):104-13.

Kolias A. G., Sen J., Belli A. 2009. Pathogenesis of cerebral vasospasm following aneurysmal subarachnoid hemorrhage: putative mechanisms and novel approaches. *J NeurosciRes*. 87(1):1-11.

Korishettar A. M., Nishijima Y., Wang Z., Xie Y., Fang J., Wilcox D. A., et al. 2021. Endothelin-1 potentiates TRPV1-mediated vasoconstriction of human adipose arterioles in a protein kinase C-dependent manner. *Br J Pharmacol*. 178(3):709-25.

Kwon K. Y., Jeon B. C. 2001. Cytokine levels in cerebrospinal fluid and delayed ischemic deficits in patients with aneurysmal subarachnoid hemorrhage. *J Korean Med Sci*. 16(6):774-80.

Lamkanfi M., Dixit V. M. 2014. Mechanisms and functions of inflammasomes. *Cell*. 157(5):1013-22.

Lan C., Das D., Wloskowicz A., Vollrath B. 2004. Endothelin-1 modulates hemoglobin-mediated signaling in cerebrovascular smooth muscle via RhoA/Rho kinase and protein kinase C. *Am J Physiol Heart Circ Physiol*. 286(1):H165-73.

Lenski M., Huge V., Briegel J., Tonn J. C., Schichor C., Thon N. 2017. Interleukin 6 in the Cerebrospinal Fluid as a Biomarker for Onset of Vasospasm and VentriculitisAfter Severe Subarachnoid Hemorrhage. *World Neurosurg*. 99:132-9.

Li P. L., Zhang D. X., Zou A. P., Campbell W. B. 1999. Effect of ceramide on KCa channel activity and vascular tone in coronary arteries. *Hypertension*. 33(6):1441-6.

Liu L., Zhang P., Zhang Z., Hu Q., He J., Liu H., et al. 2019. LXA4 ameliorates cerebrovascular endothelial dysfunction by reducing acute inflammation after subarachnoid hemorrhage in rats. *Neuroscience*. 408:105-14.

Longstreth W. T. Jr., Nelson L. M., Koepsell T. D., vanBelle G. 1993. Clinical course of spontaneous subarachnoid hemorrhage: a population-based study in King County, Washington. *Neurology*. 43(4):712-8.

Luo Y., Lu J., Ruan W., Guo X., Chen S. 2019. MCC950 attenuated early brain injury by suppressing NLRP3 inflammasome after experimental SAH in rats. *Brain Res Bull.* 146:320-6.

Lupfer C., Kanneganti T. D. 2013. Unsolved Mysteries in NLR Biology. *Front Immunol.* 4:285.

Man S. M., Kanneganti T. D. 2015. Regulation of inflammasome activation. *Immunol Rev.* 265(1): 6-21.

Mathiesen T., Andersson B., Loftenius A., vonHolst H. 1993. Increased interleukin-6 levels in cerebrospinal fluid following subarachnoid hemorrhage. *J Neurosurg.* 78(4):562-7.

McMahon C. J., Hopkins S., Vail A., King A. T., Smith D., Illingworth K. J., et al. 2013. Inflammation as a predictor for delayed cerebral ischemia after aneurysmal subarachnoid haemorrhage. *J Neurointerv Surg.* 5(6):512-7.

Meguro T., Chen B., Lancon J., Zhang J. H. 2001. Oxyhemoglobin induces caspase-mediated cell death in cerebral endothelial cells. *J Neurochem.* 77(4):1128-35.

Mellor H., Parker P. J. 1998. The extended protein kinase C superfamily. *Biochem J.* 332 (Pt 2):281-92.

Miller B. A., Turan N., Chau M., Pradilla G. 2014. Inflammation, vasospasm, and brain injury after subarachnoid hemorrhage. *Biomed Res Int.* 2014:384342.

Muroi C., Bellut D., Coluccia D., Mink S., Fujioka M., Keller E. 2011. Systemic interleukin-6 concentrations in patients with perimesencephalic non-aneurysmal subarachnoid hemorrhage. *J ClinNeurosci.* 18(12):1626-9.

Muroi C., Hugelshofer M., Seule M., Tastan I., Fujioka M., Mishima K., et al. 2013. Correlation among systemic inflammatory parameter, occurrence of delayed neurological deficits, and outcome after aneurysmal subarachnoid hemorrhage. *Neurosurgery.* 72(3):367-75, discussion 75.

Nakura T., Osuka K., Inukai T., Takagi T., Takayasu M. 2011. Soluble gp130 regulatess interleukin-6 in cerebrospinal fluid after subarachnoid haemorrhage. *J Neurol Neurosurg Psychiatry.* 82(9):952-4.

Newton A. C. 2018. Protein kinase C: perfectly balanced. Crit Rev Biochem *Mol Biol.* 53(2):208-30.

Ni W., Gu Y. X., Song D. L., Leng B., Li P. L., Mao Y. 2011. The relationship between IL-6 in CSF and occurrence of vasospasm after subarachnoid hemorrhage. *Acta Neurochir Suppl.* 110(Pt 1):203-8.

Nishikawa K., Yamamoto S., Nagumo H., Kato R. 1997. Activation of phorbol ester responsive form of protein kinase C zeta in association with Ca(2+)-induced differentiation of primary cultured mouse epidermal cells. *Jpn J Pharmacol.* 73(2):171-4.

Nishizawa S., Obara K., Nakayama K., Koide M., Yokoyama T., Yokota N., et al. 2000. Protein kinase cdelta and alpha are involved in the development of vasospasm after subarachnoid hemorrhage. *Eur J Pharmacol.* 398(1):113-9.

Nishziawa S. 2011. Roles of signal transduction mechanisms in cerebral vasospasm following subarachnoid hemorrhage: overview. *Acta Neurochir Suppl.* 110(Pt 1):27-30.

O'Shea J. J., Murray P. J. 2008. Cytokine signaling modules in inflammatory responses. *Immunity.* 28(4):477-87.

Parker B. L., Larsen M. R., Edvinsson L. I., Povlsen G. K. 2013. Signal transduction in cerebral arteries after subarachnoid hemorrhage-a phosphoproteomic approach. *J Cereb Blood Flow Metab*. 33(8):1259-69.

Parrella E., Porrini V., Benarese M., Pizzi M. 2019. The Role of Mast Cells in Stroke. *Cells*. 8(5).

Peeyush Kumar T., McBride D. W., Dash P. K., Matsumura K., Rubi A., Blackburn S. L. 2019. Endothelial Cell Dysfunction and Injury in Subarachnoid Hemorrhage. *Mol Neurobiol*. 56(3):1992-2006.

Perry D. M., Newcomb B., Adada M., Wu B. X., Roddy P., Kitatani K., et al. 2014. Defining a role for acid sphingomyelinase in the p38/interleukin-6 pathway. *J Biol Chem*. 289(32):22401-12.

Pickard J. D., Murray G. D., Illingworth R., Shaw M. D., Teasdale G. M., Foy P. M., et al. 1989. Effect of oral nimodipine on cerebral infarction and outcome after subarachnoid haemorrhage: British aneurysm nimodipine trial. *BMJ*. 298(6674): 636-42.

Pradilla G., Chaichana K. L., Hoang S., Huang J., Tamargo R. J. 2010. Inflammation and cerebral vasospasm after subarachnoid hemorrhage. *Neurosurg Clin N Am*. 21(2): 365-79.

Pyne-Geithman G. J., Nair S. G., Caudell D. N., Clark J. F. 2008. PKC and Rho in vascular smooth muscle: activation by BOXes and SAH CSF. *Front Biosci*. 13:1526-34.

Rabelo N. N., daSilva Brito J., daSilva J. S., deSouza N. B., Coelho G., Brasil S., et al. 2021. The historic evolution of intracranial pressure and cerebrospinal fluid pulse pressure concepts: Two centuries of challenges. *SurgNeurol Int*. 12:274.

Ramzy D., Rao V., Tumiati L. C., Xu N., Sheshgiri R., Miriuka S., et al. 2006. Elevated endothelin-1 levels impair nitric oxide homeostasis through a PKC-dependent pathway. *Circulation*. 114(1 Suppl):I319-26.

Rasmussen R., Bache S., Stavngaard T., Møller K. 2019. Plasma Levels of IL-6, IL-8, IL-10, ICAM-1, VCAM-1, IFNγ, and TNFα are not Associated with Delayed Cerebral Ischemia, Cerebral Vasospasm, or Clinical Outcome in Patients with Subarachnoid Hemorrhage. *World Neurosurg*. 128:e1131-e6.

Ridwan S., Grote A., Simon M. 2021. Interleukin 6 in cerebrospinal fluid is a biomarker for delayed cerebral ischemia (DCI) related infarctions after aneurysmal subarachnoid hemorrhage. *Sci Rep*. 11(1):12.

Rodriguez-Rodriguez A., Egea-Guerrero J. J., Ruiz de, Azua-Lopez Z., Murillo-Cabezas F. 2014. Biomarkers of vasospasm development and outcome in aneurysmal subarachnoid hemorrhage. *J Neurol Sci*. 341(1-2):119-27.

Rosenberg G. A., Estrada E. Y., Dencoff J. E., Stetler-Stevenson W. G. 1995. Tumor necrosis factor-alpha-induced gelatinase B causes delayed opening of the blood-brain barrier: an expanded therapeutic window. *Brain Res*. 703(1-2):151-5.

Ryba M., Grieb P., Bidzinski J., Pastuszko M., Dziewiecki C., Iwanska K. 1991. Cyclosporine A for the prevention of neurological deficit following subarachnoid hemorrhage. *Stroke*. 22(4):531.

Sabri M., Ai J., Knight B., Tariq A., Jeon H., Shang X., et al. 2011. Uncoupling of endothelial nitric oxide synthase after experimental subarachnoid hemorrhage. *J Cereb Blood Flow Metab*. 31(1):190-9.

Sasaki T., Kassell N. F., Zuccarello M., Nakagomi T., Fijiwara S., Colohan A. R., et al. 1986. Barrier disruption in the major cerebral arteries during the acute stage after experimental subarachnoid hemorrhage. *Neurosurgery*. 19(2):177-84.
Sato M., Tani E., Matsumoto T., Fujikawa H., Imajoh-Ohmi S. 1997. Generation of the catalytic fragment of protein kinase C alpha in spastic canine basilar artery. *J Neurosurg*. 87(5):752-6.
Schoch B., Regel J. P., Wichert M., Gasser T., Volbracht L., Stolke D. 2007. Analysis of intrathecal interleukin-6 as a potential predictive factor for vasospasm in subarachnoid hemorrhage. *Neurosurgery*. 60(5):828-36, discussion -36.
Serhan C. N., Savill J. 2005. Resolution of inflammation: the beginning programs the end. *Nat Immunol*. 6(12):1191-7.
Serhan C. N. 2006. Novel chemical mediators in the resolution of inflammation: resolvins and protectins. *Anesthesiol Clin*. 24(2):341-64.
Shimada K., Furukawa H., Wada K., Korai M., Wei Y., Tada Y., et al. 2015. Protective Role of Peroxisome Proliferator-Activated Receptor-γ in the Development of Intracranial Aneurysm Rupture. *Stroke*. 46(6):1664-72.
Shimokawa H. 2000. Cellular and molecular mechanisms of coronary artery spasm: lessons from animal models. *Jpn Circ J*. 64(1):1-12.
Swanson K. V., Deng M., Ting J. P. 2019. The NLRP3 inflammasome: molecular activation and regulation to therapeutics. *Nat Rev Immunol*. 19(8):477-89.
Takuwa Y., Matsui T., Abe Y., Nagafuji T., Yamashita K., Asano T. 1993. Alterations in protein kinase C activity and membrane lipid metabolism in cerebral vasospasm after subarachnoid hemorrhage. *J Cereb Blood Flow Metab*. 13(3):409-15.
Tang Q. F., Lu S. Q., Zhao Y. M., Qian J. X. 2015. The changes of von willebrand factor/a disintegrin-like and metalloprotease with thrombospondin type I repeats-13 balance in aneurysmal subarachnoid hemorrhage. *Int J Clin Exp Med*. 8(1):1342-8.
Vergouwen M. D., Etminan N., Ilodigwe D., Macdonald R. L. 2011. Lower incidence of cerebral infarction correlates with improved functional outcome after aneurysmal subarachnoid hemorrhage. *J Cereb Blood Flow Metab*. 31(7):1545-53.
Wang L., Gao Z. 2018. Expression of MMP-9 and IL-6 in patients with subarachnoid hemorrhage and the clinical significance. *Exp Ther Med*. 15(2):1510-4.
Wajima D., Hourani S., Dodd W., Patel D., Jones C., Motwani K., et al. 2020. Interleukin-6 Promotes Murine Estrogen Deficiency-Associated Cerebral Aneurysm Rupture. *Neurosurgery*. 86(4):583-92.
Weir B., Grace M., Hansen J., Rothberg C. 1978. Time course of vasospasm in man. J *Neurosurg*. 48(2):173-8.
White R. P., Robertson J. T. 1983. Comparison of piroxicam, meclofenamate, ibuprofen, aspirin, and prostacyclin efficacy in a chronic model of cerebral vasospasm. *Neurosurgery*. 12(1):40-6.
Williams D. A., Becker P. L., Fay F. S. 1987. Regional changes in calcium underlying contraction of single smooth muscle cells. *Science*. 235(4796):1644-8.
Wolburg H., Noell S., Mack A., Wolburg-Buchholz K., Fallier-Becker P. 2009. Brain endothelial cells and the glio-vascular complex. *Cell Tissue Res*. 335(1):75-96.

Won S. M., Lee J. H., Park U. J., Gwag J., Gwag B. J., Lee Y. B. 2011. Iron mediates endothelial cell damage and blood-brain barrier opening in the hippocampus after transient forebrain ischemia in rats. *ExpMol Med*. 43(2):121-8.

Wu W., Guan Y., Zhao G., Fu X. J., Guo T. Z., Liu Y. T., et al. 2016. Elevated IL-6 and TNF-α Levels in Cerebrospinal Fluid of Subarachnoid Hemorrhage Patients. *Mol Neurobiol*. 53(5):3277-85.

Xiong X. Y., Liu L., Yang Q. W. 2016. Functions and mechanisms of microglia/macrophages in neuroinflammation and neurogenesis after stroke. *Prog Neurobiol*. 142:23-44.

Yamaura I., Tani E., Saido T. C., Suzuki K., Minami N., Maeda Y. 1993. Calpain-calpastatin system of canine basilar artery in vasospasm. *J Neurosurg*. 79(4):537-43.

Yatsushige H., Yamaguchi M., Zhou C., Calvert J. W., Zhang J. H. 2005. Role of c-Jun N-terminal kinase in cerebral vasospasm after experimental subarachnoid hemorrhage. *Stroke*. 36(7):1538-43.

Zhang H., Weir B. K., Macdonald R. L., Marton L. S., Solenski N. J., Kwan A. L., et al. 1996. Mechanisms of [Ca++]i elevation induced by erythrocyte components in endothelial cells. *J Pharmacol Exp Ther*. 277(3):1501-9.

Zhang L. L., Chen B., Fan X. Y., Wu S. S., Zhang S. Q., Wu H. M. 2016. LPS Cooperates with Poly-L-Arginine to Promote IL-6 and IL-8 Release via the JNK Signaling Pathway in NCI-H292 Cells. *J Immunol Res*. 2016:3421060.

Zhang T., Huang L., Peng J., Zhang J. H., Zhang H. 2021. LJ529 attenuates mast cell-related inflammation via A. *Exp Neurol*. 340:113686.

Zhang X., Connelly J., Levitan E. S., Sun D., Wang, J. Q. 2021. Calcium/Calmodulin-Dependent Protein Kinase II in Cerebrovascular Diseases. *Transl Stroke Res*. 12(4): 513-29.

Zhou C., Yamaguchi M., Colohan A. R., Zhang J. H. 2005. Role of p53 and apoptosis in cerebral vasospasm after experimental subarachnoid hemorrhage. *J Cereb Blood Flow Metab*. 25(5):572-82.

Zhou K., Enkhjargal B., Xie Z., Sun C., Wu L., Malaguit J., et al. 2018. Dihydrolipoic Acid Inhibits Lysosomal Rupture and NLRP3 Through Lysosome-Associated Membrane Protein-1/Calcium/Calmodulin-Dependent Protein Kinase II/TAK1 Pathways After Subarachnoid Hemorrhage in Rat. *Stroke*. 49(1):175-83.

Chapter 3

Aneurysmal Subarachnoid Hemorrhage: From Diagnosis to Treatment

Irina A. Savvina[1,2,*], DScMed,
Yulia M. Zabrodskaya[2], DScMed,
Larisa V. Rozhchenko[3], PhD,
Sergey A. Goroshchenko[3], PhD,
Elena G. Potemkina[4], DScMed,
Anna O. Petrova[1], PhD
and Konstantin A. Samochernykh[3], DScMed

[1]Department of Anesthesiology and Intensive Care, Almazov National Medical Research Centre of Ministry of Health Care of Russian Federation, Saint Petersburg, Russian Federation
[2]Department of Pathomorphology of Nervous System, Russian Polenov Scientific Research Neurosurgical Institute – branch of the Almazov National Medical Research Centre of Ministry of Health Care of Russian Federation, Saint Petersburg, Russian Federation
[3]Department of Neurosurgery of Cerebral Vessels, Russian Polenov Scientific Research Neurosurgical Institute – branch of the Almazov National Medical Research Centre of Ministry of Health Care of Russian Federation, Saint Petersburg, Russian Federation
[4]Department of Radiation Diagnostics, Russian Polenov Scientific Research Neurosurgical Institute – branch of the Almazov National Medical Research Centre of Ministry of Health Care of Russian Federation, Saint Petersburg, Russian Federation

---

[*]Corresponding Author's Email: irinasavvina@mail.ru.

In: Aneurysmal Subarachnoid Hemorrhage
Editor: Irina Savvina
ISBN: 979-8-88697-251-1

Abstract

The most dangerous type of acute cerebrovascular disease accompanied by high mortality is ruptured cerebral aneurysms with subarachnoidal hemorrhage (SAH).

This chapter will focus on the mechanisms of development of SAH when a cerebral aneurysm is ruptured and the etiological factors, e.g., the role of connective tissue dysplasia in the development of aneurysms. We will cover the etiopathogenetic classification of aneurysms, the concept of aneurysmal brain disease, and the clinical and anatomical variants of the course. There will be presented the anatomical characteristics of SAH after rupturing of aneurysms (localization, prevalence, volume).

Diagnostics of aneurysmal SAH will include neurological examination and instrumental radiation methods: CT angiography, cerebral angiography, and MRI imaging. This chapter will cover complications of cerebral aneurysm rupture including SAH, cerebral vasospasm, intracranial hemorrhage, intraventricular hemorrhage, acute hydrocephalus, intracranial hypertension, and cerebral edema, hyponatremia. We will describe the clinical picture of complications of cerebral aneurysm rupture with SAH such as paroxysmal sympathetic hyperactivity syndrome (PSH syndrome), neurogenic stress cardiomyopathy, Takotsubo syndrome, and neurogenic pulmonary edema. Treatment of aneurysmal SAH will include surgical methods: operations for aneurysm clipping, ventricular drainage operations, decompressive craniotomy, and endovascular neurosurgical interventions. There will be presented the pharmacological methods of cerebral protection, neurovegetative stabilization, and therapeutic hypothermia for correction of intracranial hypertension.

Keywords: aneurysmal subarachnoid hemorrhage (SAH), cerebral vasospasm, etiopathogenesis and pathomorphology of aneurysmal brain diseases (ABD), pathophysiology, diagnostics and treatment of aneurysmal SAH

Abbreviations

ABD – aneurysmal brain disease
ACB– arterial circle of the brain
ACA – anterior cerebral artery
BI – bifurcation insufficiency
BNP – brain natriuretic peptide

CCA – common carotid artery
CT – Computer Tomography
CT-AG – computer tomography-angiography
CTD– connective tissue dysplasia
ICA – internal carotid artery
ICD– international classification of diseases
ICP – intracranial pressure
IVH – intraventricularhaemorrhage
FrFSE PS – fast –recovery Fast Spin Echo Pulse Sequences
FLAIR PS – Fluid Attenuated Inversion Recovery Pulse Sequences
MCA – middle cerebral artery
MIP –Maximum Intensive Projection
MPR – Multiplanar Reconstruction
MRI –Magnetic Resonance Imaging
NO – nitrous oxide
$NSAID_s$ –non-steroid anti-inflammation drugs
NT-proBNP–N-terminal pro-brain natriuretic peptide
PCA – posterior cerebral artery
PEEP – positive end-expiratory pressure
PICA– posterior inferior cerebellar artery
PSH –Paroxysmal Sympathetic Hyperactivity syndrome
PXE – Pseudoxanthoma elasticum
SAH–subarachnoidhaemorrhage
SCT – Spiral Computer Tomography
T1WI – T1weighted images
T2WI – T2weighted images
VA – vertebral artery
VAS – visual analog scale
VBB – vertebrobasilar basin
VRT –volume rendering technique

Introduction

Cerebral aneurysms are the most common cause of subarachnoid hemorrhage (SAH) excluding trauma. A SAH destroys cerebrovascular autoregulation and induces intracranial and very serious systemic complications, such as intracranial hypertension, cerebral vasospasm, acute neurogenic stress cardiomyopathy, and Takotsubo syndrome, paroxysmal sympathetic hyperactivity syndrome (PSH syndrome), neurogenic pulmonary edema, with high mortality. Neurologists, neurosurgeons, anesthesiologists, and doctors of general practice need to know the etiopathogenesis, pathophysiology, and treatment of SAH resulting from a cerebral aneurysm. In this chapter basic knowledge, clinical symptoms and complications, diagnostics of cerebral aneurysm and SAH, and also treatment including surgical and pharmacological methods are reviewed.

Etiology of Subarachnoid Hemorrhage

SAH in the Structure of Aneurysmal Brain Disease

In the ICD, in the section of cerebrovascular diseases, SAH is directly associated with a ruptured aneurysm of the main arteries of the brain. Aneurysmal SAH, in addition to a clear etiology, has a characteristic pathogenesis, pathomorphological and clinical manifestations and can be considered as an independent nosology unit - aneurysmal brain disease (ABD) (Medvedev 1993, 7–10).

Aneurysm formation is part of the pathogenesis of ABD associated with the realization of undifferentiated connective tissue dysplasia (CTD) in the form of SAH and its consequences.

Etiopathogenesis of Cerebral Aneurysms

The aneurysms in question are always localized within the arterial circle of the large brain, located in the places of branching arteries.

A term was proposed for their designation – "bifurcation-hemodynamic aneurysms," or more simply – "bifurcation" (Medvedev and Zabrodskaya 2000, 167).

It has long been proven that cerebral aneurysms are not congenital, as previously thought, but like any aneurysms – acquired, developing with damage or weakening of the strength of the wall in the area of bifurcations.

A turning point in understanding the etiopathogenesis of bifurcation aneurysms of the brain was the discovery of the segmental structure of the arterial circle of the brain (ACB) with the presence of micro-anatomical structures - joints at the site of branching arteries (Figure 1).

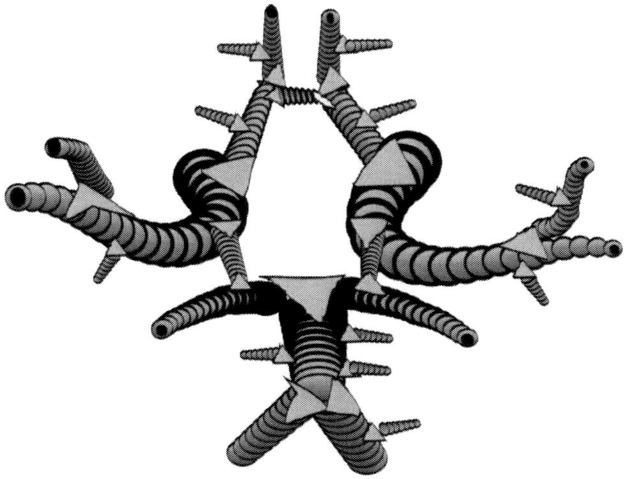

Figure 1. Scheme of the segmental structure of the ACB. In the area of bifurcations, the muscular segments of the arteries are connected to each other by means of junctions (light triangles).

The segments representing the muscular metameres (the working organ of the artery) are covered from the outside with adventitia, and from the inside with intima. The articulation formed from adventitia (outside) and intima with an internal elastic membrane (inside) is a fibrous-elastic ring (semicircle) 250-300 microns wide (Figure 2). At the same time, there is no muscular membrane (t. media) in this place. At one time, this phenomenon was regarded as a media defect. In some cases (13.5%), the articulation area is covered from the inside by the intimate cushion (muscular-elastic hyperplasia of intima). The frequency of such joints increases sharply in persons suffering from hypertension and in old age (up to 31%). Intimate pads strengthen the contact points of the segments where the middle shell is absent. They protrude into the lumen of the artery and become an integral part of the ligamentous apparatus. Articulations do not always have a "complete" structural design, and in some cases, muscle segments are intertwined by smooth muscle cells and their bundles (plexiform articulation), forming fairly strong points that fix metameres and allow them to perform a contractile function. Along the perimeter of the same vessel, different variants of the above-described compounds can be found (Medvedev and Bersnev 1998, 9-17).

Articulation of arteries in the bifurcations of the base of the brain is the target organ of aneurysmatic transformation.

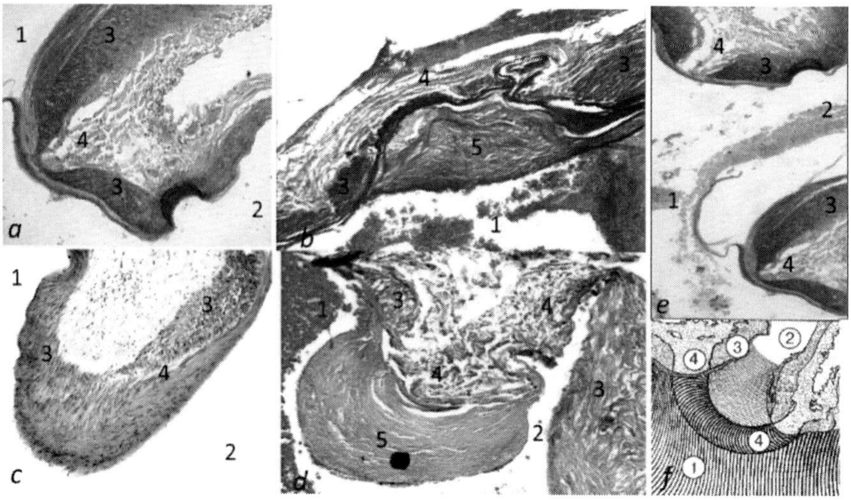

Figure 2. Histological structure of juncture of branching.
a -The juncture of the segments is formed by a fibrous-elastic ring. Toluidine staining. x100;
b - Fibrous-elastic ring in combination with an intimate pad covering the juncture from the inside. Orsein staining. x100;
c - The connection is carried out by intertwining bundles of muscle cells that come into direct contact – (plexiform type). H&E. x 200;
d - Combination of a fiber-elastic ring and intimate pad. Orsein staining. x 100;
e - Histotopogram of bifurcation. Toluidine staining. x100;
f - Reconstruction of the bifurcation (Figure 2e).
Designations: 1- vessel lumen I, 2–vessel lumen II, 3 –media, 4 – junction, 5 - intimate pad.

Connective Tissue Dysplasia (CTD) and Cerebral Aneurysms

In recent years, most researchers have associated the development of ACB aneurysms with a defect in collagen synthesis underlying CTD.

It is believed that aneurysms are more often formed sporadically, and hereditary forms are less common. Variants of hereditary connective tissue pathology involving collagen (polycystic kidney disease inherited by autosomal dominant type, incomplete osteogenesis, Ehlers-Danlo syndrome types I/II, IV, new hereditary variants of small vessel pathology associated with type IV collagen abnormalities), elastic fibers (Pseudoxanthoma elasticum - PXE) are associated with the occurrence of aneurysms, as well as RHE-like syndrome, Marfan, Loys—Dietz syndromes, bicuspid aortic valve with ascending aortic aneurysm, arterial tortuosity syndrome, supra-valvular aortic stenosis, diseases with generalized connective tissue involvement (English: disorders with generalized connective tissue involvement), spontaneous dissection of vertebral arteries, hereditary hemorrhagic telangiectasia, fibromuscular dysplasia (Vanakker 2011, 1-18).

CTD is a genetically determined condition characterized by defects in fibrous structures and the basic substance of connective tissue. Unlike rare monogenic disorders of connective tissue, such as Marfan syndrome, Ehlers-Danlo, Williams, etc., nonspecific disorders of connective tissue, grouped into a group of undifferentiated CTD, are widespread in the population (Glesby and Pyeritz 1989, 523-528; Colombi and Dordoni 2015, 6-22).

Studies are being conducted to identify genes associated with vascular diseases, but only a few are at risk of developing aneurysms. Most of the studies conducted were primarily focused on functional genes that may play a role in the formation of connective tissue, such as collagen, elastin, matrix metalloproteinases, and their tissue inhibitors, endoglin and fibrillin (Hitchcock and Gibson 2017, 21-31).

According to several foreign authors, representatives of the Caucasian race are subject to mutations in chromosome 8q (rs10958409) of the SOX17 gene, which plays a crucial role in the production of endothelial stem cells and hematopoietic lines, changes that lead to multiple vascular anomalies and endothelial remodeling, closely associated with the formation of intracranial aneurysms (Lee and Kim 2015, 995-1005). According to another study, a mutation in chromosome 4q31.23 encoding the endothelin A receptor, which is responsible for vasoconstriction and vasodilation after a hemorrhagic stroke, is crucial. Deactivation of endothelin A as a result of gene mutation contributes to the development of aneurysms after injury and concussion at a young age (Low and Takahashi 2012, 2102-2110).

The results of one of the meta-analyses report mutations in the COL1A2 rs42524 gene located on chromosome 7q22.1 in a cohort of patients with ruptured aneurysms. This gene is responsible for the elastic layer of the arteries of the brain, in particular the synthesis of type 1 collagen, which provides the strength of the vessel wall (Yasuno and Bakırcıoğlu 2011, 19707-19712).

The risk of aneurysms is associated with two single nucleotide polymorphisms of the elastin gene: rs2071307 and rs2856728. In addition, the minor allele rs2071307 (allele A) was also associated with rupture of aneurysms and the development of SAH (Shuaifeng and Tinghua 2013, 454-8).

Disabling ADAMTS15 and overexpression of ADAMTS15p.E133Q accelerates the migration of endothelial cells, thereby suggesting that ADAMTS15 may have antiangiogenic activity. Based on the study, it was concluded that ADAMTS15 is a candidate gene for aneurysms (Hitomi and Habu 2013, 13-19).

Genome-wide studies of associations based on the susceptibility of loci indicate that some loci may contain one or more predisposing genes.

There have been studies on the effect of sex hormones on collagen, there is an assumption that a decrease in circulating levels of estrogen and cerebrovascular estrogen receptors may contribute to an increased risk of aneurysm pathogenesis and rupture in women during and after menopause (Harrod and Batjer 2006, 736-756).

Bifurcation Insufficiency (BI)

As a result of CTD caused by genetic and epigenetic events, the strength of collagen and, accordingly, the resistive properties of the joints decrease, which leads to the functional failure of the arteries in the area of their branching - bifurcation insufficiency (BI). Thus, the presence of BI is the cause of aneurysm formation.

BI is a clinical and morphological symptom complex caused by undifferentiated connective tissue dysplasia in the articulation area, manifested by disorganization of connective tissue with mucoid edema of the main substance, violation of the structural organization of collagen and elastic fibers, an increase in the length of joints and leading to a weakening of the resistive properties of joints with the formation of aneurysms in the outcome (Medvedev and Zabrodskaya 2012, 59-62).

When assessing the prevalence of the above-mentioned changes, there is a "vulnerability," a special sensitivity of the arteril junctions (joints) in bifurcations associated with the basin of the internal carotid artery in deceased patients suffering from ABD, regardless of gender and age.

Morphogenesis: Stretching of the Joints of the ACB

The formation of aneurysms goes through several stages, strictly linked to the junctions of the arteries, the connective tissue of which is subject to disorganization (Medvedev and Zabrodskaya 2000, 167) (Figure 3).

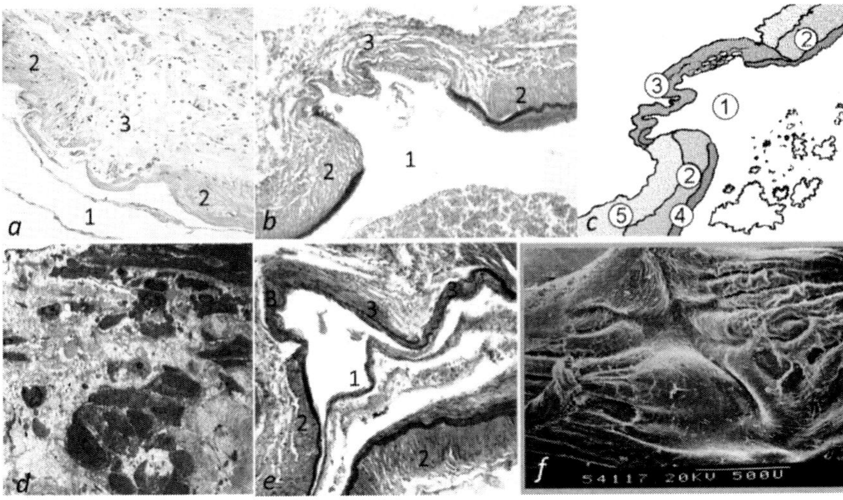

Figure 3. Morphogenesis: pre- aneurysmal stage (diverticula).
a - stretching junction. The joint is stretched (340 microns), collagen disorganization, reactive inflammation, fragmentation of the internal elastic membrane H&E, x200;
b - pre-aneurysm. Junction (3) overstretched (670 microns), thinned, sclerosed, deformed, rupture of the internal elastic membrane (4), compensatory focal muscle-elastic hyperplasia junction. Orsein staining, x 100;
c - reconstruction of a bifurcation with a pre-aneurysmal change (Figure b);
d - stretching junction. Collagen disorganization, myocyte dystrophy and necrosis. Electron microscopy.x 750;
e – evagination (bulging) junction. Stable protrusion of the overgrown (880 microns), compensatory muscle-elastic hyperplasia of juncture with formation of a newly elastic membrane, ruptured internal elastic membrane.Mallory staining, x 100;
f - evagination in area of junction. Scanning electron microscopy.
Designations (Figures a, b, c, e): 1 -vessel lumen, 2 - media 3-junction, 4 -internal elastic membrane, 5–adventitia.

A complex of general pathological, mainly alternative processes develops in the joint, characteristic of formations consisting mainly of connective tissue (collagen and elastic fibers, the main substance, sedentary fibrocyte cells). The totality of these changes (progressive, regressive and recurrent) includes the entire spectrum of mesenchymal dystrophies (edema, mucoid edema, fibrinoid necrosis with collagen breakdown, hyalinosis, sclerosis), as well as inflammation (macrophage reaction, infiltration by leukocytes, lymphoplasmacytic cells). They lead to thinning, weakening of resistive properties, and stretching of joints, which can bulge outward under the influence of pulsating blood flow, forming sac-like aneurysm-like formations with their subsequent evolution up to rupture (Figure 4). According to the morphogenetic feature, this disease was named by us as stretching (overstretching) of the junctions of the ACB.

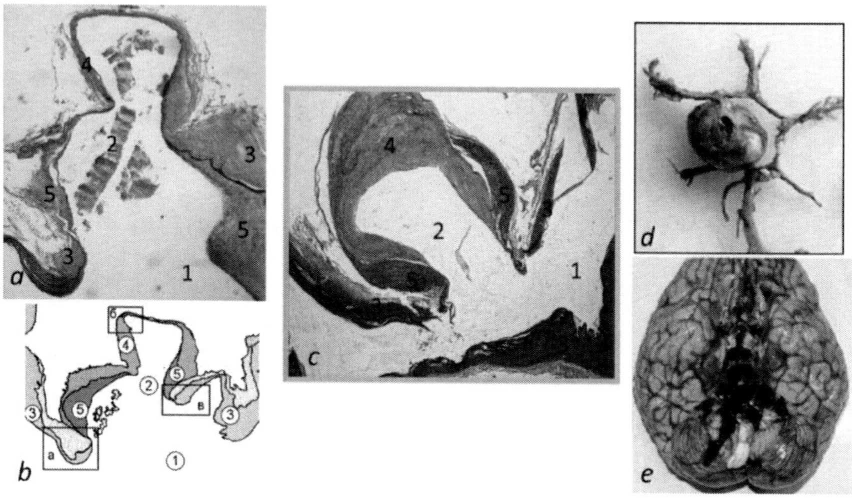

Figure 4. Morphogenesis: stages of aneurysm formation (diverticula).
a - immature aneurysm (diverticulum). Junction 3000 microns, protrusion, deformation, sclerosis, sharp thinning of the articulation (b), fragments of internal elastic membrane, muscle-elastic hyperplasia form rollers at the mouth of the aneurysm. Orsein staining, x100;
b - reconstruction of the bifurcation with immature aneurysm (Figure a). Designations: 1 - vessel lumen, 2 - lumen of the aneurysm, 3 - the wall of adjacent arteries, 4 - aneurysm wall, 5 – muscle-elastic hyperplasia at the mouth of the aneurysm;
c - mature aneurysm (diverticulum). Joint diverticulum (d 1cm), densely packed collagen fibers with secondary dystrophic changes (hyalinos, scleros). Toluidine staining. x 100;
d – ruptured aneurysm. Macropreparation;
e - aneurysmal basal subarachnoid hemorrhage. Macropreparation.

Bifurcation aneurysms, being a protrusion of a hollow organ (articulation), is more correct to call a diverticulum (*diverticulum* (Latin) - a move to the side). Aneurysms, or rather diverticula, are an optional manifestation of the described disease, which can exist by itself (without diverticula) (Medvedev and Zabrodskaya 2012, 59-62).

Pathogenesis: Hemodynamic Factor

BI is realized in aneurysmal protrusion under certain structural and hemodynamic conditions. Based on the theory of the acquired origin of aneurysms, the condition initiating aneurysm formation at first is the hemodynamic factor. The articulation of the arteries is in a state of incessant workload and is constantly subjected to mechanical stress, regardless of whether it is "sick" or not. The joints in this case are subjected to a direct "shock" of the pulse wave, the strength of which increases sharply with systemic arterial hypertension, as well as with changes in local hemodynamic conditions during stenotic processes in the arteries (atherosclerosis, fibromuscular hyperplasia, etc.). Well-known anatomical features of the arteries, often combined with aneurysms (trifurcation, obtuse angle of bifurcation, asymmetric anatomical variants of the ACB, persistent embryonic arteries, etc.) also increase hemodynamic stress in the area of compromised bifurcations (Can and Du 2016, 510-520).

Pathogenesis and morphogenesis are based on the weakening of the resistive properties of joints against the background of local or systemic conditions of blood flow, leading to micro-injuries, degenerative processes that, under conditions of hemodynamic stress, lead to increased disorganization of connective tissue and stretching of joints with the formation of an aneurysm and further intracranial hemorrhage as a result of rupture of an aneurysm (ABD) (Figure 5).

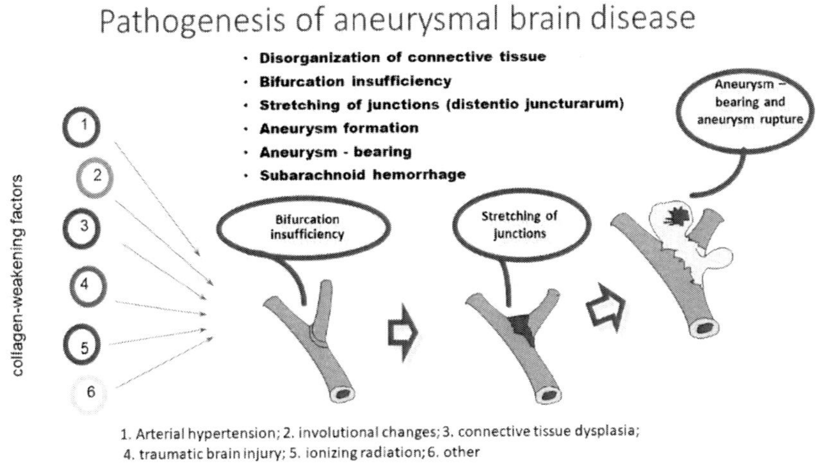

Figure 5. Pathogenesis of aneurysmal brain disease.

Mechanisms of Aneurysm Rupture

The mechanisms of aneurysm ruptures were deciphered, while it was noted that about 50% of aneurysm ruptures occur in the neck area, the rest in the bottom area.

Morphological analysis showed that cases of ruptures in the cervical region are preceded by autoimmune inflammation, which is not surprising since at this point the "healthy" tissue of the adjacent arterial segment contacts essentially with the extracellular "dead" material of the aneurysmal sac (Medvedev and Zabrodskaya 2000, 167; Medvedev and Bersnev 1998, 9-17).

The Constitution and the Risk of Developing SAH

The great importance of the constitutional features of a person in the predisposition to the development of various diseases is known. Works that consider aneurysm as a constitutional pathology are of interest (Razmologova and Medvedev 2009, 33-35).

Taking into account their correlation with the constitutional type of physique and the variant of ACB, the results of the study allowed us to identify two risk groups for the development of ABD and variants of the course (Table 1).

Two variants of the course of ABD have been identified in individuals with pronounced phenotypic manifestations of CTD syndrome (dysembrioplastic variant) and with mild CTD syndrome in combination with hypertensive angiopathy (involution-hypertensive).

In individuals with a dysembrioplastic variant of aneurysmal brain disease, connective tissue dysplasia is a leading factor in the etiopathogenesis of BI. In individuals with an involution-hypertensive variant of ABD, the formation of BI is due to a combination of CTD and hypertensive arteriopathy.

The determination of constitutional features in combination with manifestations of connective tissue dysplasia syndrome makes it possible to identify risk groups. And when verifying ABD, predict the possible course of the disease (Medvedev and Panuntsev 2012, 22-28).

Table 1. Options characteristics of variants of the course of ABD

Option Indicator	Dysembrioplastic	Involution-hypertensive
Age	40,2 ± 6,1 лет	53,4 ± 3,6 лет
Body type Height	Asthenic 178,5 ± 3 CM	Hypersthenic 163 ± 2 см
Type of ACB vessels	hypoplastic	hyperplastic
Changes in the vascular wall when stained with toluidine blue	Metachromasia of collagen fibers in t.media	Metachromasia of collagen fibers t.intima
Connective tissue dysplasia syndromebyGlesby et al. (1989)	Moderately and strongly expressed (from 10 points and above)	Weakly expressed (up to 10 points)
Hypertension	Is not present or isolated episodes of blood pressure rise to 140 mmHg.	2 - 3 stage, long-term course
The onset of the disease (aneurysm rupture, SAH)	On the background of health, after physical or psychoemotional stress	In the background of a hypertensive crisis
The cause of death	Ischemic cerebral infarction on the background of vasospasm (according to clinical data during dopplerography, according to morphological data, the presence of constrictive stenotic arteriopathy)	Massive, more often repeated intracranial hemorrhages

A Group with Bright Phenotypic Manifestations of CTD

Young and middle-aged persons - up to 50 years old, asthenic, less often normosthenic physique with hypoplastic vessels (ACB and aorta), not suffering from hypertension, but having manifestations of moderate or severe connective tissue dysplasia syndrome. The disease develops after physical or psycho-emotional stress. The death of patients occurs as a result of total ischemic cerebral infarction caused by vasospasm (according to clinical data during dopplerography, according to morphological data – the presence of vasospasm) of initially narrow vessels.

A Group with Mild Manifestations of CTD in Combination with Hypertension

Persons over 50 years of age, hypersthenic or normosthenic physique, suffering from hypertension, with a hyperplastic type of ACB vessels. The onset of the disease is associated with a hypertensive crisis, and the cause of death in most cases is massive, more often repeated against the background of increased blood pressure, and intracranial hemorrhage.

Prevention of SAH

Taking into account the established pathogenesis of ABD and its connection with CTD, it is necessary to conduct preventive therapy within the framework of CTD treatment standards.

Diagnosis of Aneurysmal Subarachnoid Hemorrhage

Neurological Assessment of Patients with SAH

Non-traumatic subarachnoid hemorrhage (SAH) most often (up to 80%) (Go and Mozaffarian 2014) is a consequence of a cerebral aneurysm rupture and is a reason for 3-5% of cerebral strokes and the cause of high rates of disability and mortality (15 and 35%, respectively) (Muehlschlegel 2018). From 10 to 20% of patients with SAH die before reaching the hospital, and 25% die within the first 24 hours (van Gijn and Kerr 2007).

Samoilov V.I. (1990) in his monography identified 7 types of non-traumatic subarachnoid hemorrhage depending on the etiological factor:

- aneurysmal etiology;
- hypertensive etiology;
- atherosclerotic etiology;
- infectious and toxic etiology;
- blastomatous etiology;
- pathogenic etiology;
- unidentified etiology (Samoilov 1990).

The clinical picture of an intracranial aneurysm rupture usually corresponds to the first type of SAH, however, it may be atypical and correspond to other forms.

Aneurysm rupture occurs suddenly and is provoked by some factors that can be divided into modifiable and unmodified. Modifiable factors include hypertension, alcohol abuse, the use of sympathomimetics (e.g., cocaine), and NSAIDs.

The unmodified ones include the patient's age (most often SAH develops in the fifth and sixth decades of the patient's life), female gender, ethnicity to Spaniards, Africans, Finns, and Japanese, family history of SAH, autosomal dominant polycystic kidney disease, Ellers-Danlo syndrome type 4, sickle cell anemia, as well as the presence of a cerebral aneurysm 7 and > mm in diameter (Suarez 2015).

According to Samoilov V.I. (1990), the most frequent manifestation of an aneurysm rupture is the SAH syndrome, which consists of cerebral and meningeal symptoms, in rare cases focal symptoms may be noted (Samoilov 1990).

The general cerebral symptoms include headache, vomiting, impaired consciousness, epileptic seizures, etc.

Headache is the most constant symptom (up to 97%) and usually has the character of "unbearable" (Linn and Wijdicks 1994; Fine and Singh 2012). Some patients describe it as "the worst pain in life" (Muehlschlegel 2018). The pain develops sharply and reaches its maximum by the end of 1 minute (Ducros and Bousser 2013). Only a small number of patients have moderate headache without a combination with other neurological symptoms, as a result of which this group of patients can tolerate hemorrhage "on their feet," seeking medical help late, and as a result of the incorrect or untimely diagnosis, the risk of recurrent hemorrhage increases (van Gijn and Kerr 2007; Edlow and Malek 2008; Lawton and Vates 2017). It should be noted that if there is only an isolated headache in the clinical picture, an erroneous diagnosis is made in 12-51% of cases, which can significantly worsen the results of treatment of these patients (Kowalski and Claassen 2004; Adams and Jergenson 1980; Mayer and Awad 1996; Vannemreddy and Nanda 2001; Chan and Dorsch1991; Kassell and Kongable 1985; Schievink and van der Werf 1988; Neil-Dwyer and Lang 1997; Fridriksson and Hillman 2001; Edlow and Caplan 2000). At the same time, some authors note that the localization of headache may coincide with the side of the aneurysm location in about 30% of cases. For example, when an aneurysm of the internal carotid artery ruptures, homolateral pain in the frontal-orbital region is often observed (Samoilov 1990; Linn and Wijdicks 1994; Gorelick and Hier 1986).

Often, a few weeks before the development of a massive SAH, from 30 to 50% of patients suffer a "small" or so-called "sentinel" ("guard") hemorrhage that is not treated for medical help (Linn and Wijdicks 1994; Polmear 2003). In all likelihood, such a condition can be regarded as a "leak" of blood from an aneurysm (Linn and Wijdicks 1994).

Headache can often be combined with nausea and vomiting, while vomiting has the character of "central," i.e., not related to food intake and not combined with dyspeptic symptoms and does not bring relief (Samoilov 1990).

Less typical symptoms may be loss of consciousness, seizures, and in some cases, an acute subdural hematoma is detected in the patient, both with a history of trauma and without it, which in turn makes it difficult to correctly and timely diagnose SAH (Edlow and Malek 2008).

An epileptic syndrome is considered characteristic of SAH and occurs in about 6-20% of cases. The seizure can be either generalized or partial and develop both during SAH and after some time after it (van Gijn and Kerr 2007; Schievink 1997; Butzkueven and Evans 2000; Gilmore and Choi 2010).

Often, patients with SAH develop psychomotor agitation, which some authors associate with the spread of blood into the subarachnoid space of both the brain and spinal cord (Gorelick and Hier 1986; Butzkueven and Evans 2000; Konovalov 1973; Suarez and Tarr 2006; Landtblom and Fridriksson 2002; Morgenstern and Luna-Gonzales 1998; Harling and Peatfield 1989; Linn and Rinkel 1998; Carpenter and Hussain 2016).

Both seizures and loss of consciousness at the time of manifestation of SAH are associated with a 2.8-fold increase in disability and mortality, compared with patients whose manifestation of the disease was not accompanied by these symptoms (Butzkueven and Evans 2000; Suwatcharangkoon and Meyers 2015).

Focal symptoms of aneurysm rupture are most often represented by damage to the oculomotor nerves (Samoilov 1990). Focal symptoms associated with damage to the brain substance are relatively rare and occur during the formation of parenchymal hemorrhage, the mass effect of a giant aneurysm, as well as postictal prolapses after developing convulsive syndrome (Jomin and Lesoin 1984; Creissard and Freger 1985; Borges and Facure 1987; Voth 1987).

Meningeal symptoms in aneurysmal SAH can be direct and indirect and are caused by irritation of the outpouring of blood of the meninges. It can be represented by symptoms of Kernig and Brudzinsky, Burdenko-Kramer syndrome, as well as photophobia and sonophobia, hyperesthesia of the skin, pin in the percussion of the zygomatic arches (Gorelick and Hier 1986; Boullin and Tagari 1983; Sasaki and Asano 1984).

If the clinical picture is atypical, an ophthalmic examination may be useful. Intraocular hemorrhage caused by SAH (Terson syndrome) occurs in about 40% of cases, is caused by a short-term pronounced increase in intracranial pressure, and directly correlates with an increase in mortality (Hassan and Lanzino 2011).

Also, patients with SAH may have non-cerebral symptoms, such as fever, increased blood pressure and ECG changes - inversion of the T wave and ST segment changes, QT prolongation, which is associated with massive catecholamines entering the bloodstream, or increased arterial wall tone (Chatterjee 2011; Petridis and Kamp 2017). An increase in troponin and myocardial dysfunction without coronary angiospasm may also be detected (Jeon and Chang 2009; Naidech and Kreiter 2005). According to some authors, cardiac changes reflect the severity of neurological damage, but they can be reversible (Mashaly and Provencio 2008; Ibrahim and Macdonald 2012; Jain and Deveikis 2004; Kono and Morita 1994).

The presence of fever in these patients is associated with an increase in ICP, and an increase in brain edema and is a predictor of an unfavorable outcome (Tam and Ilodigwe 2010). One of the rare symptoms of SAH may be neurogenic pulmonary edema, which is associated with severe sympathicotonia as a result of damage to the central nervous system and is associated with global left ventricular dysfunction (Mayer and Fink 1994). Such a symptom complex can cause hospitalization in a cardiological hospital and lead to a delay in the verification of the SAH. The development of this condition is an extremely unfavorable prognostic sign (Muroi and Keller 2008; Davison and Terek 2012).

Complications caused by subarachnoid hemorrhage can be divided into two large groups: complications developing directly in the "acute" period of hemorrhage and complications developing in the long-term period. The first group includes dislocation syndrome associated with the formation of intracerebral or subdural hematoma; acute occlusion of the cerebrospinal fluid pathways associated with the spread of blood into the ventricular system of the brain and leading to the development of acute occlusive hydrocephalus, as well as repeated hemorrhage from an aneurysm. The second group includes constrictive-stenotic arteriopathy (cerebral vasospasm), leading to delayed cerebral ischemia, as well as hypo- and aresorptive chronic hydrocephalus, associated, most often, with impaired absorption of cerebrospinal fluid by pachyonic granulations (Bu and Chen 2016).

The Hunt and Hess scale has been used widely as a preoperative neurological symptom grading scale (Table 2).

Table 2. Hunt and Hess grading scale (Hunt and Hess 1968)

Grade	
I	Asymptomatic or minimal headache and slight nuchal rigidity
II	Moderate to severe headache, nuchal rigidity, no neurological deficit other than cranial nerve palsy
III	Drowsiness, confusion, or mild focal deficit
IV	Stupor, moderate to severe hemiparesis, possibly early decerebrate rigidity, and vegetative disturbances
V	Deep coma, decerebrate rigidity, moribund appearance

As the World Federation of Neurological Surgeons (WFNS) grading scale is based on the Glasgow coma scale (GCS), the scale is designed more simply and clinically estimates the prognosis by combining the GCS with major focal neurological deficits (aphasia, hemiparesis, or hemiplegia) (Table 3).

Table 3. World Federation of Neurological Surgeons (WFNS) grading scale (Drake 1988)

WFNS Grade	GCS score	Motor deficit
I	15	Absent
II	14 - 13	Absent
III	14 - 13	Present
IV	12 - 7	Present or absent
V	6 - 3	Present or absent

SAH Imaging

The rapid development of imaging techniques over the past decades has contributed to a significant change in the algorithm of diagnosis and treatment of patients with non-traumatic subarachnoid hemorrhage (SAH). The etiological factor of non-traumatic SAH in 90% of cases is the rupture of a cerebral aneurysm. Before the introduction of modern neuroimaging methods into clinical practice, cerebral angiography was the main method of diagnosing the etiology of hemorrhage, but it required strict indications for implementation. Recommendation protocol for the management of patients with subarachnoid hemorrhage due to rupture of cerebral aneurysms (Konovalov and Krylov 2006; Brian and Ranliang 2019).

Currently, it is believed that SCT is the leading diagnostic method that allows the diagnosis of the majority of both traumatic and non-traumatic SAC quickly, including in patients with artificial life support systems.

MRI, due to its high resolution and sensitivity, has several advantages for examining patients with SAC but is not included in the algorithm of the examination protocol because of the duration of the procedure, the lack of life support equipment compatible with magnetic resonance imaging does not allow us SCT-characteristic of hematomas depending on the stage of hemoglobin breakdown to take full advantage of this method (Trufanov 2006).

X-ray Spiral Computed Tomography (SCT)

The sensitivity of spiral computed tomography in the first 12 hours after SAH reaches 98% and persists the same for the first three days from the onset of the disease. Further, due to the resorption of blood from subarachnoid spaces, the diagnostic informativeness of SCT is significantly reduced (Zyablova and Porkhanov 2021).

The standard SCT technique begins with the execution of a tomogram designed to determine the level of the initial slice, and then the entire scanning area, the orbitomeatal line (the line connecting the outer corner of the eye and the external auditory canal) serves as a guideline for marking. A standard study is conducted according to the BRAIN program.

To obtain images in the sagittal and frontal planes, multiplanar reconstruction (MPR) is used, and volumetric images (VRT) are used for a detailed study of contrasted vessels.

During the analysis of the study, a change in the width and level of the window is carried out to consistently determine the size and volume of the detected intracranial changes, and densitometry is carried out to identify "fresh" blood having a HU density close to the brain substance.

In the acute stage, on CT scans, the blood of hyperdense density is localized in cisterns and subarachnoid spaces, while leveling of the interdigital cistern suggests the presence of isodense blood. The smaller the size of the hemorrhage, the more diagnostic difficulties it causes when interpreting the results. The determination of the limitation of SAH requires knowledge of changes in density characteristics during the interpretation of the process at the stages of evolution (Table 4).

Table 4. SCT characteristics of hematomas depend on the stage of hemoglobin breakdown

Stage	Composition	CT-density
Super acute (<24 hours)	oxyhemoglobin	+60… +80 HU
Acute (1-3 days)	deoxyhemoglobin	+60… +80 HU
Early subacute(3-7 days)	intracellular methemoglobin	+40…+70 HU
Late subacute(1-2 weeks)	extracellular methemoglobin	+30…+40 HU
Chronic(more than 2 weeks)	hemosiderin	+4…+15 HU

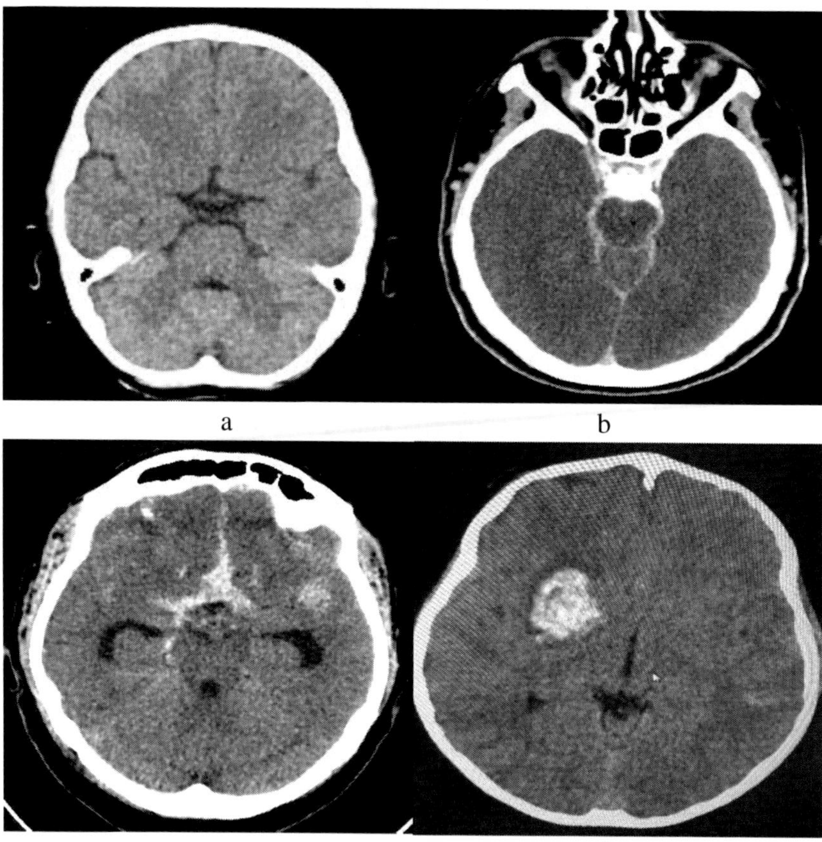

a b

c d

Figure 6. The degree and distribution of hemorrhage in basal cisterns in SAH on the scale of Fisher C. et al. (1980).
a – Grade 1; b – Grade 2; c – Grade 3; d – Grade 4.

In 1980 to assess the severity of hemorrhage according to SCT data the Fisher scale was developed. According to it, localized clots or diffuse hemorrhage with a layer of more than 1 mm are risk factors for the development of cerebral vasospasm and an unfavorable outcome. The degree and distribution of hemorrhage in basal cisterns in SAH on the scale of Fisher C. et al. (1980) are presented in Figure 6:

- Grade 1 - there is no subarachnoid and ventricular hemorrhage, and the probability of vasospasm is 21%;
- Grade 2 - diffuse subarachnoid hemorrhage < 1 mm thick, the probability of vasospasm is 25%;
- Grade 3 - local clots and/or a layer of blood more than > 1 mm thick, the probability of vasospasm is 37%;
- Grade 4 - intracerebral or intraventricular hemorrhage with or without diffuse subarachnoid, the probability of vasospasm is 31%.

With the help of CT, according to the localization of blood in the brain cisterns and the location of the parenchymal component in 90% of cases, it is possible to assume the localization of an aneurysm or other source of SAH, these data are very important when planning an angiographic examination.

With the localization of blood in the temporal lobe or parenchyma of the basal nuclei, it is possible to assume the presence of an aneurysm of the middle cerebral or internal carotid artery, posterior connective artery, and when there is blood in the lateral cleft of the brain - aneurysm M1-M2 segments of the middle cerebral artery. Blood in the lower-medial parts of the frontal lobe and the anterior divisions of the interhemispheric fissure indicates an aneurysm of the anterior cerebral and anterior connective artery, the ophthalmic segment of the internal carotid artery, blood in the cavity of the transparent septum - an aneurysm of the anterior connective artery. Localization of blood in the corpus callosum does not allow to exclude an aneurysm of the pericallosal artery. Isolated intraventricular hemorrhage implies an aneurysm of the anterior choroidal artery. Isolated accumulation of blood in the fourth ventricle and subarachnoid spaces of the cerebellum – aneurysm of the posterior inferior cerebellar artery. The accumulation of blood in the periarticular cisterns with a slight spread into the lateral slits of the brain does not exclude the rupture of the aneurysm of the bifurcation of the basilar artery or the posterior connective artery.

With native CT (without a contrast agent), it is possible to diagnose only aneurysms with a diameter of more than 10 mm. The aneurysm is visualized as a rounded area of increased density with fairly clear contours near the vessels of the arterial circle, the walls of the aneurysm may be partially calcified (Figure 7).

With volumetric exposure, an aneurysm can deform the adjacent parts of the ventricular system and the cisterns of the base of the brain. However, the information obtained is insufficient to determine the tactics of surgical treatment of this pathology.

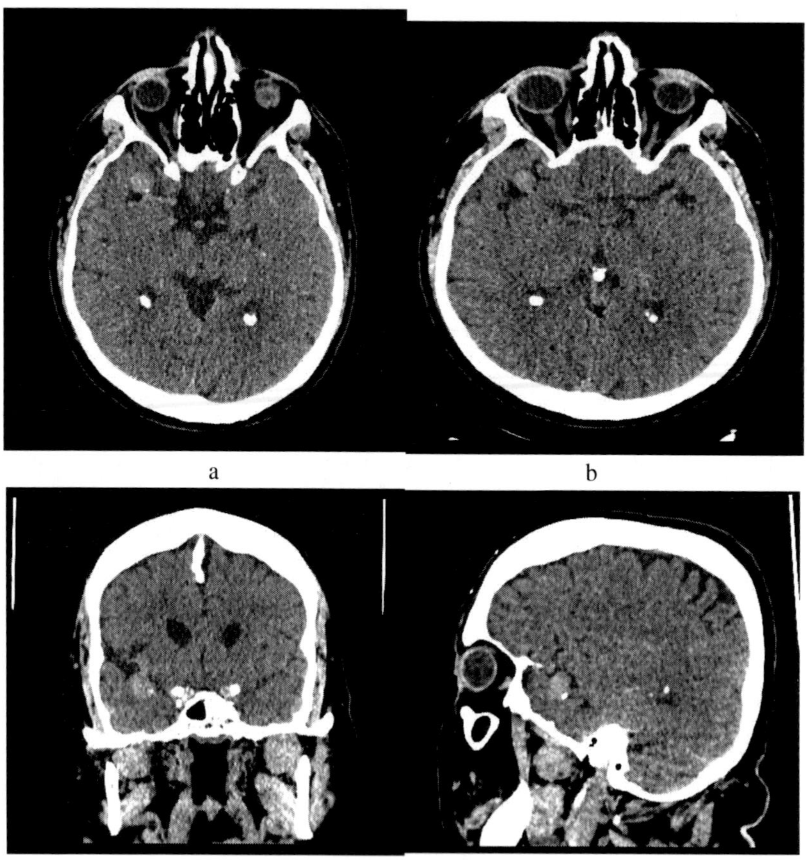

a b

c d

Figure 7. Saccular aneurysm of the right MCA bifurcation. On the SCT of the brain, an additional vascular shadow of a rounded shape, measuring 13x12x14mm, is traced in the projection of the right lateral slit of the brain. Axial projection (a, b), MPR in coronary (c) and sagittal (d) projections.

CT Angiography

CT angiography significantly increases the capabilities of CT in the diagnosis of cerebral aneurysms and SAH, contributes to solving several tasks when planning treatment tactics, and allows to get results closest to cerebral angiography. Depending on the technical capabilities of the X-ray computed tomography with CT-AG, it is possible to detect cerebral aneurysms of 2-3 mm or more in size. Most of these aneurysms are located in the anterior parts of the arterial circle of the large brain, only 20% of them are in the posterior parts.

The technique of performing SCT-AG involves rapid intravenous bolus administration of a radiopaque drug in an amount of 100 ml at a rate of 4 ml/s. Scanning of the anatomical area of interest is performed during the period of the greatest contrast enhancement of the vessel lumen, as a rule, during the first passage of the bolus of the contrast agent for 15-18 seconds.

The data obtained with CT-AG include images not only of vessels but also of other anatomical structures, as with conventional native CT. Arterial and venous structures are displayed simultaneously. To analyze the received data, the following is used: MIP (maximum intensity projection) is a three-dimensional image of predominantly high-density structures; MPR (multiplanar reconstruction) is planar images of structures in planes other than axial planes; VRT (volume rendering technique) is a three-dimensional image of the surfaces of the structures under study (Figure 8) (Zyablova and Porkhanov 2021).

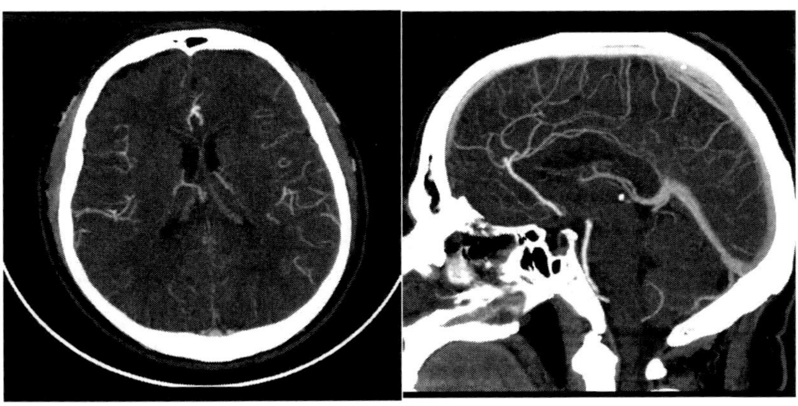

a b

Figure 8. (Continued)

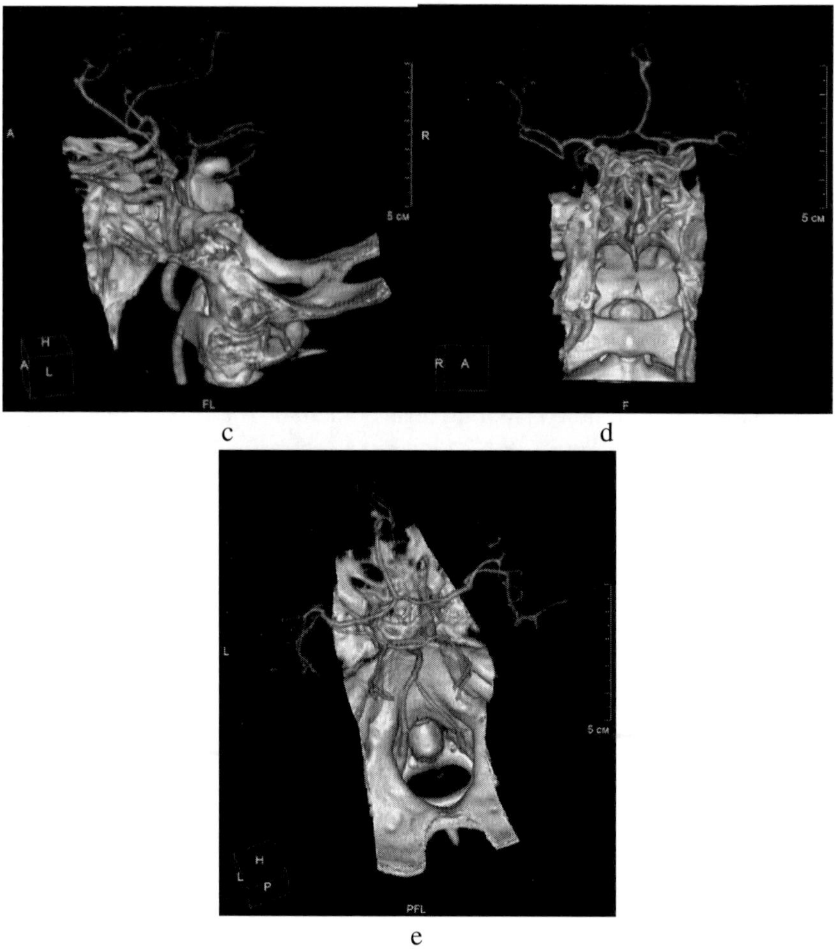

Figure 8. Saccular aneurysm of the A2-A3 segments of the right ACA. There is a saccular aneurysm of the A2-A3 segments of the right ACA with a size of 2.5x2.4 m, oriented anteriorly and upward, a neck of 1.9 mm. The anatomical feature of both ACA at the A2 segment level is that they depart with a single trunk. MIP (a, b) axial and sagittal planes, VRT (c - e).

On CT-AG, a saccular aneurysm is visualized as a rounded or irregularly shaped vascular formation associated with one of the branches of the cerebral arteries, and a fusiform aneurysm as an extended fusiform expansion of the vessel lumen (Grigorieva and Polunina 2017; Zyablova and Tkachev 2021).

The intensity of the aneurysm contrast depends on the degree of thrombosis in its cavity, if the aneurysm is partially thrombosed, in this case only its filled part is contrasted (Figure 9).

When interpreting the results of the study, the localization of the sac aneurysm relative to the segment of the artery and the defect of the artery wall (anterior, posterior, medial, and lateral), the position and direction of the aneurysm dome, the size of the filled and/or thrombosed part of the aneurysm, the size of the aneurysm neck, structural changes in the aneurysm sac wall are evaluated. In the presence of a wide neck, measurements are made of the diameter of the vessel distal and proximal to the aneurysm sac, the distance between the changing diameters, and marking under the stent is performed when modeling surgical treatment.

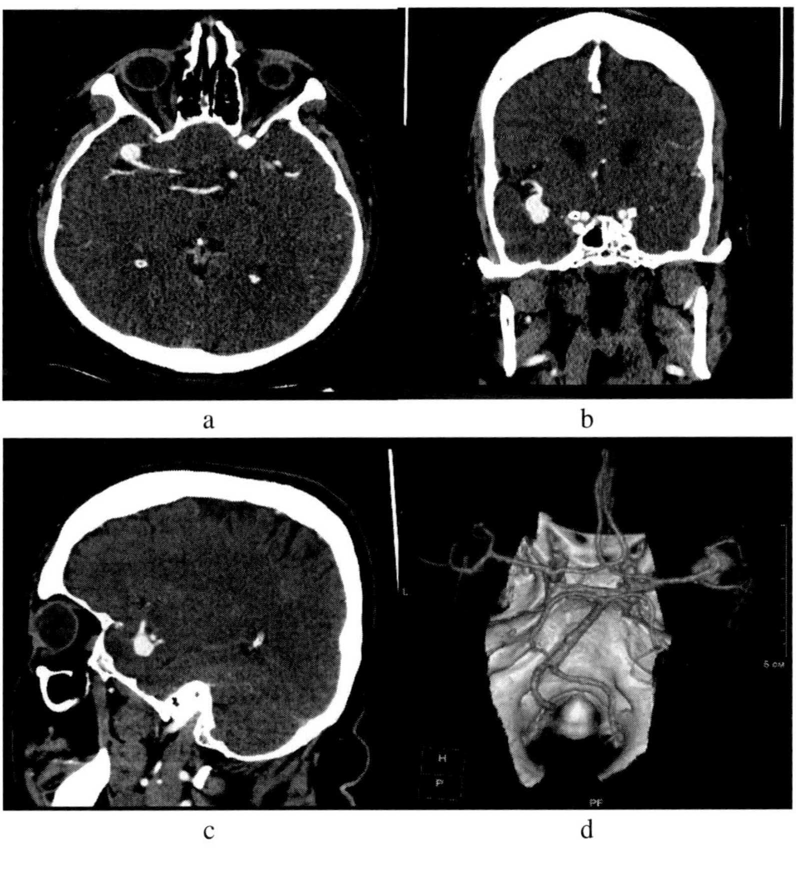

a b

c d

Figure 9. (Continued)

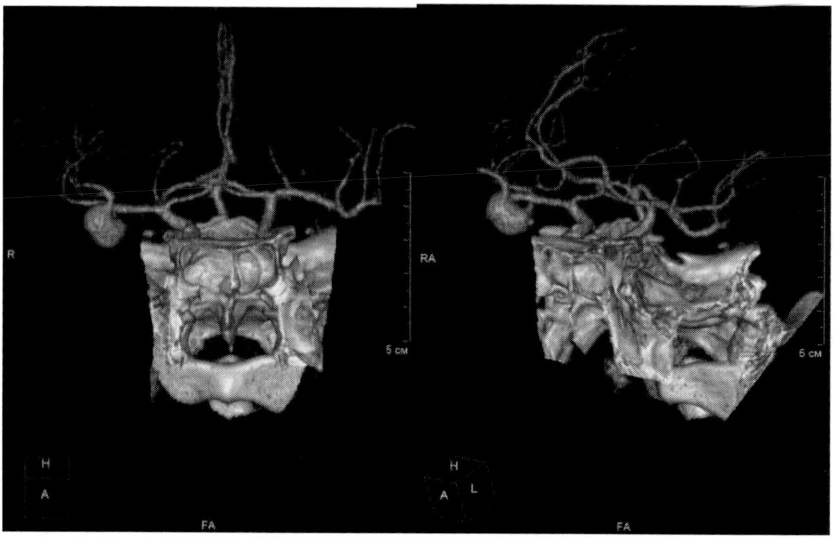

e f

Figure 9. Saccular aneurysm of the right MCA bifurcation. A saccular aneurysm of the right MCA bifurcation measuring 14x9x9mm, with small calcifications of the wall, oriented anteriorly and downwards, the neck is 8mm, one of the branches of the MCA departs from the aneurysm sac. MPR (a - c) axial, coronary and sagittal planes, VRT (d - f).

Difficulties in the diagnosis of cerebral aneurysms by the CT-AG method are associated with the small size of aneurysms (<2 mm) and the close diligence of other vascular structures.

Magnetic Resonance Imaging

MRI is less sensitive than CT in the acute stage of hemorrhage (less than 24 hours) since non-magnetic intracellular oxyhemoglobin does not have unpaired electrons and the signal from the blood clot approaches the normal brain, that is, iso- or weakly hypointense on T1 and weakly hyperintense on T2. MRI is recommended to be performed if clinical data do not correspond to CT data, especially in comatose patients, to detect hemorrhages of atypical localization and isodense density (according to SCT data).

To obtain approximate slices of the brain in the axial, sagittal and frontal planes, a search program (Localizer) is performed, the scanning time of which does not exceed 20 seconds.

After receiving the targeting images, a standard set of pulse sequences is performed: frFSE PS with obtaining T2WI in the axial plane, T2 FLAIR PS in the axial plane, and T1 FLAIR PS in the sagittal and frontal planes. On MRI-tomograms using standard programs, SAH in the acute stage gives a signal identical to the signal of the brain on T1WI and T2WI, this may obscure the diagnosis. The use of FLAIR PS in this situation makes it possible to identify small elements of SAH, in the form of a hypertensive signal along the course of the subarachnoid spaces of the brain, which are not visible on other pulse sequences.

Subarachnoid and intraventricular hemorrhages are easy to differentiate from parenchymal hemorrhages since they are mixed with cerebrospinal fluid, bloody cerebrospinal fluid looks hyperintense on FLAIR PS.

When interpreting the results of MRI, the localization, size, and volume of the detected hemorrhagic changes are determined.

Diagnosis of SAH and parenchymal hemorrhage in the brain requires knowledge of changes in the MR signal during the interpretation of hemorrhage at the stages of evolution.

In the acute phase (1-3 days) there is a hypo-signal on T1 and T2WI, early subacute phase (3-7 days) hyperintense signal on T1WI and hypo- on T2WI, late subacute phase (2 weeks) hyperintense signal on T1 and T2WI, chronic stage (more than 3 weeks) hypo- on T1 and T2WI and the rim of hemosiderin (Table 5).

Table 5. MR characteristics of hematomas depend on the stage of hemoglobin breakdown (Cementis S.A., 2005)

Stage	Composition	MR signal	
		T1	T2
Super acute (<24 hours)	Oxyhemoglobin	↑↓	↑
Acute (1-3 days)	Deoxyhemoglobin	↓	↓
Early subacute (3-7 days)	Intracellular methemoglobin	↑	↓
Late subacute (1-2 weeks)	Extracellular methemoglobin	↑	↑
Chronic (more than 2 weeks)	Hemosiderin	↓ at the edge (hemosiderin) ↑in the center	↓ at the edge (hemosiderin) ↑in the center

MRI has a high soft–tissue resolution and allows for visualizing the relationship between aneurysm and brain structures, to identify volumetric effects in parenchymal hemorrhages and structural changes in the substance of the brain adjacent to the aneurysm (Figure 10). Extrapontine myelinolysis developed after aneurysmal subarachnoid hemorrhage (case from practice and literature review) (Goroshchenko and Ivanov 2016).

According to MRI data, aneurysms are defined as formations of a rounded or oval shape, as a zone of the absence of an MR signal (due to the effect of "washing out"), with clear contours adjacent to the vessel wall, with dimensions of 3 mm or more (Figure 11).

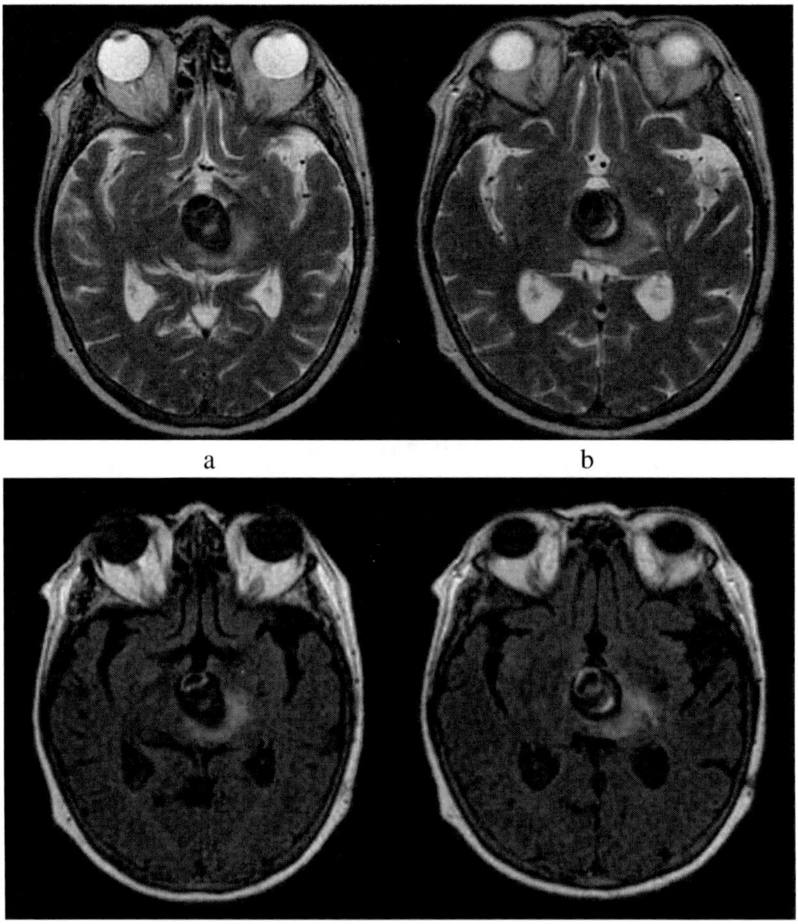

a b

c d

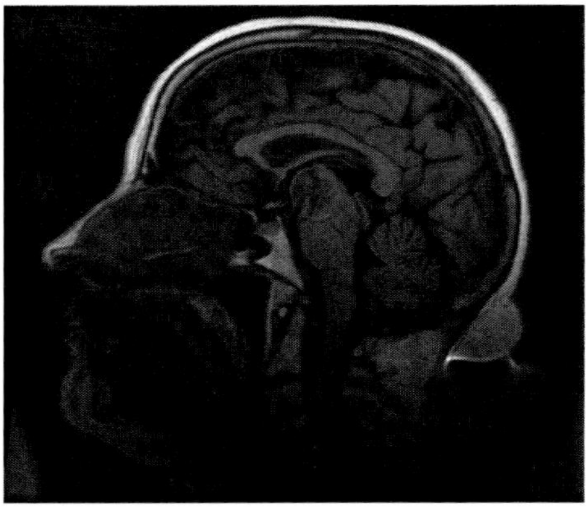

e

Figure 10. Giant saccular aneurysm of the basilar artery bifurcation. On a series of MRI scans of the brain T2WI and FLAIR IP in axial projection (a-d) and sagittal (e) in the interdigital cistern, an additional vascular shadow is revealed, oval in shape with clear contours, heterogeneous structure, size 26x18x23mm, the interdigital cistern is compressed, the lower parts of the 3rd ventricle are deformed. In the left half of the pons and the left brain stem, there is a 27x14mm hyperintensive signal zone on T2WI (mass effect from an aneurysm).

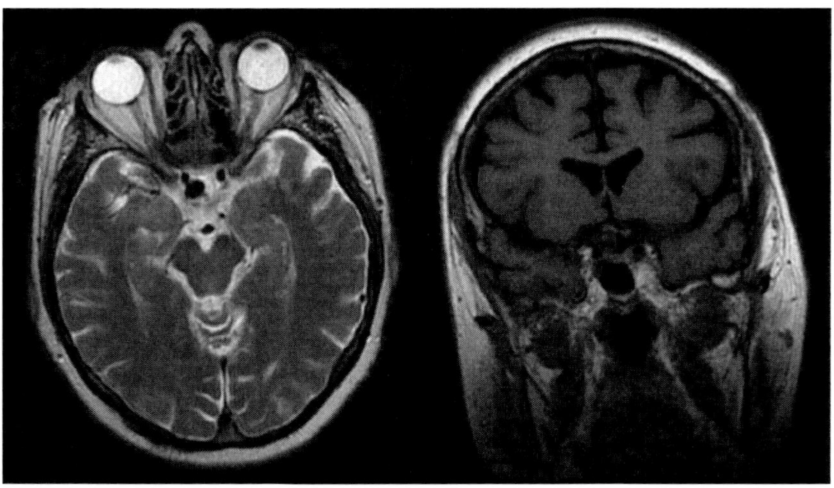

a b

Figure 11. (Continued)

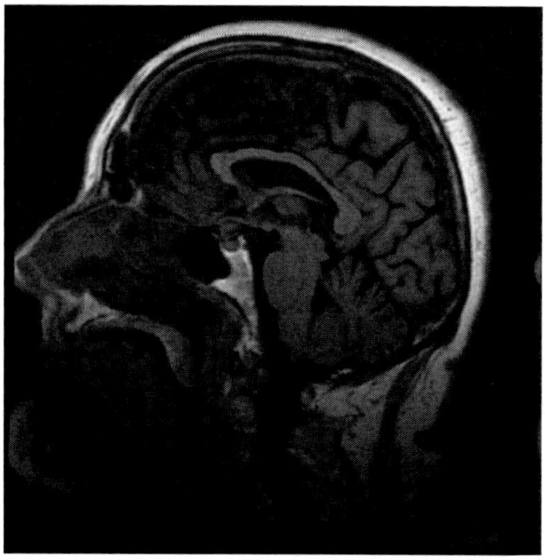

c

Figure 11. Saccular aneurysm of the supraclinoid section of the right ICA. On a series of MRI scans of the brain T2WI in axial projection (a), T1WI coronary (b) and sagittal (c) in the suprasellar cistern on the right, an additional vascular shadow, round, 7x8mm in size, deforming the right half of the chiasm, the pituitary funnel is shifted slightly to the left.

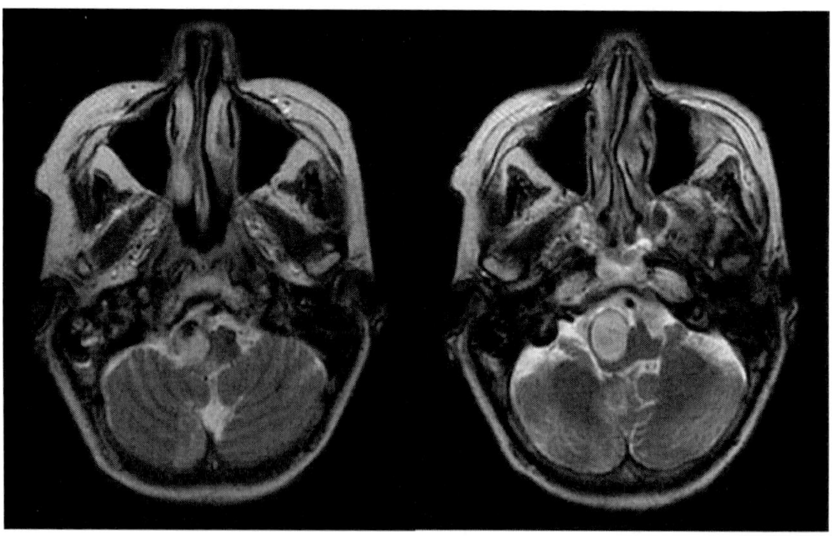

a b

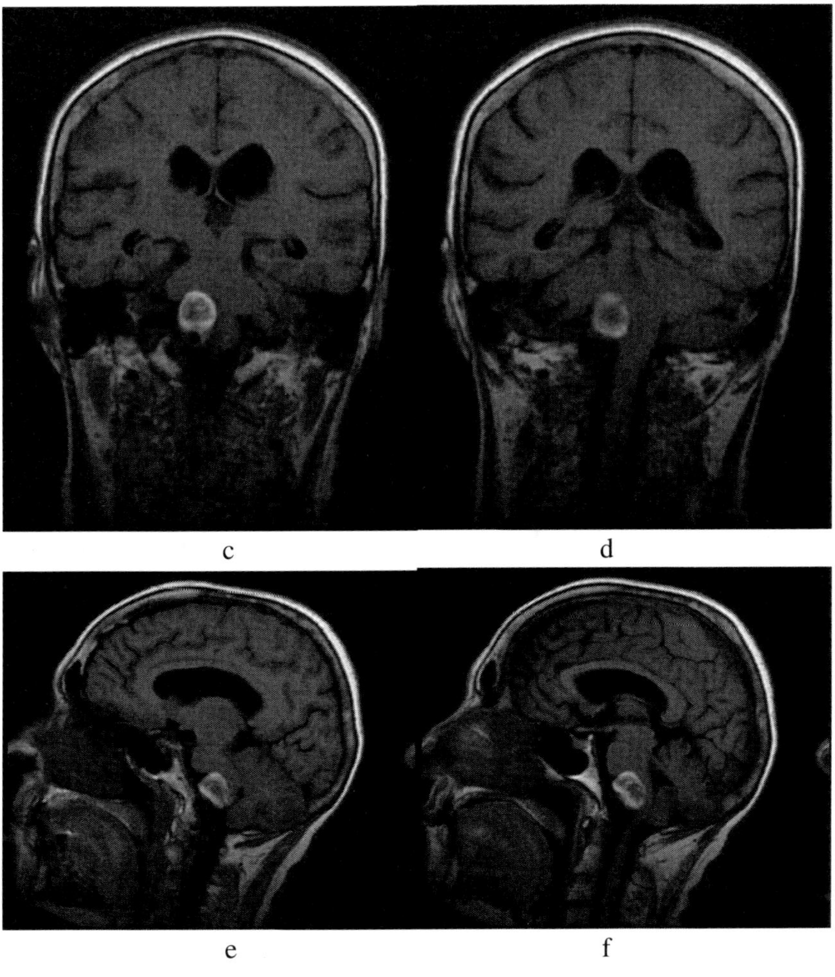

Figure 12. Partially thrombosed giant saccular aneurysm of the right PICA. The condition after installing a flow-redirecting stent in the right VA. On a series of MRI T2WI in axial projection (a, b), T1WI coronary (c, d) and sagittal (e, f) projections in the pre-pontine cistern on the right, an additional vascular shadow, round shaped, size 14x22x14mm, exerts a volumetric effect on the adjacent parts of the medulla oblongata and the pons.

MRI capabilities allow detecting the presence of a blood clot in the aneurysm body, depending on the presence of hemoglobin breakdown products in it. A thrombus is defined as a zone of hypo-, iso-, or hyperintense signal on T1 and T2WI compared to the absence of an MR signal from the non-thrombosed part of the aneurysm, and with large aneurysm sizes, it causes some "layering" of the MR signal (Figure 12).

MR Angiography

The use of MR angiography makes it possible to detect medium and large aneurysms of any localization. Detection of small aneurysms causes the greatest difficulties, which are explained by the low intensity of the MR signal due to the small blood flow in the body of a small aneurysm. It is also difficult to assess the departure of vascular branches from the dome and the cervical part of the aneurysm, and visualization of the compacted calcified aneurysm wall.

On MR angiograms, a saccular aneurysm is defined as an area of increased intensity of the MR signal, rounded in shape with clear contours, adjacent to the cerebral vessels, and a fusiform aneurysm as an extended spindle-shaped area of increased intensity of the MR signal (Figure 13).

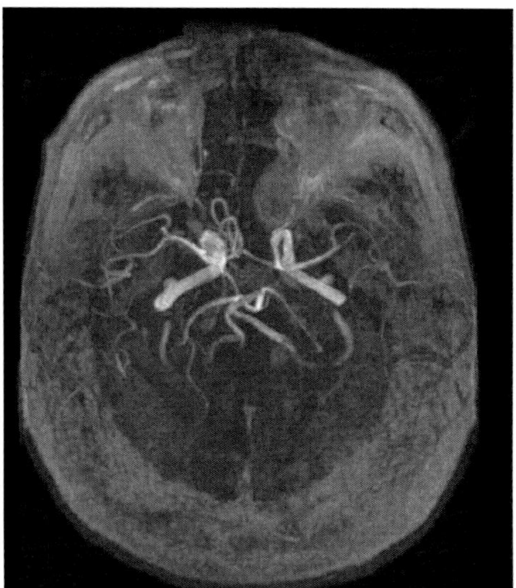

Figure 13. Saccular aneurysm of the right MCA bifurcation. On MR-angiograms of the brain, the main vessels are passable. The Willis circle is open in the projection of the left PCA. A saccular aneurysm of the right MCA bifurcation with a size of 2x1.2 mm, oriented laterally, is revealed.

Thus, an arterial aneurysm of medium and large size can be diagnosed using MRI and MR angiography, which can be screened at the initial stage of examination, but the lack of a detailed assessment of the morphology of the aneurysm does not allow using these methods in preoperative planning without performing CT or cerebral angiography.

Cerebral Angiography

Cerebral angiography provides the most reliable information about the size of the aneurysm, its configuration, the width of the neck, and the interaction of the aneurysm and blood vessels (Marcolini and Hine 2019). This method also allows you to identify the multiple nature of the lesion, arterial spasm, its severity and extent, and assess the functioning of a large circle of the base of the brain (blood flow through the anterior and posterior communicant arteries).

Saccular aneurysms on angiograms are defined as the limited protrusion of the artery wall, and fusiform ones as a uniform expansion of the artery in a limited area. Fusiform or atherosclerotic aneurysms are associated with atherosclerotic dilation of the basilar and/or vertebral arteries.

The angiographic signs of partial aneurysm thrombosis include unevenness and indistinctness of the aneurysm wall. Signs of a ruptured aneurysm on angiograms may be uneven and sometimes fuzzy contours of the aneurysm wall, spasm of adjacent segments of cerebral arteries, and displacement of vessels carrying the aneurysm.

For optimal visualization of the anatomical structure of the aneurysm, it is necessary to use not only standard projections (straight and lateral) but also oblique atypical styling, allowing to bring the neck of the aneurysm in the best projection, to identify perforating branches (which may be located in the aneurysm dome), to assess collateral circulation and concomitant pathology, vasospasm and mass effect. The use of three-dimensional rotational angiography makes it possible to facilitate and shorten this complex process (Figure 14).

A sign of ongoing aneurysmal hemorrhage on angiograms is the presence of extravasation of a contrast agent of various shapes located near the contrasted vessel. Hemorrhages can also occur when the artery is dissected (pseudoaneurysms, dissections) (Marcolini and Hine 2019).

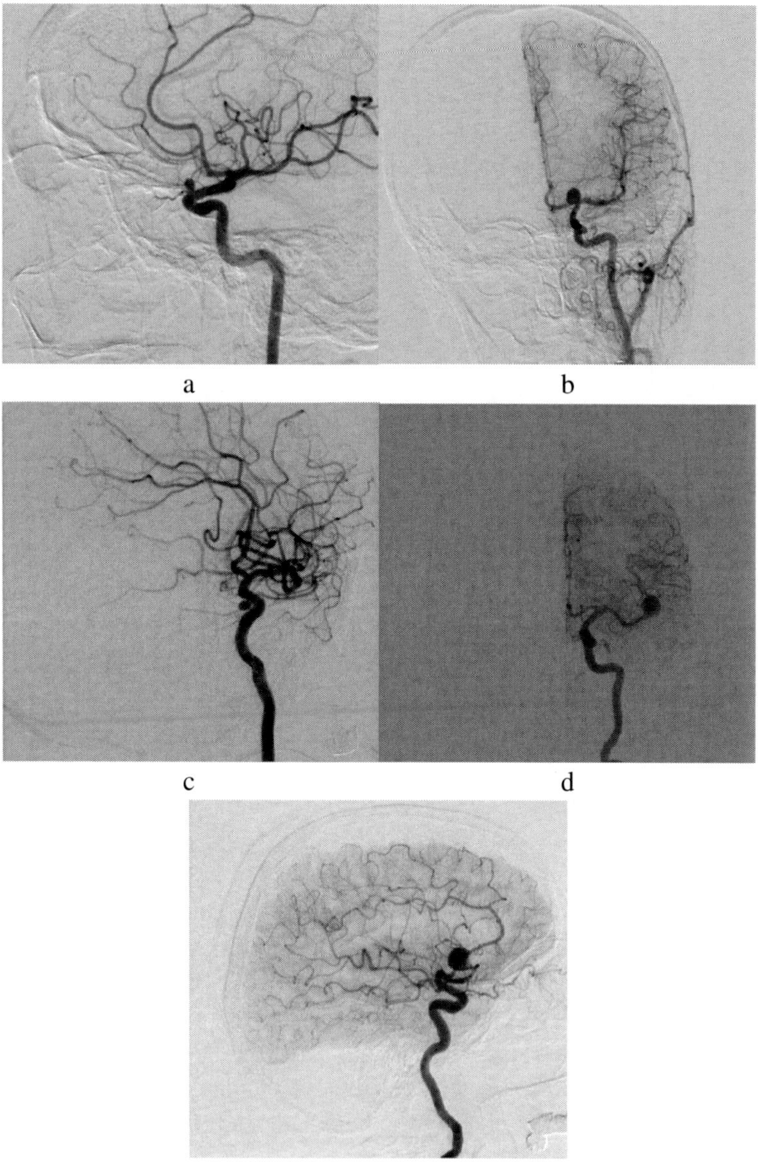

a b c d e

Figure 14. Cerebral angiography. Saccular aneurysm of the ophthalmic segment of the right ICA, lateral projection (a). Saccular aneurysm of the left ICA bifurcation, direct projection (b). Saccular aneurysm of the communicant segment of the left ICA, oblique projection (c). Saccular aneurysm M1-M2 of the segments of the left MCA, direct and lateral projections (d, e).

An important point in the evaluation of angiograms is the determination of intra-aneurysmal blood flow, which is one of the constituent factors in the preoperative planning of endovascular occlusion. Assessment of collateral blood flow is necessary when planning destructive interventions. During carotid angiography, it is necessary to perform finger compression of the contralateral CCA and evaluate the flow of contrast agents along the anterior communicant and posterior communicant arteries.

Thus, if it is possible to use CT-AG or MRI, it is not recommended to use cerebral angiography exclusively for diagnostic purposes.

Complications of Aneurysm Rupture

Complications caused by subarachnoid hemorrhage can be divided into two large groups: complications developing directly in the "acute" period of hemorrhage and complications developing in the long-term period. The first group includes dislocation syndrome associated with the formation of intracerebral or subdural hematoma; acute occlusion of the cerebrospinal fluid pathways associated with the spread of blood into the ventricular system of the brain and leading to the development of acute occlusive hydrocephalus, as well as repeated hemorrhage from an aneurysm. The second group includes constrictive-stenotic arteriopathy (cerebral vasospasm), leading to delayed cerebral ischemia, as well as hypo- and aresorptive chronic hydrocephalus, associated, most often, with impaired absorption of cerebrospinal fluid by pachyonic granulations (Bu and Chen 2016).

Cerebral Vasospasm

Cerebral vasospasm is a frequent complication of SAH and can develop in 50-90% of patients (Zubkov and Nikiforov 1984; Dorsch and King 1994). Analysis conducted by Fergusen S. et al. (2007), revealed that brain infarction caused by vasospasm develops within 6 weeks in 26% of patients, which directly correlates with an unfavorable outcome (Fergusen and MacDonald 2007). Today, the cumulative risk of disability and mortality due to vasospasm alone is 10%, but it remains one of the main causes of poor treatment outcomes in patients with aneurysmal SAH (Kassell and Tomer 1990; Broderick and Brott 1994; Proust and Hannequin 1995).

The most significant predictor of vasospasm development is the volume of blood poured into the subarachnoid space, as well as the rate of its elimination (Friedman and Goerss 2002; Reilly and Amidei 2004). Loss of consciousness during the manifestation of the disease, the presence of severe neurological symptoms upon admission to the hospital, smoking, diabetes mellitus, as well as arterial hypertension increase the likelihood of vasospasm development (Harrod and Bendok 2005; de Rooij and Rinkel 2013; de Rooij and Greving 2013). Also, the development of vasospasm can be influenced by factors such as young age, female gender, and localization of aneurysm. According to Abla A. et al. (2014), the incidence of vasospasm was significantly higher with rupture of an aneurysm of the anterior connective artery (Abla and Wilson 2014). It has also been suggested that the Japanese population, as well as cocaine use, increases the risk of vasospasm in patients with aneurysmal SAH (Mocco and Ransom 2006, Conway and Tamargo 2001).

There is evidence that intravascular intervention on an aneurysm reduces the risk of vasospasm, compared with microsurgical clipping (Rabinstein and Pichelmann 2003; Gross and Rosalind 2014; Ibrahim and Morgan 2014). According to some data, a violation of cerebral autoregulation, assessed by transcranial Dopplerography and detected early after SAH, is also a predictor of the development of vasospasm (Otite and Mink 2014).

Cerebral vasospasm – at the beginning of its development, this is a prolonged narrowing of the cerebral artery caused by a contraction of the smooth muscles of the vascular wall. The release of hemoglobin from blood clots trapped in the subarachnoid space triggers the release of calcium and subsequent activation of calcium/calmodulin-dependent kinase of the myosin light chain, which, in turn, leads to phosphorylation of the myosin light chain and induces actin and myosin cross-links, causing smooth muscle contraction. Such a reduction requires adenosine triphosphate and calcium, and vascular smooth muscles are more dependent on extracellular calcium reserves, which come through potential-dependent and receptor-controlled calcium channels. Contractile proteins, kinase C, and protein tyrosine kinase involve the corresponding signal transmission pathways in vasospasm models (Koide and Nishizawa 2002, Hansen-Schwartz and Vajkoczy 2007). This continuous stage of "chronic" vasospasm is less reversible with the help of pharmacological agents, both in animal models (Megyesi and Vollrath 1999) and in humans.

Sustained vasoconstriction is associated not only with the functional state of vasospasm but also with a violation of the structure of the vascular wall:

damage to the layers of the vascular wall, including vacuolization of endothelial cells, rupture of the internal elastic plate, and the development of mosaic myonecrosis in the arterial wall (Megyesi and Vollrath 1999; Medvedev and Zakaryavichus 2002). Also, autoxidation of hemoglobin contained in blood clots surrounding cerebral arteries produces the release of methemoglobin and superoxide radicals, which in turn activate lipid peroxidation (Sasaki and Wakai 1981; Kamezaki and Yanaka 2002). Hydroxyl radicals and peroxide lipids penetrate the vascular wall, damaging endothelial and smooth muscle cells (Ohta and Satoh 1992; Foley and Takenaka 1994).

Endothelial damage plays a key role in the development of vasospasm either due to a decrease in the synthesis of endothelial NO, which is a powerful vasodilator; or due to excessive production of endothelin, which is a vasoconstrictor peptide (Iuliano and Pluta 2004).

Although vasospasm is not a type of vasculitis, there is evidence of the activation of inflammatory mechanisms after SAH is involved in its formation. These are an increase in the plasma content of complement C3a, soluble molecules of intercellular adhesion-1, and an increased level of intrathecal cytokines (Mack and Ducruet 2007; Mocco and Mack 2002) leading to vasoconstriction and the development of changes in the phenotype of smooth muscle cells – the so-called "vascular remodeling" (Dumont and Dumont 2003).

Early brain damage as a result of blood pressure spikes, and global cerebral ischemia due to aneurysm rupture can trigger a cascade of pathological processes, including inflammation, capillary thrombosis, blood-brain barrier dysfunction, brain edema, and apoptosis of neurons (Rowland and Hadjipavlou 2012; Chen and Feng 2014; Zubkov 1989). In combination with vasospasm, these processes underlie the progressive deterioration of the condition in patients with aneurysmal SAH.

The first clinical signs of vasospasm in most patients are observed 3-4 days after the rupture of the aneurysm and reach their maximum severity by 7-11 days (Zubkov and Khilko 1982).

V.V. Krylov et al. (1988), based on an angiographic assessment, 4 types of vascular spasm were identified:

- *Type 1* is unexpressed and non-widespread, with a degree of narrowing of the arteries less than 50% of the normal diameter and extending to 1-2 segments of the artery.
- *Type 2* is pronounced non-widespread, with a degree of narrowing of the arteries by 50% or more and extending to 1-2 arterial segments.

- *Type 3* is unexpressed and widespread, with a degree of narrowing of the arteries less than 50% and spreading to 3 segments or more.
- *Type 4* is pronounced and widespread, with a degree of narrowing of the arteries by 50% or more and extending to 3 segments or more (Zubkov and Khilko 1982; Sanchez-Porras and Zheng 2013; Topkoru and Egemen 2017; Lebedev and Krylov 1996). However, it should be noted that there is not always a correspondence between the localization and prevalence of vasospasm and its clinical manifestations, which can be explained by the safety and adequacy of collateral blood flow (Kaye and Tagari 1984).

The symptoms of cerebral vasospasm, as a rule, are delayed, and therefore careful monitoring of the patient's condition is necessary for at least 2 weeks after the development of SAH.Vasospasm, more often, manifests itself gradually and may be accompanied by an increase in headache, drowsiness, or, conversely, arousal of the patient, a change in his behavior (Fisher and Roberson 1977). In the future, focal symptoms due to developing cerebral ischemia may join (Findlay and Nisar 2016).

Thus, with the development of ischemia in the middle cerebral artery basin, the appearance of mono- or hemiparesis, sensory, and motor aphasia can be observed. With the predominance of ischemia in the basin of the anterior cerebral artery, patients experience weakness in the legs, confusion, impoverishment of speech, and the development of apathetic-abulic syndrome is possible in the future. An increase in ischemia in the vertebrobasilar basin often causes primary depression of consciousness (Findlay and Nisar 2016).

Paroxysmal Sympathetic Hyperactivity Syndrome (PSH)

The stimulation of the higher cortical center of the sympathetic nervous system - the insular cortex - with blood spilled due to SAH is realized in a sympathetic "storm" or Paroxysmal Sympathetic Hyperactivity syndrome (PSH). PSH is associated with the development of secondary complications, a longer stay of the patient in the ICU, and higher disability and mortality (Compton 2018; Perks and Bagley 2010).

Timely and adequate prevention and therapy of the syndrome improve the functional result (Savvina and Zabrodskaya 2021). Criteria for PSH syndrome are present in Table 6 (Savvina and Zabrodskaya 2021).

Table 6. Criteria for PSH syndrome (Savvina and Zabrodskaya 2021)

Indicators/points	0	1	2	3
Main criteria				
Pulse rate	<100	110-119	120-139	>140
BP syst	<140	140-159	160-179	>180
Breath rate	<18	18-23	24-29	>30
Kerdo index	0	+1-+10	+10-+20	>+21
T C	<37	37-37,9	38-38,9	>40
Increased muscle tone(points)	0	1-2	3	4-5
Frequency of episodes of vegetativeinstability (in 24 hours)	no	3	6	>6
Additional criteria				
Level of consciousness (points) (GCS)	15-14	14-13	12-10	<10
Hyperhidrosis	No	+	++	+++
Skin hyperemia	no	+	++	+++
Albumin g/l	34-48	28-34	22-28	<22
EEG signsof irrigation of diencephalic structures	no	+	++	+++

Interpretation of results:

0-no;

1-7 p according to the main criteria, no more than 5p according to additional criteria – weakly expressed PSH syndrome;

8-14 p according to the main criteria, no more than 10 p according to additional criteria – moderate PSH syndrome;

15-21 p according to the main criteria, 10-15 p according to additional criteria - pronounced PSH syndrome.

Neurogenic Stress Cardiomyopathy and Takotsubo Syndrome

SAH has been correlated with syndrome described as neurogenic stress cardiomyopathy and mimics acute coronary syndrome (Rasputina and Rutkovsky 2019; Lampropoulos and Giannoulis 2017; Lee and Oh 2006; Murthy and Shah 2015; Malik and Gross 2015; Kadooka and Hadeishi 2017). Neurogenic stunned myocardium was another term to describe the cardiac dysfunction after SAH (Lampropoulos and Giannoulis 2017; Lee and Oh 2006; Murthy and Shah 2015; Malik and Gross 2015; Kadooka and Hadeishi 2017). Usually, patients with sudden and grave SAH immediately get complicated by a neurogenic cardiac disease with fatal heart rhythm abnormalities (Murthy and Shah 2015; Malik and Gross 2015; Kadooka and Hadeishi 2017).

Takotsubo cardiomyopathy is characterized by acute and profound, but transient regional left ventricular dysfunction in the absence of obstructive coronary disease (Samuels 2007; Nanda and Bhatt 2008). Takotsubo cardiomyopathy was first described in the early 1990s in Japan (Ono and Falcao 2016). Its Japanese name was derived from the characteristic appearance of the left ventricle as evidenced by ventriculography during diagnostic coronary angiography for evaluation of an acute coronary syndrome. This classic left ventricular shape had a round bottom and narrow neck due to the stunning of the apical ventricular segments, thus resembling a Japanese octopus trap known as a takotsubo, explaining why Takotsubo syndrome is also known as a "transient apical ballooning syndrome" (Ono and Falcao 2016).

Transitory adrenergic activation and an exaggerating sympathetic stimulation can explain the occurrence of Takotsubo syndrome (Samuels 2007; Nanda and Bhatt 2008). Many authors reported a general increase in the circulating catecholamine levels or local augmentation in the coronary system (Murthy and Shah 2015; Malik and Gross 2015; Kadooka and Hadeishi 2017). Usually, patients with sudden and grave SAH immediately get complicated by a neurogenic cardiac disease with fatal heart rhythm abnormalities (Murthy and Shah 2015; Malik and Gross 2015; Kadooka and Hadeishi 2017; Samuels 2007; Nanda and Bhatt 2008). Metabolic disorders in the myocardium after a high level of catecholamines have been proposed for the mechanisms of Takotsubo syndrome (Nanda and Bhatt 2008). Biomarkers of myocardial injury, such as creatine kinase, creatine kinase-MB, and troponin, are elevated in most patients with Takotsubo syndrome. However, the extent of these biomarkers is disproportionately low when compared with the extent of wall motion abnormality (Templin and Ghardi 2015). During the acute phase of Takotsubo syndrome, serum cardiac BNP or NT-proBNP (N-terminal pro-brain natriuretic peptide) is often notably elevated compared with patients with the acute coronary syndrome (Ahmed and Madhavan 2012).

Neurogenic Pulmonary Edema

In 1997, it has been reported that intracerebral high pressure leads to an upregulation of the sympathetic system to assure brain perfusion (Brambrink and Dick 1997).

Neurogenic pulmonary edema is caused by systemic and lung vasoconstriction-induced massive adrenergic discharge (Theodore and Robin 1976). To determine whether the lung edema is neurogenic, it has to be distinguished from iatrogenic lung edema caused by excessive infusion of crystalloid or transfusion of blood, edema resulting from heart or renal failure, and aspiration pneumonia. Treatment includes airway management, oxygenation, positive end-expiratory pressure (PEEP), administration of adreno-cortical hormone, and diuretic drugs.

Hyponatremia

Hyponatremia occurs commonly after SAH. It is regarded as being induced by the cerebral salt-wasting syndrome (CSWS) rather than by the syndrome of inappropriate secretion of antidiuretic hormone (SIADH) (Nelson and Seif 1981). CSWS brings about excessive natriuresis through atrial natriuretic peptide (ANP) from the hypothalamus, and therefore we must treat to replace the sodium deficit with salt, using either normal or hypertonic (3%) saline. Recently, brain natriuretic peptide (BNP) (MacGirt and Mavropoulos 2003) or Dendroaspis natriuretic peptide (DNP) (Kurana and Wijdicks 2004) has been suggested as giving rise to hyponatremia.

Intracerebral Hemorrhage

Intracerebral hemorrhage, as a consequence of aneurysm rupture, occurs in 10-38% of cases of SAH. Although clinically significant hematoma occurs only in 4-17% of patients with aneurysmal SAH, its presence complicates the course of the disease and is directly associated with an increase in the frequency of adverse outcomes (Tokuda and Inagawav 1995; Shimoda and Oda 1997; Niemann and Wills 2003; Liu and Rinkel 2011; Nemoto and Masuda 2018; and Nguyen 2013; Jabbarli and Reinhard 2016; Darkwah and Skowronek 2018; Abbed and Ogilvy 2003). There is some data, that suggests that patients with intracerebral hematoma initially have a poorer clinical condition, as well as an increased risk of recurrent hemorrhage (Nemoto and Masuda 2018; Jabbarli and Reinhard 2016; Bohm and Hugosson 1978). The mass effect caused by intracerebral hematoma leads to an increase in intracranial pressure and serves as one of the causes of early brain damage (Wheelock and Weir 1983).

Localization of aneurysm is considered to be one of the main risk factors for the formation of intracerebral hemorrhage. Thus, the most significant localizations for intracerebral hematoma are considered to be the location of the aneurysm on the middle cerebral artery (Tokuda and Inagawa1 995; Niemann and Wills 2003; Jabbarli and Reinhard 2016; Bohm and Hugosson

1978) and, to a lesser extent, on the anterior connective artery (Darkwah and Skowronek 2018). About 1% are intracerebral hematomas formed during the rupture of vertebrobasilar aneurysms (Darkwah and Skowronek 2018). Risk factors for the formation of hematoma also include smoking, diabetes mellitus, hypertension, as well as taking antiplatelet therapy (Shimoda and Oda 1997; Niemann and Wills 2003; Nemoto and Masuda 2018; Wheelock and Weir 1983).

The clinical picture of an intracerebral hemorrhage depends on the localization, the volume of the hematoma, the severity of the mass effect, and the magnitude of intracranial pressure.Thus, when a hematoma is located in the frontal and temporal lobes, contralateral mono- and hemiparesis, aphasia phenomena may be noted. When a hematoma is localized in the frontal lobes (with aneurysms of the anterior connective artery), mental disorders prevail in the clinical picture (de Rooij and Rinkel 2013). It should be noted that in the case of a serious condition of the patient, the clinical picture of intracerebral hemorrhage can be erased by the symptoms of dislocation syndrome.

Intraventricular Hemorrhage

One of the formidable complications of SAH is the spread of blood into the ventricular system. Isolated intraventricular hemorrhage (IVH) in aneurysmal SAH is rare but is associated with high mortality (Wheelock and Weir 1983). Thus, according to Verma A. (1987), the presence of IVH led to a fatal outcome in 47.5% of patients (Wheelock and Weir 1983). Most often, aneurysms of the anterior connective artery, as well as aneurysms of the communicant segment of the internal carotid artery, leading to intraventricular blood distribution. There have also been described cases of IVH with rupture of aneurysms of the lenticular-striate artery (Wan and Jaja 2016; Anagnostopoulos and Chamilos 2019; Verma and Maheshwari 1987; Srivastava and Sannegowda 2013; Killeen and Wanke 2014; Yoneoka and Ezuka 1998; Gordon 1976).

Before the advent of neuroimaging methods, the diagnosis of IVH was established based on the development of sudden depression of consciousness to coma, often with a fatal outcome (Graeb and Robertson 1982; McDonald 1962; Ojemann 1963; Plum and Posner 1972), this condition was associated with massive haemo-tamponade of the ventricular system. At present, when an aneurysm ruptures, the presence of blood in the ventricular system is detected with SCT of the brain even in the absence of a classical clinical picture (Ojemann 1963; Plum and Posner 1972; Baker and Campbell 1974; Jacobs and Kinkel 1976).

The classical clinical picture in IVH is similar to that in SAH – there is a pronounced headache, and meningeal symptoms. In the presence of blood in the III ventricle, the patient may experience water-electrolyte disturbances and diencephalic symptoms associated with irritation of the bottom of the III ventricle. With massive haemo-tamponade, depression of consciousness, seizures, and suppression of the function of the respiratory and cardiovascular centers are noted (Steiner and Gomori 1984).

Acute Hydrocephalus

Acute hydrocephalus developing against the background of aneurysmal SAH is a complication that occurs in 20-67% of cases of SAH, characterized by an expansion of the ventricular system detected by CT examination (Giray and Sen 2009; Arboix and García-Eroles 2012; Black 1986; Graff-Radford and Torner 1989; Hasan and Tanghe 1992; Hasan and Vermeulen 1989; Rozhchenko 1995; Mehta and Holness 1996; MacDonald and Weir 2004; Hellingman and van den Bergh 2007; Germanwala and Huang 2010; van Asch CJ and van der Schaaf 2010; Hasan and Lindsay 1991) while being the cause of death in 5-10% of patients (Mura and Rojas-Zalazar 2007). This condition was first described by Bagley in 1928 (Vale and Bradley 1997). Female patients have an increased risk of developing occlusive hydrocephalus after SAH (MacDonald and Weir 2004; van Gijn and Rinkel 2001; Kongable and Lanzino 1996; Longstreth and Koepsell 1985; Rothwell and Coull 2005). At the same time, there is no proven relationship between the incidence of acute dropsy and the age of the patient (Black 1986; Hasan and Vermeulen 1989).

Acute hydrocephalus occurs in the first 72 hours after SAH. It is believed that its development is associated with the spread of blood into the subarachnoid space, basal cisterns, and ventricles of the brain, which prevents the outflow of cerebrospinal fluid due to exposure to the midbrain, plumbing, Monroe holes (Verma and Maheshwari 1987; Hellingman and van den Bergh 2007; Germanwala and Huang 2010; van Asch and van der Schaaf 2010). SAH from aneurysms of the internal carotid, middle cerebral arteries, as well as from aneurysms of the posterior circulatory circle is more often accompanied by the development of acute hydrocephalus due to obstruction of the outflow of cerebrospinal fluid at the level of 4 ventricles (van Asch and van der Schaaf 2010; Mura and Rojas-Zalazar 2007; Dupont Rabinstein 2013).

According to Mehta V. et al. (1996), rupture of an aneurysm of VBB was also significantly more often accompanied by the development of hydrocephalus (Hasan and Vermeulen 1989).

This condition can lead to a decrease in cerebral perfusion pressure due to an increase in ICP even in awake patients (Hasan and Tanghe 1992; Yasargil and Yonekawa 1973). Several studies on the measurement of cerebral blood flow in patients with aneurysmal SAH have revealed a decrease in perfusion pressure in such patients (Del Bigio 1993; Hayashi and Kobayashi 1984; Menon and Weir 1981).

Patients with acute hydrocephalus do not have specific symptoms, and the clinical picture is represented by severe headache, vomiting, symptoms of irritation of the meninges, impaired movement of the eyeballs, as well as depression of consciousness (Hasan and van Peski 1991). Some researchers suggest that the development of acute hydrocephalus is a poor prognostic sign, but its effect on the development of secondary cerebral ischemia has not been proven (Lu and Ji 2012). According to Dupont S. et al. (2013), the presence of acute hydrocephalus after SAH also negatively affects the long-term functional outcome of treatment, worsening it (Longstreth and Koepsell 1985). There is evidence that about half of the patients undergo independent rehabilitation of the ventricular system within 24 hours (Mehta and Holness1996; Vermeij and Hasan 1994). This is the reason for the recommendations of wait-and-see tactics in patients who are not in a sopor or comatose state (van Gijn and Kerr 2007) due to the high risk of infectious complications after implantation of external ventricular drainage (Kongable and Lanzino 1996, Wong and Poon 2002). The possibility of repeated hemorrhage from an aneurysm after the installation of external ventricular drainage is also discussed in the literature (MacDonald and Weir 2004; McIver and Friedman 2002; Ruijs and Dirven 2005; Cagnazzo and Gambacciani 2017).

Treatment of the Aneurysmal SAH

Surgical Methods of Treatment

"Open" Neurosurgical Operations of Aneurysm Clipping

The volume of the operation in the acute period of the SAC involves clipping of the aneurysm. Indications for microsurgical aneurysm clipping in the acute period of SAC are determined by many factors, among which are:

- age of the patient;
- the severity of the condition on admission to the hospital;
- localization of aneurysm;
- anatomical and morphological features of an aneurysm;
- the presence and volume of intracranial hematoma;
- the presence of occlusive hydrocephalus;
- the presence of dislocation syndrome;
- the presence of ICH refractory to therapy exceeding 20 mmHg (Guimond and Chagnon 2012; Eliava 2019).

Patients with complicated somatic status, a severe condition corresponding to the IV-V gradations on the Hunt & Hess scale, with localization of aneurysm in the VBB, or proximal to the distal dural ring, in the absence of occlusive hydrocephalus or large intracerebral hematoma causing dislocation of the median structures of the brain, intravascular intervention aimed at turning off the aneurysm from the bloodstream is indicated (Molyneux and Kerr 2002; Molyneux and Kerr 2005).

Patients in a state corresponding to grades I-III on the Hunt&Hess scale, young, as well as patients with large intracerebral hematoma, occlusive hydrocephalus, or dislocation syndrome clinic, in the presence of a partially thrombosed aneurysm, with localization of an aneurysm in the anterior parts of the circle of Willis located distal to the distal dural ring, an open intervention aimed at turning off the aneurysm from the bloodstream, removal of intracerebral hematoma is indicated, if necessary, it is possible to sanitize the basal cisterns from blood clots (Macdonald 2007; Johnson and Potter 1958; Klimo and Kestle 2004), as well as perform three-ventriculostomy by perforating the terminal plate, or applying external ventricular drainage (Suarez and Tarr 2006; Rothwell and Coull 2005, Chung and Olson 2019; Sarica and Tanrikulu 2018; Lu and Ji 2012; Kassell and Torner 1990; Mitchell and Kerr 2008). If necessary, the operation can also be supplemented by performing decompressive craniotomy (Konovalov and Belousova 2016; Pilipenko and Konovalov 2018; Schirmer and Hoit 2007; Wang and Ye 2014).

According to the indications, other surgical interventions and manipulations aimed at improving and stabilizing their condition, such as external ventricular drainage, external decompression with dura mater plastic, removal of intracerebral hematoma without turning off the aneurysm, installation of a sensor for monitoring intracranial pressure, can be performed in patients whose severity of the condition does not allow surgical intervention on the aneurysm (Konovalov and Krylov 2012).

Ventricular Drainage Operations

As mentioned above, acute hydrocephalus occurring against the background of SAH is a life-threatening condition, which in some cases (depression of consciousness) may require an emergency neurosurgical aid (Wong and Poon 2002; McIver and Friedman 2002; Gigante and Hwang 2010). The risk of developing acute hydrocephalus increases with age and is more often formed when aneurysms of the posterior sections of the Willis circle rupture (Rivero Rodríguez and Matamoros 2017; Lanzino and Kassell 1996; de Rooij and Linn 2007). Almost half of the hemorrhages corresponding to Fisher IV lead to the need for external ventricular drainage (Sanusi and McLarnon 2020).

Among the main surgical interventions performed for acute hydrocephalus after SAH, external ventricular drainage and three-ventriculostomy surgery performed during aneurysm clipping can be distinguished (Chung and Mayer 2018; Fukuhara and Shimizu 2009).

Implantation of external ventricular drainage is a standard neurosurgical procedure for the treatment of acute hydrocephalus in patients with SAH (Olson and Batjer 2014) and was first described in 1973 by Kusske J. A. et al. (Kusske and Turner 1973).

The advantages of this procedure are:

- the possibility of monitoring intracranial pressure;
- can prevent secondary cortical damage, improve the neurological status of the patient and facilitate open surgery on an aneurysm;
- can be used for intrathecal administration of drugs (Fountas and Kapsalaki 2006; Bratton and Chestnut 2007; Gambardella and De Blasi 1998; Mack and King 2003).

There is evidence that drainage of cerebrospinal fluid by external drainage of the ventricular system reduces the likelihood of vasospasm (Della Pepa and Scerrati 2014).

The disadvantages of external drainage are considered:

- increased risk of recurrent hemorrhage (with a functioning aneurysm) (Molyneux and Kerr 2002; Fukuhara and Shimizu 2009; Olson and Batjer 2014);
- risks of infectious complications;
- formation of a drainage-dependent state (Hasan and Tanghe 1992; Lozier and Sciacca 2002; Hirashima and Kurimoto 2005; Krylov and Burov 2009).

In case of massive hemorrhage into the lateral ventricles, a combination of external drainage with local fibrinolysis of blood clots (provided the aneurysm is turned off from the bloodstream) or their endoscopic removal is possible, which accelerates the rehabilitation of the ventricular system from blood (Krylov and Dashyan 2014; Krylov and Dashyan 2016; Chung and Leslie-Mazwi 2017). Possibly faster drainage removal, as well as intermittent drainage, in comparison with the constant removal of cerebrospinal fluid, reduces the risks of both infectious complications and the frequency of the formation of a drainage-dependent condition, which leads to a reduction in the patient's stay in the hospital (Palasz and D'Antona 2021; Bing and Rabinstein 2015).

Decompressive Craniotomy

Aneurysmal subarachnoid hemorrhage is a devastating disease with high mortality and disability, which reach 40% in some clinics (Bing and Rabinstein 2015; Connolly and Rabinstein 2012). In addition to the primary manifestations of aneurysm rupture, such as the formation of intracerebral (Niemann and Wills 2003), intraventricular hemorrhage (Macdonald 2014), or acute hydrocephalus, numerous subsequent pathophysiological processes, such as early brain damage (Wheelock and Weir 1983), symptomatic vasospasm (Jabbarli and Reinhard 2016), and delayed cerebral ischemia (Frontera and Fernandez 2009) complicate the course of SAH. All these conditions can eventually lead to a persistent increase in intracranial pressure (ICP).

Decompressive craniotomy (DCT) is an effective treatment option for patients with a refractory increase in ICP caused by malignant ischemic infarction (Vergouwen and Vermeulen 2010; Hofmeijer and Kappelle 2009; Jüttler and Schwab 2007; Jüttler and Unterberg 2014; Vahedi and Hofmeijer 2007; Vahedi and Vicaut 2007; Cooper and Rosenfeld 2011), as well as traumatic brain injury (Hutchinson and Kolias 2016, Alotaibi and Elkarim 2017). The available data are rather ambiguous concerning the DCT in SAH (Alotaibi and Elkarim 2017; Rangel-Castillo and Gopinath 2008; Krylov and Petrikov 2012; Dashyan and Levchenko 2015). According to various authors, the need for decompression in patients with SAH is present in 7-20% of patients (Fisher and Ojemann 1994; Buschmann and Yonekawa 2007; Dorfer and Frick 2010; Güresir and Schuss 2012; Dereeper and Berré 2002).

There are two types of DCT:

- primary, it is also preventive, when clipping or embolization of an aneurysm is accompanied by decompression in the presence of intracerebral hematoma, or the presence of signs of intracranial hypertension, determined before the intervention on the aneurysm (Güresir and Schuss 2012);
- secondary, when decompressive intervention is performed 24 hours or more after the primary intervention on an aneurysm due to an increase in ICP (Lu and Ji 2012; Frontera and Fernandez 2009, Kim and Park 2008; Nelson and Powell 1982; Gupta and Connolly 2004; Smith and Carter 2002).

The optimal size of decompressive trepanation of the skull is considered to be 9-15 cm, this size is designed to reduce ICP by 50-60% of the original (Konovalov and Belousova 2016; Dorfer and Frick 2010; Güresir and Schuss 2012; Dereeper and Berré 2002).

Some authors prefer primary DCT, believing that it leads to a better outcome in patients in serious conditions (Krylov and Petrikov 2012). According to the data of Pilipenko Yu. V. et al. (2016), the conduct of DCT is most justified and effective in the first days after SAH in patients with signs of intracranial hypertension, which is also confirmed by the data of other authors (Mitchell and Kerr 2008).

The main indications for primary DCT in patients with aneurysmal SAH are considered to be the severe condition of the patient upon admission to the hospital, corresponding to the IV-V gradation on the Hunt& Hess scale, the presence of intracranial hematoma causing lateral dislocation of the brain, visual signs of cerebral edema intraoperatively (Konovalov and Belousova 2016).

Secondary DCT in patients without a large intracerebral hematoma is performed when signs of compression of the oculomotor nerve (anisocoria), midbrain (mydriasis), with stable intracranial hypertension (more than 20 mmHg), are recorded by hardware and refractory to conservative treatment methods (Schirmer and Hoit 2007; Dorfer and Frick 2010; Dereeper and Berré2002; Kim and Park 2008; Nelson and Powell 1982; Gupta and Connolly 2004; Smith and Carter 2002; Otani and Takasato 2008). Signs of the effectiveness of DCT are the prolapse of the medulla into the trepanation defect by more than 5 mm, a decrease in the dislocation of the median structures of the brain in the postoperative period to less than 5 mm, and a decrease in elevated ICP (Smith and Carter 2002).

Endovascular Interventions

The use of an intravascular treatment may have priority in cases of aneurysms of localization that are difficult to access for microsurgical intervention (cavernous internal carotid artery, para-clinoid localization, vertebrobasilar basin); in elderly people (over 75 years old); in patients in serious condition; with fusiform and delaminating aneurysms (Otani and Takasato 2008; Uozumi and Sakowitz 2014; Diaz and Ohaegbulam 1989; van der Schaaf and Brilstra 2002; van Rooij 2012; Kim and Cha 2013; Gonzalez and Dusick 2010).

The use of intravascular treatment is indicated in the following cases:

- if it was not possible to clip the aneurysm during an open operation
- if the surgeon (assessing his experience) predicts serious technical difficulties or the impossibility of clipping the aneurysm.

And also in cases of:

- small aneurysms with a diameter of < 2 mm;
- large and giant aneurysms, except in cases when a stationary occlusion of the carrier artery is planned;
- an aneurysm with a wide neck (neck diameter more than 4 mm, dome/neck ratio < 2).

In cases of intravascular occlusion of aneurysms with a wide neck, various assisting techniques are used (intravascular stents, balloon assistance, the usc of flow-bending stents) (van Rooij 2012; Kim and Cha 2013).

Patients who, after endovascular treatment, have a residual filling of the cerebral aneurysm, need repeated endovascular intervention performed in the "cold" period, and if it is impossible or unsuccessful, an open operation aimed at completely turning off the aneurysm from the bloodstream (Gonzalez and Dusick 2010; Lobsien and Clajus 2021; Roh and Kim 2019).

Neurovegetative Stabilization

Neurovegetative stabilization in the intensive care program for cerebral vasospasm and acute cerebral injury due to aneurysmal rupture and massive SAH implies the creation of conditions for the absence of debilitating sympathicotonia and the implementation of long-term economical adaptation associated with the predominance of the parasympathetic tone of the autonomic nervous system (Savvina and Zabrodskaya 2021). It includes intravenous administration of the opioid analgesic fentanyl 0.5-1 mcg/kg / h, alpha-2 adrenoagonists (clonidine 0.2-0.7 mcg/kg/h or dexmedetomidine 0.2-0.5 mcg/kg/h), sodium thiopental 2-4 mg/kg/h (Kondratyev and Tsentsiper 2014).

In the diagnosis of cerebral vasospasm of II - III degree and PSH syndrome (Table 6) in patients with SAH, conservative treatment is carried out:

- Mild PSH syndrome (1 - 7 points) - pharmacotherapy: beta-blockers, phenytoin, NSAIDs; physical methods-therapeutic hypothermia.
- Moderate PSH syndrome (8 - 14 points) - pharmacotherapy: beta-blockers, phenytoin, alpha-2 adrenoagonist, NSAIDs; physical methods-therapeutic hypothermia.
- Severe PSH syndrome (14 - 21 b) - neurovegetative stabilization (opioid analgesic, alpha-2aadrenoagonist, hypnotics); physical methods - therapeutic hypothermia (craniocerebral hypothermia).

The duration of therapy is determined individually, after a repeated assessment of the patient's condition.

Therapeutic Hypothermia

Apply physical cooling methods to maintain normothermia: craniocerebral hypothermia, which consists in lowering the temperature of the scalp to 5-8° with the help of helmets cooled by circulating fluid, to maintain the skin temperature at a constant level during the entire cooling session. The cooling duration is from 12 hours to 7 days, with an increase in temperature after the cooling is stopped repeat the procedure, carry out until a stable normothermia is achieved, and do not allow the body temperature to drop below 35.5°C; it is permissible to use other cooling methods to maintain normothermia (Shevelev and Grechko 2019).

Multimodal Analgesia

Intense headache after SAH is usually 8,0±1,9 points according to VAS (Bayalieva and Shpaner 2017). Several authors demonstrated that the intensity of headache depends on the amount of blood in the subarachnoid space according to CT data (Bayalieva and Shpaner 2017). Multimodal analgesia without excessive oppression of consciousness is achieved with gabapentin and $NSAID_s$ to prevent irritation of the meninges and nociceptive stimulation from the bloodshed (Bayalieva and Shpaner 2017). Gabapentin together with transdermal fentanyl leads to depression of consciousness (2 points on the Richmond scale) (Bayalieva and Shpaner 2017).

Vasospasm is more pronounced on the side of the aneurysm and in the vessels carrying the aneurysm. All patients must receive infusion therapy with the calcium channel blocker nimodipine (60 mg every 4 hours). As the degree and prevalence of vasospasm increases, the outcomes worsen, but this does not reach a significant degree, since the cause of fatal and unsatisfactory outcomes in patients with ICH is mainly the volume effect of hematoma, edema, and dislocation of the brain.

Correction of Intracranial Hypertension and Brain Swelling

Treatment to decrease the ICP includes maintaining a head-up position (15 - 30^0) and augmenting hyperventilation ($PaCO_2$ of 25 - 30 mmHg) during a short period (5 - 15 minutes).

Barbiturates, which suppress cerebral metabolism and reduce cerebral blood flow, can also be used to decrease the ICP. Thiopental, a 5 mg/kg bolus infusion followed by a 3-5 mg/kg continuous infusion, maybe a conventional prescription. Mannitol (0, 5 - 1, 0 g/kg), an osmotic diuretic, reduces cerebral volume beginning 5 - 10 min after infusion. Rapid administration or large doses of mannitol cause several side effects, including hypotension, hyponatremia, and hyperosmotic serum. Furosemide (0,5-1,0 mg/kg), a diuretic metabolism and reduce cerebral blood flow, can also be used to decrease the ICP.

Neurovegetative stabilization is the main treatment strategy for patients with intracranial hypertension, edema of the brain, and dislocation syndrome. Alpha2-adrenoagonists (clonidine or dexmedetomidine continuous infusion 0, 2 - 1, 0 mcg/kg/h) are very important to support the mechanisms of autoregulation of cerebral blood flow under the condition of a decrease in cerebral perfusion pressure by targeting the central adrenergic structures of the brainstem and in particular locus coeruleus.

Conclusion

SAH is a dangerous complication of the rupture of a cerebral aneurysm which is associated with high mortality and disability. However, the vascular catastrophe may resolve with the return of the patient to a full-fledged social life if early diagnosis and timely treatment including modern approaches based on pathophysiological knowledge will be applied. This chapter is devoted to the description of these clinically relevant and important features of supervision of patients with aneurysmal SAH.

Acknowledgments

This chapter is devoted to the memory of the Pioneer of Endovascular Neurosurgery; Professor Yuriy N. Zubkov worked in the Russian Polenov Scientific Research Neurosurgical Institute in Saint Petersburg, Russia, and the University of Mississippi Medical Center of Jackson, the U. S. A. in 1990-1997 yy.

References

Abbed KM, Ogilvy CS., 2003 "Intracerebral hematoma from aneurysm rupture." *Neurosurg Focus*. Oct 15;15(4): E4. doi: 10.3171/foc.2003.15.4.4.

Abla AA, Wilson DA, Williamson RW, Nakaji P, McDougall CG, Zabramski JM, Albuquerque FC, Spetzler RF., 2014 "The relationship between ruptured aneurysm location, subarachnoid hemorrhage clot thickness, and incidence of radiographic or symptomatic vasospasm in patients enrolled in a prospective randomized controlled trial." *J Neurosurg*. Feb;120(2):391-7.

Adams HP, Jergenson DD, Kassell NF, Sahs AL., 1980 "Pitfalls in the recognition of subarachnoid hemorrhage." *JAMA*. 244:794–6.

Ahmed KA, Madhavan M, Prasad A, 2012 "Brain natriuretic peptide in apical ballooning syndrome (Takitsubo/stress cardiomyopathy): comparison with acute myocardial infarction." *Coron Artery Dis*. 23:259-64.

Alotaibi NM, Elkarim GA, Samuel N, Ayling OGS, Guha D, Fallah A, Aldakkan A, Jaja BNR, de Oliveira Manoel AL, Ibrahim GM, Macdonald RL., 2017 "Effects of decompressive craniectomy on functional outcomes and death in poor-grade aneurysmal subarachnoid hemorrhage: a systematic review and meta-analysis." *J Neurosurg*. Dec;127(6):1315-1325.

Anagnostopoulos C, Chamilos C, Hadjigeorgiou GF, Petsanas A., 2019 "Isolated massive intraventricular haemorrhage without subarachnoid haemorrhage due to rupture of a posterior communicating artery aneurysm." *Br J Neurosurg*. Oct;33(5):597-598.

Arboix A, García-Eroles L, Vicens A, Oliveres M, Massons J., 2012 "Spontaneous primary intraventricular hemorrhage: clinical features and early outcome." *ISRN Neurol*. 498303. doi: 10.5402/2012/498303.

Baker HL Jr, Campbell JK, Houser OW, Reese DF, Sheedy PF, Holman CB., 1974 "Computer-assisted tomography of the head. An early evaluation." *Mayo Clin Proc*. Jan;49(1):17-27.

Bayalieva AZh, Shpaner RYa, Ganeeva IR, Nasunov SYu, 2017 " Looking for optimal treatment of headache at non-traumatic subarachnoid hemorrhage." *Anesthesiology and Reanimatology [In Russ.]*.62(2):149-152.

Bing Z, Rabinstein AA, Murad MH, Lanzino G, Panni P, Brinjikji W., 2015 "Surgical and endovascular treatment of poor-grade aneurysmal subarachnoid hemorrhage: a systematic review and meta-analysis." *J NeurosurgSci*.

Black PM., 1986 "Hydrocephalus and vasospasm after subarachnoid hemorrhage from ruptured intracranial aneurysms." *Neurosurgery*. 18:12–6.

Bohm E, Hugosson R., 1978 "Experiences of surgical treatment of 400 consecutive ruptured cerebral arterial aneurysms." *Acta Neurochir* 40:33–43.

Bohnstedt BN, Nguyen HS, Kulwin CG, Shoja MM, Helbig GM, Leipzig TJ, Payner TD, Cohen-Gadol AA., 2013 "Outcomes for clip ligation and hematoma evacuation associated with 102 patients with ruptured middle cerebral artery aneurysms. *World Neurosurg*. Sep-Oct;80(3-4):335-41. doi: 10.1016/j.wneu.2012.03.008.

Borges G, Facure NO, Facure JJ., 1987. "KlinischeWechselbeziehung der Gefässspasmen in der Chirurgie der Aneurysmen" [Clinical correlations of vascular spasms in the surgery of aneurysms]. *ZentralblNeurochir*. 48(3):219-21. German.

Boullin DJ, Tagari P, du Boulay G, Aitken V, Hughes JT., 1983 "The role of hemoglobin in the etiology of cerebral vasospasm. An in vivo study of baboons." *J Neurosurg.* Aug;59(2):231-6.

Brambrink AM, Dick WF, 1997 " Neurogenic pulmonary edema. Pathogenesis, clinical picture and therapy." *Anaesthesist.* 46:953-63.

Bratton SL, Chestnut RM, Ghajar J, McConnell Hammond FF, Harris OA, Hartl R, Manley GT, Nemecek A, Newell DW, Rosenthal G, Schouten J, Shutter L, Timmons SD, Ullman JS, Videtta W, Wilberger JE, Wright DW., 2007 "Brain Trauma Foundation; American Association of Neurological Surgeons; Congress of Neurological Surgeons; Joint Section on Neurotrauma and Critical Care, AANS/CNS, Guidelines for the management of severe traumatic brain injury. VII. Intracranial pressure monitoring technology." *J Neurotrauma.* 24 Suppl 1:S45-54.

Brian M. Howard, Ranliang Hu, Jack W., 2019. "Barrow and Daniel L. Comprehensive review of imaging of intracranial aneurysms and angiographically negative subarachnoid hemorrhage." *Neurosurg Focus.* 47 (6): E20. doi:10.3171/2019.9. FOCUS19653.

Broderick JP, Brott TG, Duldner JE, Tomsick T, Leach A., 1994 "Initial and recurrent bleeding are the major causes of death following subarachnoid hemorrhage." *Stroke.* 25:1342-7.

Bu Y, Chen M, Gao T, Wang X, Li X, Gao F., 2016 "Mechanisms of hydrocephalus after intraventricular haemorrhage in adults." *Stroke Vasc Neurol.* Feb 16;1(1):23-27.

Buschmann U, Yonekawa Y, Fortunati M, Cesnulis E, Keller E., 2007 "Decompressive hemicraniectomy in patients with subarachnoid hemorrhage and intractable intracranial hypertension." *Acta Neurochir* (Wien). Jan;149(1):59-65.

Butzkueven H, Evans AH, Pitman A, Leopold C, Jolley DJ, Kaye AH, Kilpatrick CJ, Davis SM., 2000 "Onset seizures independently predict poor outcome after subarachnoid hemorrhage." *Neurology.* Nov 14;55(9):1315-20. doi: 10.1212/wnl.55.9.1315.

Cagnazzo F, Gambacciani C, Morganti R, Perrini P., 2017 "Aneurysm rebleeding after placement of external ventricular drainage: a systematic review and meta-analysis." *Acta Neurochir (Wien).* Apr;159(4):695-704.

Can A, Du R., 2016 "Association of Hemodynamic Factors With Intracranial Aneurysm Formation and Rupture: Systematic Review and Meta-analysis." *Neurosurgery.* 78(4):510-520.

Carpenter CR, Hussain AM, Ward MJ, Zipfel GJ, Fowler S, Pines JM, Sivilotti ML., 2016. "Spontaneous Subarachnoid Hemorrhage: A Systematic Review and Meta-analysis Describing the Diagnostic Accuracy of History, Physical Examination, Imaging, and Lumbar Puncture With an Exploration of Test Thresholds." *Acad Emerg Med.* Sep;23(9):963-1003.

Chan BS, Dorsch NW, 1991. "Delayed diagnosis in subarachnoid haemorrhage." *Med J Aust.* 154:509–11.

Chatterjee S., 2011 "ECG changes in subarachnoid haemorrhage: a synopsis." *Neth Heart J* 19(1):31–4.

Chen S, Feng H, Sherchan P, Klebe D, Zhao G, Sun X, Zhang J, Tang J, Zhang JH, 2014. "Controversies and evolving new mechanisms in subarachnoid hemorrhage." *Prog Neurobiol.* Apr;115:64-91.

Chung DY, Leslie-Mazwi TM, Patel AB, Rordorf GA., 2017 "Management of External Ventricular Drains After Subarachnoid Hemorrhage: A Multi-Institutional Survey." *Neurocrit Care.* Jun;26(3):356-361.

Chung DY, Mayer SA, Rordorf GA., 2018 "External Ventricular Drains After Subarachnoid Hemorrhage: Is Less More?" *Neurocrit Care.* Apr;28(2):157-161.

Chung DY, Olson DM, John S, Mohamed W, Kumar MA, Thompson BB, Rordorf GA., 2019 "Evidence-Based Management of External Ventricular Drains." *Curr Neurol Neurosci Rep.* Nov 26;19(12):94.

Colombi M, Dordoni C, Chiarelli N, Ritelli M. 2015. "Differential diagnosis and diagnostic flow chart of joint hypermobility syndrome/Ehlers-Danlos syndrome hypermobility type compared to other heritable connective tissue disorders." *Am J Med Genet Part* C, 169C:6–22.

Compton E. Syndrome Of Paroxysmal Sympathetic Hyperactivity After Traumatic brain injury. *Nurses Clin North Am.* 2018 September;53(3):459-467. doi: 10.1016/j. cnur. 2018. 05. 003.

Connolly ES Jr, Rabinstein AA, Carhuapoma JR, Derdeyn CP, Dion J, Higashida RT, Hoh BL, Kirkness CJ, Naidech AM, Ogilvy CS, Patel AB, Thompson BG, Vespa P., 2012 "American Heart Association Stroke Council; Council on Cardiovascular Radiology and Intervention; Council on Cardiovascular Nursing; Council on Cardiovascular Surgery and Anesthesia; Council on Clinical Cardiology. Guidelines for the management of aneurysmal subarachnoid hemorrhage: a guideline for healthcare professionals from the American Heart Association/American Stroke Association." *Stroke.* Jun;43(6):1711-37.

Conway JE, Tamargo RJ., 2001 "Cocaine use is an independent risk factor for cerebral vasospasm after aneurysmal subarachnoid hemorrhage." *Stroke.* Oct;32(10):2338-43.

Cooper DJ, Rosenfeld JV, Murray L, Arabi YM, Davies AR, D'Urso P, Kossmann T, Ponsford J, Seppelt I, Reilly P, Wolfe R., 2011 "DECRA Trial Investigators; Australian and New Zealand Intensive Care Society Clinical Trials Group. Decompressive craniectomy in diffuse traumatic brain injury." *N Engl J Med.* Apr 21;364(16):1493-502.

Creissard P, Freger P, Houtteville JP, Toumi K, Baumgartner J, Plas JY, Guy G, Mercier P, Massini B, Fischer G., 1985 "L'opérationprécoce des anévrysmesrompus. Un facteur de prévention de l'ischémie" [Early surgery of ruptured aneurysms. A factor in preventing ischemia]. *Neurochirurgie.* 31(4):251-4. French.

Darkwah Oppong M, Skowronek V, Pierscianek D, Gembruch O, Herten A, Saban DV, Dammann P, Forsting M, Sure U, Jabbarli R., 2018 "Aneurysmal intracerebral hematoma: Risk factors and surgical treatment decisions." *Clin Neurol Neurosurg.* Oct;173:1-7.

Dashyan VG, Levchenko OV, Hayrapetyan AA, Lukyanchikov VA, Tokarev AS, Shatokhin TA, Kalinkin AA, Sharifulin FA, Krylov VV, 2015 "Decompressive craniotomy in surgery of ruptured brain aneurysms." *The Russian Neurosurgical Journal named after prof. A.L. Polenov.* 4:17-24205.

Davison DL, Terek M, Chawla LS., 2012 "Neurogenic pulmonary edema." *Crit Care.* 16:212.

de Rooij N, Greving J, Rinkel G, Frijins CJ., 2013 "Early prediction of delayed cerebral ischemia after subarachnoid hemorrhage: development and validation of a practical risk chart." *Stroke.* 44(5):1288-94.

de Rooij N, Rinkel G, Danbaar J, Frijins CJ., 2013 "Delayed cerebral ischemia after subarachnoid hemorrhage: a systematic review of clinical, laboratory, and radiological predictors." *Stroke.* 44:43-54.

de Rooij NK, Linn FH, van der Plas JA, Algra A, Rinkel GJ., 2007 "Incidence of subarachnoid haemorrhage: a systematic review with emphasis on region, age, gender and time trends." *J Neurol Neurosurg Psychiatry.* 2007 Dec;78(12):1365-72.

Del Bigio MR., 1993 "Neuropathological changes caused by hydrocephalus." *Acta Neuropathol* 85:573–85.

Della Pepa GM, Scerrati A, Albanese A, Marchese E, Maira G, Sabatino G., 2014 "Protective effect of external ventricular drainage on cerebral vasospasm. A retrospective study on aneurysmal SAH treated endovascularly." *Clin Neurol Neurosurg.* Sep;124:97-101.

Dereeper E, Berré J, Vandesteene A, Lefranc F, Vincent JL., 2002 "Barbiturate coma for intracranial hypertension: clinical observations." *J Crit Care.* Mar;17(1):58-62.

Diaz FG, Ohaegbulam S, Dujovny M, Ausman JI., 1989 "Surgical alternatives in the treatment of cavernous sinus aneurysms." *J Neurosurg.* Dec;71(6):846-53.

Dorfer C, Frick A, Knosp E, Gruber A., 2010 "Decompressive hemicraniectomy after aneurysmal subarachnoid hemorrhage." *World Neurosurg.* Oct-Nov;74(4-5):465-71. doi: 10.1016/j.wneu.2010.08.001.

Dorsch NWC, King MT., 1994 "A review of cerebral vasospasm in aneurysmal subarachnoid haemorrhage: I. Incidence and effects." *J Clin Neurosci.* 1:19-26.

Drake CG., 1988 "Report of the world federation of neurological surgeons committee on a universal subarachnoid hemorrhage grading scale. *J Neurosurg* 68:985-986.

Ducros A, Bousser MG., 2013 "Thunderclap headache." *BMJ* 346:e8557.

Dumont AS, Dumont RJ, Chow MM, Lin CL, Calisaneller T, Ley KF, Kassell NF, Lee KS., 2003 "Cerebral vasospasm after subarachnoid hemorrhage: putative role of inflammation." *Neurosurgery.* Jul;53(1):123-33; discussion 133-5.

Dupont S, Rabinstein AA., 2013 "Extent of acute hydrocephalus after subarachnoid hemorrhage as a risk factor for poor functional outcome." *Neurol Res.* Mar;35(2):107-10.

Edlow JA, Caplan LR., 2000 "Avoiding pitfalls in the diagnosis of subarachnoid hemorrhage." *N Engl J Med.* 342:29–36.

Edlow JA, Malek AM, Ogilvy CS., 2008 "Aneurysmal subarachnoid hemorrhage: update for emergency physicians."*J Emerg Med* 34(3):237–251.

Eliava, Shalva Sh. 2019. *Surgical treatment of brain aneurysms in the acute period of hemorrhage.* Moscow: Publishing house individual enterpreneur Alekseeva.

Fergusen S, MacDonald RL., 2007 "Predictors of cerebral infarction in patients with aneurysmal subarachnoid hemorrhage." *Neurosurgery.* 60:658-67.

Findlay JM, Nisar J, Darsaut T., 2016 "Cerebral Vasospasm: A Review." *Can J Neurol Sci.* Jan;43(1):15-32.

Fine B, Singh N, Aviv R, Macdonald RL., 2012 "Decisions: does a patient with a thunderclap headache need a lumbar puncture?" *CMAJ.* Mar 20;184(5):555-6.

Fisher CM, Ojemann RG., 1994 "Bilateral decompressive craniectomy for worsening coma in acute subarachnoid hemorrhage. Observations in support of the procedure." *Surg Neurol.* Jan;41(1):65-74.

Fisher CM, Roberson GH, Ojemann RG., 1977 "Cerebral vasospasm with ruptured saccular aneurysm—the clinical manifestations." *Neurosurgery.* 1:245-58.

Foley PL, Takenaka K, Kassell NF, Lee KS., 1994 "Cytotoxic effects of bloody cerebrospinal fluid on cerebral endothelial cells in culture." *J Neurosurg.* 81:87-92.

Fountas KN, Kapsalaki EZ, Machinis T, Karampelas I, Smisson HF, Robinson JS., 2006 "Review of the literature regarding the relationship of rebleeding and external ventricular drainage in patients with subarachnoid hemorrhage of aneurysmal origin." *Neurosurg Rev* 29:14–18; discussion 9–20.

Fridriksson S, Hillman J, Landtblom AM, Boive J., 2001 "Education of referring doctors about sudden onset headache in subarachnoid hemorrhage: a prospective study." *Acta Neurol Scand.* 103: 238–42.

Friedman JA, Goerss SJ, Meyer FB, Piepgras DG, Pichelmann MA, McIver JI, Toussaint LG 3rd, McClelland RL, Nichols DA, Atkinson JL, Wijdicks EF., 2002 "Volumetric quantification of Fisher Grade 3 aneurysmal subarachnoid hemorrhage: a novel method to predict symptomatic vasospasm on admission computerized tomography scans." *J Neurosurg.* Aug;97(2):401-7.

Frontera JA, Fernandez A, Schmidt JM, Claassen J, Wartenberg KE, Badjatia N, Connolly ES, Mayer SA., 2009 "Defining vasospasm after subarachnoid hemorrhage: what is the most clinically relevant definition?" *Stroke.* Jun;40(6):1963-8.

Fukuhara T, Shimizu T, Namba Y., 2009 "Limited efficacy of endoscopic third ventriculostomy for hydrocephalus following aneurysmal subarachnoid hemorrhage." *Neurol Med Chir (Tokyo).* Oct;49(10):449-55.

Gambardella G, De Blasi F, Caruso G, Zema A, Turiano F, Collufio D. Intracranial pressure, cerebral perfusion pressure, and SPECT in the management of patients with SAH Hunt and Hess grades I-II. *Acta Neurochir Suppl* 1998;71:215–218.

Germanwala AV, Huang J, Tamargo RJ., 2010 "Hydrocephalus after aneurysmal subarachnoid hemorrhage." *Neurosurg Clin N Am.* Apr;21(2):263-70.

Gigante P, Hwang BY, Appelboom G, Kellner CP, Kellner MA, Connolly ES., 2010 "External ventricular drainage following aneurysmal subarachnoid haemorrhage." *Br J Neurosurg.* 24:625–32.

Gilmore E, Choi HA, Hirsch LJ, Claassen J., 2010 "Seizures and CNS hemorrhage: spontaneous intracerebral and aneurysmal subarachnoid hemorrhage." *Neurologist.* May;16(3):165-75.

Giray S, Sen O, Sarica FB, Tufan K, Karatas M, Goksel BK, Yerdelen D, Cekinmez M, Can U., 2009 "Spontaneous primary intraventricular hemorrhage in adults: clinical data, etiology and outcome." *Turk Neurosurg.* Oct;19(4):338-44.

Glesby MJ, Pyeritz RE. 1989 "Association of mitral valve prolapse and systemic abnormalities of connective tissue: A phenotypic continuum." *JAMA*, 262:523–528.

Go AS, Mozaffarian D, Roger VL, Benjamin EJ, Berry JD, Blaha MJ, Dai S, Ford ES, Fox CS, Franco S, Fullerton HJ, Gillespie C, Hailpern SM, Heit JA, Howard VJ, Huffman MD, Judd SE, Kissela BM, Kittner SJ, Lackland DT, Lichtman JH, Lisabeth LD, Mackey RH, Magid DJ, Marcus GM, Marelli A, Matchar DB, McGuire DK, Mohler

ER 3rd, Moy CS, Mussolino ME, Neumar RW, Nichol G, Pandey DK, Paynter NP, Reeves MJ, Sorlie PD, Stein J, TowfighiA, Turan TN, Virani SS, Wong ND, Woo D, Turner MB, 2014. "American Heart Association Statistics Committee and Stroke Statistics Subcommittee. Heart disease and stroke statistics--2014 update: a report from the American Heart Association." *Circulation* Jan 21;129(3):e28-e292.

Gonzalez NR, Dusick JR, Duckwiler G, Tateshima S, Jahan R, Martin NA, Viñuela F., 2010 "Endovascular coiling of intracranial aneurysms in elderly patients: report of 205 treated aneurysms." *Neurosurgery.* Apr;66(4):714-20; discussion 720-1.

Gordon A, 1976 "Primary ventricular hemorrhage. Further contribution to a characteristic symptom group." *Arch Neurol Psychiatry.* 39: 1272-1276.

Gorelick PB, Hier DB, Caplan LR, Langenberg P., 1986 "Headache in acute cerebrovascular disease." *Neurology.* Nov;36(11):1445-50.

Goroshchenko SA, Ivanov AYu, Rozhchenko LV, 2016 "Extrapontine myelinosis developed after aneurysmal subarachnoid hemorrhage (case study and review of the literature)" *Problems of neurosurgery of N.N. Burdenko.* 80(6): 82-87.

Graeb DA, Robertson WD, Lapointe JS, Nugent RA, Harrison PB., 1982 "Computed tomographic diagnosis of intraventricular hemorrhage. Etiology and prognosis." *Radiology.* Apr;143(1):91-6.

Graff-Radford NR, Torner J, Adams HP Jr, Kassell NF., 1989 "Factors associated with hydrocephalus after subarachnoid hemorrhage. A report of the Cooperative Aneurysm Study." *Arch Neurol.* 46:744–52.

Grigorieva EV, Polunina NA, Lukyanchikov VA, Krylov VV, 2017 "Features of CT angiography and construction of 2-D and 3-D reconstructions of preoperative planning in patients with intracranial aneurysms." *Neurosurgery.* 3: 88-95.

Gross BA, Rosalind Lai PM, Frerichs KU, Du R., 2014 "Treatment modality and vasospasm after aneurysmal subarachnoid hemorrhage." *World Neurosurg.* Dec;82(6):e725-30. doi: 10.1016/j.wneu.2013.08.017.

Guimond JG, Chagnon PM, Bojanowski MW., 2012 "Clipping vs. coiling in acute aneurysmal subarachnoid haemorrhage: Should the patient's medical condition influence treatment modality?" *Neurochirurgie.* Apr-Jun;58(2-3):115-24. English, French.

Gupta R, Connolly ES, Mayer S, Elkind MS., 2004 "Hemicraniectomy for massive middle cerebral artery territory infarction: a systematic review." *Stroke.* Feb;35(2):539-43.

Güresir E, Schuss P, Seifert V, Vatter H., 2012 "Decompressive craniectomy in children: single-center series and systematic review." *Neurosurgery.* Apr;70(4):881-8; discussion 888-9.

Hansen-Schwartz J, Vajkoczy P, Macdonald RL, Pluta RM, Zhang JH., 2007 "Cerebral vasospasm: looking beyond vasoconstriction." *Trends Pharmacol Sci.* 28:252-6.

Harling DW, Peatfield RC, Van Hille PT, Abbott RJ., 1989 "Thunderclap headache: is it migraine?" *Cephalalgia.* Jun;9(2):87-90.

Harrod CG, Batjer HH, Bendok BR 2006 "Deficiencies in estrogen-mediated regulation of cerebrovascular homeostasis may contribute to an increased risk of cerebral aneurysm pathogenesis and rupture in menopausal and postmenopausal women." *Med Hypotheses.* 66(4):736–756.

Harrod CG, Bendok BR, Batjer HH., 2005 "Prediction of cerebral vasospasm in patients presenting with aneurysmal subarachnoid hemorrhage: a review." *Neurosurgery.* 56:633-54.

Hasan D, Lindsay KW, Vermeulen M., 1991 "Treatment of acute hydrocephalus after subarachnoid hemorrhage with serial lumbar puncture." *Stroke* 22:190–4.

Hasan D, Tanghe HL., 1992 "Distribution of cisternal blood in patients with acute hydrocephalus after subarachnoid hemorrhage." *Ann Neurol.* 1992;31:374–8.

Hasan D, van Peski J, Loeve I, Krenning EP, Vermeulen M., 1991 "Single photon emission computed tomography in patients with acute hydrocephalus or with cerebral ischemia after subarachnoid haemorrhage." *J Neurol Neurosurg Psychiatry.* Jun;54(6):490-3.

Hasan D, Vermeulen M, Wijdicks EF, Hijdra A, van Gijn J., 1989 "Management problems in acute hydrocephalus after subarachnoid hemorrhage." *Stroke.* 20:747–53.

Hassan A, Lanzino G, Wijdicks EF, Rabinstein AA, Flemming KD., 2011 "Terson's syndrome." *Neurocrit Care.* Dec;15(3):554-8.

Hayashi M, Kobayashi H, Kawano H, Yamamoto S, Maeda T., 1984 "Cerebral blood flow and ICP patterns in patients with communicating hydrocephalus after aneurysm rupture." *J Neurosurg.* Jul;61(1):30-6.

Hellingman CA, van den Bergh WM, Beijer IS, van Dijk GW, Algra A, van Gijn J, Rinkel GJ., 2007 "Risk of rebleeding after treatment of acute hydrocephalus in patients with aneurysmal subarachnoid hemorrhage." *Stroke.* Jan;38(1):96-9.

Hirashima Y, Kurimoto M, Hayashi N, Umemura K, Hori E, Origasa H, Endo S., 2005 "Duration of cerebrospinal fluid drainage in patients with aneurysmal subarachnoid hemorrhage for prevention of symptomatic vasospasm and late hydrocephalus." *Neurol Med Chir (Tokyo).* Apr;45(4):177-82; discussion 182-3.

Hitchcock E, Gibson WT. 2017 "A Review of the Genetics of Intracranial Berry Aneurysms and Implications for Genetic Counseling." *J Genet Couns.* 26(1):21-31.

Hitomi, T, Habu, T, Kobayashi, H, Okuda, H, Harada, KH, Osafune, K, Taura, D, Sone, M, Asaka, I, Ameku, T, Watanabe, A, Kasahara, T, Sudo, T, Shiota, F, Hashikata, H, Takagi, Y, Morito, D, Miyamoto, S, Nakao, K, & Koizumi, A. 2013 "Down-regulation of Securin by the variant RNF213 R4810K (rs112735431, G>A) reduces the angiogenic activity of induced pluripotent stem cell-derived vascular endothelial cells from moyamoya patients." *Biochem Biophys Res Commun.* 438:13–19.

Hofmeijer J, Kappelle LJ, Algra A, Amelink GJ, van Gijn J, van der Worp HB., 2009 "HAMLET investigators. Surgical decompression for space-occupying cerebral infarction (the Hemicraniectomy After Middle Cerebral Artery infarction with Life-threatening Edema Trial [HAMLET]): a multicentre, open, randomized trial." *Lancet Neurol.* Apr;8(4):326-33.

Hunt WE, Hess RM, 1968 " Surgical risk as related to the time of intervention in the repair of intracranial aneurysms. *J Neurosurg* 28:14-20.

Hutchinson PJ, Kolias AG, Timofeev IS, Corteen EA, Czosnyka M, Timothy J, Anderson I, Bulters DO, Belli A, Eynon CA, Wadley J, Mendelow AD, Mitchell PM, Wilson MH, Critchley G, Sahuquillo J, Unterberg A, Servadei F, Teasdale GM, Pickard JD, Menon DK, Murray GD, Kirkpatrick PJ., 2016 "RESCUEicp Trial Collaborators. Trial of Decompressive Craniectomy for Traumatic Intracranial Hypertension." *N Engl J Med.* Sep 22;375(12):1119-30.

Ibrahim G, Morgan B, Macdonald L., 2014 "Patient phenotypes associated with outcomes after aneurysmal subarachnoid hemorrhage." *Stroke.* 45:670-6001;32:2338-43.

Ibrahim GM, Macdonald RL., 2012 "Electrocardiographic changes predict angiographic vasospasm after aneurysmal subarachnoid hemorrhage." *Stroke.* 43:2102–2107.

Iuliano BA, Pluta RM, Jung C, Oldfield EH., 2004 "Endothelial dysfunction in a primate model of cerebral vasospasm." *J Neurosurg.* 100:287-94.

Jabbarli R, Reinhard M, Roelz R, Shah M, Niesen WD, Kaier K, Taschner C, Weyerbrock A, Van Velthoven V., 2016 "Intracerebral Hematoma Due to Aneurysm Rupture: Are There Risk Factors Beyond Aneurysm Location?" *Neurosurgery.* Jun;78(6):813-20.

Jabbarli R, Reinhard M, Roelz R, Shah M, Niesen WD, Kaier K, Taschner C, Weyerbrock A, Velthoven VV, 2016 "The predictors and clinical impact of intraventricular hemorrhage in patients with aneurysmal subarachnoid hemorrhage." *Int. J. Stroke* 11 68–76.

Jacobs L, Kinkel WR, Heffner RR Jr., 1976 "Autopsy correlations of computerized tomography: experience with 6000 CT scans." *Neurology (Minneap)* 26: 1111-1118.

Jain R, Deveikis J, Thompson BG., 2004 "Management of patients with stunned myocardium associated with subarachnoid hemorrhage." *Am J Neuroradiol.* 25:126–129.

Jeon, I-C., Chang, C-H., Choi, B-Y., Kim, M-S., Kim, S-W., & Kim, S-H. 2009. "Cardiac troponin 1 elevation in patients with aneurysmal subarachnoid hemorrhage." *J Korean NeurosurgSoc.* 46:99–102.

Johnson R, Potter JM, Reid RG., 1958 "Arterial spasm in subarachnoid haemorrhage: mechanical considerations." *J Neurol Neurosurg Psychiatr* 21.

Jomin M, Lesoin F, Lozes G., 1984 "Prognosis with 500 ruptured and operated intracranial arterial aneurysms." *Surg Neurol.* Jan;21(1):13-8.

Jüttler E, Schwab S, Schmiedek P, Unterberg A, Hennerici M, Woitzik J, Witte S, Jenetzky E, Hacke W, 2007 "DESTINY Study Group. Decompressive Surgery for the Treatment of Malignant Infarction of the Middle Cerebral Artery (DESTINY): a randomized, controlled trial." *Stroke.* Sep;38(9):2518-25.

Jüttler E, Unterberg A, Woitzik J, Bösel J, Amiri H, Sakowitz OW, Gondan M, Schiller P, Limprecht R, Luntz S, Schneider H, Pinzer T, Hobohm C, Meixensberger J, Hacke W, 2014 "DESTINY II Investigators. Hemicraniectomy in older patients with extensive middle-cerebral-artery stroke." *N Engl J Med.* Mar 20;370(12):1091-100.

Kadooka K, Hadeishi H, Kadooka K, 2017 " Delayed normalization of electrocardiograms in patients with takotsubo cardiomyopathy due to aneurismal subarachnoid hemorrhage. *World Neurosurg.*100: 467-73.

Kamezaki T, Yanaka K, Nagase S, Fujita K, Kato N, Nose T., 2002 "Increased levels of lipid peroxides as predictive of symptomatic vasospasm and poor outcome after aneurysmal subarachnoid hemorrhage." *J Neurosurg.* 97:1302-5.

Kassell NF, Kongable GL, Torner JC, Adams HP Jr, Mazuz H., 1985 "Delay in the referral of patients with ruptured aneurysms to neurosurgical attention." *Stroke.* 16:587–90.

Kassell NF, Tomer JC, Haley EC, Jr, Jane JA, Adams HP, Kongable GL., 1990 "The International Cooperative Study on the Timing of Aneurysm Surgery: I. Overall management results." *J Neurosurg.* 73:18-36.

Kassell NF, Torner JC, Jane JA, Haley EC Jr, Adams HP., 1990 "The International Cooperative Study on the Timing of Aneurysm Surgery. Part 2: Surgical results." *J Neurosurg.* Jul;73(1):37-47.

Kaye AH, Tagari PC, Teddy PJ, Adams CB, Blaso WP, Boullin DJ., 1984 "CSF smooth-muscle constrictor activity associated with cerebral vasospasm and mortality in SAH patients." *J Neurosurg.* May;60(5):927-34.

Killeen T, Wanke I, Mangiardi J, Cesnulis E., 2014 "Ruptured, fusiform, distal lenticular-striatal aneurysm causing intraventricular haemorrhage in a patient with antiphospholipid-negative Sneddon's syndrome." *Clin Neurol Neurosurg.* Jan;116:80-2.

Kim KH, Cha KC, Kim JS, Hong SC., 2013 "Endovascular coiling of middle cerebral artery aneurysms as an alternative to a surgical clipping." *J Clin Neurosci.* Apr;20(4):520-2.

Kim YI, Park SW, Nam TK, Park YS, Min BK, Hwang SN., 2008 "The effect of barbiturate coma therapy for the patients with severe intracranial hypertension: a 10-year experience." *J Korean Neurosurg Soc.* Sep;44(3):141-5.

Klimo Jr. P, Kestle JR, MacDonald JD, Schmidt RH., 2004 "Marked reduction of cerebral vasospasm with lumbar drainage of cerebrospinal fluid after subarachnoid hemorrhage." *J Neurosurg* 100:215–24.

Koide M, Nishizawa S, Ohta S, Yokoyama T, Namba H., 2002 "Chronological changes of the contractile mechanism in prolonged vasospasm after subarachnoid hemorrhage: from protein kinase C to protein tyrosine kinase." *Neurosurgery.* 51:1468-76.

Kondratyev AN, Tsentsiper LM, Kondratyeva EA, Nazarov RV. 2014 " Neurovegetative stabilization as a pathogenetic therapy of brain injury." *Anesthesiology and reanimatology [In Russ.].* 1: 82-84.

Kongable GL, Lanzino G, Germanson TP, Truskowski LL, Alves WM, Torner JC, Kassell NF., 1996 "Gender-related differences in aneurysmal subarachnoid hemorrhage." *J Neurosurg.* Jan;84(1):43-8.

Kono T, Morita H, Kuroiwa T, Onaka H, Takatsuka H, Fujiwara A., 1994 "Left ventricular wall motion abnormalities in patients with subarachnoid hemorrhage: neurogenic stunned myocardium." *J Am Coll Cardiol.* Sep;24(3):636-40.

Konovalov AN. 1973. *Surgical treatment of arterial aneurysms of the brain.* Moscow: Medicine.

Konovalov AN, Belousova OB, Pilipenko YuV, Eliava ShSh, 2016 "Decompressive trepanation of the skull in patients with intracranial hemorrhage of aneurysmal genesis." *Journal "Questions of Neurosurgery" named after N.N. Burdenko.* 80(5):144-150.

Konovalov AN, Krylov VV, Filatov YuM, 2006 "Recommendation Protocol of management of patients with subarachnoid hemorrhage due to rupture of aneurysms of cerebral vessels" *Problems of neurosurgery of N.N. Burdenko.* 3: 3-10.

Konovalov AN, Krylov VV, Filatov YuM, Eliava ShSh, Belousova BB, Tkachev VV, Parfyenov VE, et al. 2012. «Treatment of patients with subarachnoid hemorrhage due to rupture of cerebral aneurysms». *Clinical recommendations of Association of Neurosurgeons of Russian Federation. www.ruans.org*

Konstantinos Lampropoulos, Evangelos Giannoulis, George Bazoukis, Gary Tse, Epameinondas Triantafyllou, and Athanasios Triantafyllou, 2017 "Reversible stress cardiomyopathy secondary to aneurismal subarachnoid hemorrhage: a case report." *The Journal of Emergency Medicine.* P.1-3 http://dx.doi.org/10.1016/j.jemermed. 2017.08.034.

Kowalski RG, Claassen J, Kreiter KT, Bates JE, Ostapkovich ND, Connolly ES, Mayer SA., 2004 "Initial misdiagnosis and outcome after subarachnoid hemorrhage." *JAMA.* Feb 18;291(7):866-9.

Krylov, Vladimir V., and Burov S. A. 2009. *Puncture aspiration and local fibrinolysis in surgery of intracranial hemorrhages.* Moscow: Partnership of scientific publications KMK and Author's Academy.

Krylov, Vladimir V., and Dashyan V. G. 2014. *Endoscopic surgery of hemorrhagic stroke.* Moscow: Publishing house «Knowledge».

Krylov VV, Petrikov SS, Solodov AA, Talypov AE, Puras YuV, Khamidova LT, KutrovskayaNYu, 2012 "Intracranial hypertension in patients with intracranial hemorrhages. Diagnosis and treatment." *N.V. Sklifosovsky Journal Emergency Medical Care.* 4:44-50.

Krylov VV, Dashyan VG, Danilov VA, Godkov IM. 2016. «Surgical treatment of hypertensive intracerebral hematomas (Clinical recommendations)». *Neurological Journal* 3:146-151.

Kurana VG, Wijdicks EF, Heublein DM, 2004 "A pilot study of Dendroaspis natriuretic peptide in aneurismal subarachnoid hemorrhage." *Neurosurgery* 55:75-76.

Kusske JA, Turner PT, Ojemann GA, Harris AB., 1973 "Ventriculostomy for the treatment of acute hydrocephalus following subarachnoid hemorrhage." *J Neurosurg* 38:591–595.

Landtblom AM, Fridriksson S, Boivie J, Hillman J, Johansson G, Johansson I., 2002 "Sudden onset headache: a prospective study of features, incidence and causes." *Cephalalgia.* Jun;22(5):354-60.

Lanzino G, Kassell NF, Germanson TP, Kongable GL, Truskowski LL, Torner JC, Jane JA., 1996 "Age and outcome after aneurysmal subarachnoid hemorrhage: why do older patients fare worse?" *J Neurosurg.* Sep;85(3):410-8.

Lawton MT, Vates GE., 2017 "Subarachnoid hemorrhage." *N Engl J Med* 377(3):257–266. doi:10.1056/NEJMcp1605827.

Lebedev, Vyacheslav V., and Krylov V. V. 1996. *Clinic, diagnosis and treatment of intracranial arterial aneurysms in the acute period of hemorrhage.* Moscow: Antidor.

Lee VH, Oh JK, Mulvagh SL, Wijdicks EF., 2006 "Mechanisms in neurogenic stress cardiomyopathy after aneurismal subarachnoid hemorrhage." *Neurocrit. Care.*5:243-9.

Lee, S, Kim, I-K., Ahn, JS, Woo, D-C, Kim, S-T, Song, S, Koh, GY, Kim, H-S, Jeon, BH, & Kim, I.2015 "Deficiency of endothelium-specific transcription factor Sox17 induces intracranial aneurysm." *Circulation,* 131(11):995-1005.

Linn FH, Rinkel GJ, Algra A, van Gijn J., 1998 "Headache characteristics in subarachnoid haemorrhage and benign thunderclap headache." *J Neurol Neurosurg Psychiatry.* Nov;65(5):791-3.

Linn FH, Wijdicks EF, van der Graaf Y, Weerdesteyn-van Vliet FA, Bartelds AI, van Gijn J., 1994 "Prospective study of sentinel headache in aneurysmal subarachnoid haemorrhage." *Lancet.* Aug 27;344(8922):590-3.

Liu X, Rinkel GJ., 2011 "Aneurysmal and clinical characteristics as risk factors for intracerebral haematoma from aneurysmal rupture." *J Neurol.* May;258(5):862-5.

Lobsien D, Clajus C, Behme D, Ernst M, Riedel CH, Abu-Fares O, Götz FG, Fiorella D, Klisch J., 2021 "Aneurysm Treatment in Acute SAH with Hydrophilic-Coated Flow Diverters under Single-Antiplatelet Therapy: A 3-Center Experience." *AJNR Am J Neuroradiol.* Mar;42(3):508-515. doi: 10.3174/ajnr.A6942.

Longstreth WT Jr, Koepsell TD, Yerby MS, van Belle G., 1985 "Risk factors for subarachnoid hemorrhage." *Stroke.* May-Jun;16(3):377-85.

Low SK, Takahashi A, Cha PC, Zembutsu H, Kamatani N, Kubo M etal.2012. "Genome-wide association study for intracranial aneurysm in the Japanese population identifies three candidate susceptible loci and a functional genetic variant at EDNRA." *Hum. Mol. Genet.* 21 (9): 2102-2110.

Lozier AP, Sciacca RR, Romagnoli MF, Connolly ES, Jr., 2002 "Ventriculostomy-related infections: a critical review of the literature." *Neurosurgery.* 51:170–181; discussion 81–82.

Lu J, Ji N, Yang Z, Zhao X., 2012 "Prognosis and treatment of acute hydrocephalus following aneurysmal subarachnoid haemorrhage." *J Clin Neurosci.* May;19(5):669-72.

Lu J, Ji N, Yang Z, Zhao X., 2012 "Prognosis and treatment of acute hydrocephalus following aneurysmal subarachnoid haemorrhage." *J Clin Neurosci.* May;19(5):669-72.

MacDonald RL, Weir B., 2004 *Perioperative management of subarachnoid hemorrhage.* In: *Youmans Neurological Surgery,* vol. 2. 5th edition, p. 1.

Macdonald RL., 2007 "Lumbar drainage after subarachnoid hemorrhage: does it reduce vasospasm and delayed hydrocephalus?" *Neurocrit Care* 7:1–2.

Macdonald RL., 2014 "Delayed neurological deterioration after subarachnoid haemorrhage." *Nat Rev Neurol* 10:44–58.

MacGirt MJ, Mavropoulos JC, McGirt LY, 2003 " Leukocytosis as an independent risk factor for cerebral vasospasm following aneurismal subarachnoid hemorrhage." *J Neurosurg.* 98:1222-1226.

Mack WJ, Ducruet AF, Hickman ZL, Garrett MC, Albert EJ, Kellner CP, Mocco J, Connolly ES Jr., 2007 "Early plasma complement C3a levels correlate with functional outcome after aneurysmal subarachnoid hemorrhage." *Neurosurgery.* Aug;61(2):255-60; discussion 260-1.

Mack WJ, King RG, Ducruet AF, Kreiter K, Mocco J, Maghoub A, Mayer S, Connolly ES Jr., 2003 "Intracranial pressure following aneurysmal subarachnoid hemorrhage: monitoring practices and outcome data." *Neurosurg Focus.* Apr 15;14(4):e3.

Malik AN, Gross BA, Rosalind Lai PM, Moses ZB, Du R., 2015 "Neurogenic stress cardiomyopathy after aneurismal subarachnoid hemorrhage." *World Neurosurg.* 83:880-5.

Marcolini E, Hine J, 2019 "Approach to the diagnosis and management of subarachnoid hemorrhage." *West J Emerg Med.* 20 (2): 203-211.

Mashaly HA, Provencio JJ., 2008 "Inflammation as a link between brain injury and heart damage: the model of subarachnoid hemorrhage." *Cleve Clin J Med.* 75(suppl 2):S26–S30.

Mayer PL, Awad IA, Todor R, Harbaugh K, Varnavas G, Lansen TA, Dickey P, Harbaugh R, Hopkins LN., 1996 "Misdiagnosis of symptomatic cerebral aneurysm. Prevalence and correlation with outcome at four institutions." *Stroke*. Sep;27(9):1558-63.

Mayer SA, Fink ME, Homma S, Sherman D, LiMandri G, Lennihan L, Solomon RA, Klebanoff LM, Beckford A, Raps EC., 1994 "Cardiac injury associated with neurogenic pulmonary edema following subarachnoid hemorrhage." *Neurology*. May;44(5):815-20.

McDonald JV., 1962 "Midline hematomas simulating tumors of the third ventricle." *Neurology (Minneap)*. 12: 805-809.

McIver JI, Friedman JA, Wijdicks EF, Piepgras DG, Pichelmann MA, Toussaint LG 3rd, McClelland RL, Nichols DA, Atkinson JL., 2002 "Preoperative ventriculostomy and rebleeding after aneurysmal subarachnoid hemorrhage." *J Neurosurg*. Nov;97(5):1042-4.

Medvedev YuA, 1993 "Aneurysm-bearing and aneurysmal brain disease." *Arch. Pathol.* 4: 7–10.

Medvedev YuA, Bersnev VP, Zabrodskaya YuM., 1998 "About segmental structure of the arterial circle of the brain, junctures in it and previously unknown disease of these junctures." *Neurosurg.*, 2:9-17.

Medvedev YuA, Panuntsov VS, Razmologova OYu, Zabrodskaya YuM, Sivtsova EV, 2012 "Bifurcation aneurysms (diverticulae) of the Willian circle joints and clinical and morphological variants of brain aneurysmal disease." *Polenov Russian Neurosurg. J.* 1: 22-28.

Medvedev YuA, Zabrodskaya YuM. 2000 *A new concept of the origin of bifurcation aneurysms of the arteries of the base of the brain.*- Saint Petersburg: Aeskulap.

Medvedev YuA, Zabrodskaya YuM, RazmologovaOYu, Sivtsova EV. 2012 "Bifurcation diverticulae ("aneurysms") of vascular junctures of the arterial circle of the brain." *Arch. Pathol.* 1: 59–62.

Medvedev, YuA, Zakaryavichus Zh., 2002 "Refractoriness of posthemorrhagic constrictive-stenotic arteriopathy to vasodilation drug therapy (morphological aspects)." *Neurosurgery*. No. 2., pp. 16-22.

Megyesi JF, Vollrath B, Cook DA, Chen MH, Findlay JM., 1999 "Long-term effects of in vivo angioplasty in normal and vasospastic canine carotid arteries: pharmacological and morphological analyses." *J Neurosurg*. 91:100-8.

Mehta V, Holness RO, Connolly K, Walling S, Hall R.,1996 "Acute hydrocephalus following aneurysmal subarachnoid hemorrhage." *Can J Neurol Sci.* Feb;23(1):40-5.

Menon D, Weir B, Overton T., 1981 "Ventricular size and cerebral blood flow following subarachnoid hemorrhage." *J Comput Assist Tomogr* 5:328–33.

Mitchell P, Kerr R, Mendelow AD, Molyneux A., 2008 "Could late rebleeding overturn the superiority of cranial aneurysm coil embolization over clip ligation seen in the International Subarachnoid Aneurysm Trial?" *J Neurosurg*. Mar;108(3):437-42.

Mocco J, Mack WJ, Kim GH, Lozier AP, Laufer I, Kreiter KT, Sciacca RR, Solomon RA, Mayer SA, Connolly ES Jr., 2002 "Rise in serum soluble intercellular adhesion molecule-1 levels with vasospasm following aneurysmal subarachnoid hemorrhage." *J Neurosurg*. Sep;97(3):537-41.

Mocco J, Ransom ER, Komotar RJ, Mack WJ, Sergot PB, Albert SM, Connolly ES Jr., 2006 "Racial differences in cerebral vasospasm: a systematic review of the literature." *Neurosurgery.* Feb;58(2):305-14.

Molyneux A, Kerr R, Stratton I, Sandercock P, Clarke M, Shrimpton J, Holman R., 2002 "International Subarachnoid Aneurysm Trial (ISAT) Collaborative Group. International Subarachnoid Aneurysm Trial (ISAT) of neurosurgical clipping versus endovascular coiling in 2143 patients with ruptured intracranial aneurysms: a randomized trial." *Lancet.* Oct 26;360(9342):1267-74.

Molyneux AJ, Kerr RS, Yu LM, Clarke M, Sneade M, Yarnold JA, Sandercock P., 2005 "International Subarachnoid Aneurysm Trial (ISAT) Collaborative Group. International subarachnoid aneurysm trial (ISAT) of neurosurgical clipping versus endovascular coiling in 2143 patients with ruptured intracranial aneurysms: a randomized comparison of effects on survival, dependency, seizures, rebleeding, subgroups, and aneurysm occlusion." *Lancet.* Sep 3-9;366(9488):809-17.

Morgenstern LB, Luna-Gonzales H, Huber JC Jr, Wong SS, Uthman MO, Gurian JH, Castillo PR, Shaw SG, Frankowski RF, Grotta JC., 1998 "Worst headache and subarachnoid hemorrhage: prospective, modern computed tomography and spinal fluid analysis." *Ann Emerg Med.* Sep;32(3 Pt 1):297-304.

Muehlschlegel S., 2018 "Subarachnoid Hemorrhage." *Continuum (MinneapMinn)* Dec;24(6):1623-1657.

Mura J, Rojas-Zalazar D, Ruíz A., 2007 "Improved outcome in high-grade aneurysmal subarachnoid hemorrhage by enhancement of endogenous clearance of cisternal blood clots: a prospective study that demonstrates the role of lamina terminalis fenestration combined with modern microsurgical cisternal blood evacuation." *Minim Invasive Neurosurg* 50:355–62.

Muroi C, Keller M, Pangalu A, Fortunati M, Yonekawa Y, Keller E., 2008 "Neurogenic pulmonary edema in patients with subarachnoid hemorrhage." *J Neurosurg Anesthesiol.* Jul;20(3):188-92.

Murthy SB, Shah S, Rao CP, Bershad EM, Suarez JI, 2015 " Neurogenic stunned myocardium following acute subarachnoid hemorrhage: pathophysiology and practical considerations." *J Intensive Care Med.* 30:318-25.

Naidech AM, Kreiter KT, Janjua N, Ostapkovich ND, Parra A, Commichau C, Fitzsimmons BF, Connolly ES, Mayer SA., 2005 "Cardiac troponin elevation, cardiovascular morbidity, and outcome after subarachnoid hemorrhage." 2005 Nov 1; *Circulation* 112(18):2851-6.

Nanda S, Bhatt SP, Dale TH, 2008 "Tako-tsubo cardiomyopathy: an insight into pathogenesis." *Chest.* 133:583.

Neil-Dwyer G, Lang D., 1997 "Brain attack" aneurysmal subarachnoid hemorrhage: death due to delayed diagnosis." *J R Coll Physicians Lond.* 31:49–52.

Nelson E, Powell JR, Conrad K, Likes K, Byers J, Baker S, Perrier D., 1982 "Phenobarbital pharmacokinetics and bioavailability in adults." *J Clin Pharmacol.* Feb-Mar;22(2-3):141-8.

Nelson, PB, Seif, SM, Maroon, JC, & Robinson, AG. 1981 " Hyponatremia in intracranial disease: perhaps not the syndrome of inappropriate secretion of antidiuretic hormone (SIADH)." *J Neurosurg.* 55:938-941.

Nemoto M, Masuda H, Sakaeyama Y, Okonogi S, Node Y, Ueda K, Ando S, Kondo K, Harada N, Sugo N., 2018 "Clinical Characteristics of Subarachnoid Hemorrhage with an Intracerebral Hematoma and Prognostic Factors." *J Stroke Cerebrovasc Dis.* May;27(5):1160-1166.

Niemann DB, Wills AD, Maartens NF, Kerr RS, Byrne JV, Molyneux AJ., 2003 "Treatment of intracerebral hematomas caused by aneurysm rupture: coil placement followed by clot evacuation." *J Neurosurg.* Nov;99(5):843-7.

Ohta T, Satoh G, Kuroiwa T., 1992 "The permeability change of major cerebral arteries in experimental vasospasm." *Neurosurgery.* 30:331-6.

Ojemann RG., 1963 "New pf. spontaneous resolution of an intraventricular hematoma. Report of a case with recovery." *J Neurosurg.* Oct;20:899-902.

Olson DM, Batjer HH, Abdulkadir K, Hall CE., 2014 "Measuring and monitoring ICP in Neurocritical Care: results from a national practice survey." *Neurocrit Care.* 20:15–20.

Ono R, Falcao LM, 2016 "Takotsubo cardiomyopathy systematic review: pathophysiologic process, clinical presentation, and diagnostic approach to takotsubo cardiomyopathy." *Int J Cardiol.* 209:196-205.

Otani N, Takasato Y, Masaoka H, Hayakawa T, Yoshino Y, Yatsushige H, Miyawaki H, Sumiyoshi K, Chikashi A, Takeuchi S, Suzuki G., 2008 "Surgical outcome following decompressive craniectomy for poor-grade aneurysmal subarachnoid hemorrhage in patients with associated massive intracerebral or Sylvian hematomas." *Cerebrovasc Dis.* 26(6):612-617.

Otite F, Mink S, Tan CO, Puri A, Zamani AA, Mehregan A, Chou S, Orzell S, Purkayastha S, Du R, Sorond FA., 2014 "Impaired cerebral autoregulation is associated with vasospasm and delayed cerebral ischemia in subarachnoid hemorrhage." *Stroke.* Mar;45(3):677-82.

Palasz J, D'Antona L, Farrell S, Elborady MA, Watkins LD, Toma AK., 2021 "External ventricular drain management in subarachnoid haemorrhage: a systematic review and meta-analysis." *Neurosurg Rev.* Aug 26.

Perks, Ian, Bagley, Ian J, Knott, Melissa T, Menon, David K. (2010). "Reviewof paroxysmal sympathetic hyperactivity after acquired brain injury." *Annals of Neurology.* 68 (2): 126-135. doi:10.1002/ana.22066. ISSN 0364-5134.

Petridis AK, Kamp MA, Cornelius JF, Beez T, Beseoglu K, Turowski B, Steiger HJ, 2017. "Aneurysmal Subarachnoid Hemorrhage." *Dtsch Arztebl Int.* Mar 31;114(13):226-236.

Pilipenko YuV, Konovalov AN, Eliava ShSh, Belousova OB, Okishev DN, Sazonov IA, Tabasaransky TF, 2018 "Determination of the justification and effectiveness of decompressive skull trepanation in patients with subarachnoid hemorrhage after the microsurgical shutdown of aneurysms." *Journal "Questions of Neurosurgery" named after N.N. Burdenko.* 82(1):59-71.

Plum F, Posner JB., 1972 "The diagnosis of stupor and coma." *Contemp Neurol Ser.* 10:1-286.

Polmear A., 2003 "Sentinel headaches in aneurysmal subarachnoid haemorrhage: what is the true incidence? A systematic review." *Cephalalgia* 23(10):935–41.

Proust F, Hannequin D, Langlois O, Freger P, Crissard P., 1995 "Causes of morbidity and mortality after ruptured aneurysm surgery in a series of 230 patients: the importance of control angiography." *Stroke.* 26:1553-7.

Rabinstein AA, Pichelmann MA, Friedman JA, Piepgras DG, Nichols DA, McIver JI, Toussaint LG 3rd, McClelland RL, Fulgham JR, Meyer FB, Atkinson JL, Wijdicks EF., 2003 "Symptomatic vasospasm and outcomes following aneurysmal subarachnoid hemorrhage: a comparison between surgical repair and endovascular coil occlusion." *J Neurosurg.* Feb;98(2):319-25.

Rangel-Castillo L, Gopinath S, Robertson CS., 2008 "Management of intracranial hypertension." *Neurol Clin.* 26(2):521-541.

Rasputina DA, Rutkovsky RV, Mertsalov SA, Krupko TA, Gulyaev ME, Salogub ED, Savello AV, Yakovlev AN, Zverev DA, Kozlenok AV, Savvina IA, 2019 "Neurogenic stressor cardiomyopathy caused by aneurysmal subarachnoid hemorrhage." *Russian Journal of Cardiology.* 2:81-85. (In Russ.) https://doi.org/10.15829/1560-4071-2019-2-81-85.

Razmologova OYu, Medvedev YuA., 2009 "Constitutional variants of the structure of the arterial circle of the brain and their role in the development of aneurysmal disease." *Arch. Pathol.* 6: 33–35.

Reilly C, Amidei C, Tolentino J, Jahromi BS, MacDonald RL., 2004 "Clot volume and clearance rate as independent predictors of vasospasm after aneurysmal subarachnoid hemorrhage." *J Neurosurg.* 101:255-61.

Rivero Rodríguez D, Scherle Matamoros C, Fernández Cúe L, Miranda Hernández JL, Pernas Sánchez Y, Pérez Nellar J., 2017 "Factors associated with poor outcome for aneurysmal subarachnoid haemorrhage in a series of 334 patients." *Neurologia.* Jan-Feb;32(1):15-21. English, Spanish.

Roh H, Kim J, Bae H, Chong K, Kim JH, Suh SI, Kwon TH, Yoon W., 2019 "Comparison of stent-assisted and no-stent coil embolization for safety and effectiveness in the treatment of ruptured intracranial aneurysms." *J Neurosurg.* Aug 30:1-7.

Rothwell PM, Coull AJ, Silver LE, Fairhead JF, Giles MF, Lovelock CE, Redgrave JN, Bull LM, Welch SJ, Cuthbertson FC, Binney LE, Gutnikov SA, Anslow P, Banning AP, Mant D, Mehta Z., 2005 "Oxford Vascular Study. Population-based study of event-rate, incidence, case fatality, and mortality for all acute vascular events in all arterial territories (Oxford Vascular Study)." *Lancet.* Nov 19;366(9499):1773-83.

Rowland M, Hadjipavlou G, Kelly M, Westbrook J, Pattinson KT., 2012 "Delayed cerebral ischaemia after subarachnoid haemorrhage: looking beyond vasospasm." *Br J Anaesth.* 09(3):315-29.

Rozhchenko LV, 1995 "*Disorders of cerebrospinal fluid circulation in the hemorrhagic period of cerebral aneurysms, their diagnosis and correction.*" Ph.D. Diss., Saint-Petersburg.

Ruijs AC, Dirven CM, Algra A, Beijer I, Vandertop WP, Rinkel G., 2005 "The risk of rebleeding after external lumbar drainage in patients with untreated ruptured cerebral aneurysms." *Acta Neurochir (Wien).* Nov;147(11):1157-61; discussion 1161-2.

Samoilov VI. 1990. *Subarachnoid hemorrhage.* Leningrad: Medicine.

Samuels MA, 2007 " The brain-heart connection." *Circulation.* 116:77-84.

Sanchez-Porras R, Zheng Z, Santos E, Scholl M, Unterberg AW, Sakowitz OW., 2013 "The role of spreading depolarization in subarachnoid hemorrhage." *Eur J Neurol.* 20:1121-7.

Sanusi TD, McLarnon M, Abouharb A., 2020 "Risk factors of chronic shunt dependent hydrocephalus following aneurysmal subarachnoid haemorrhage." *Clin Neurol Neurosurg.* Nov;198:106095.

Sarica C, Tanrikulu B, Sahin Y, Dağçınar A, Baltacioglu F, Bayri Y., 2018 "Acute Obstructive Hydrocephalus due to a Giant Posterior Cerebral Artery Aneurysm in a Pediatric Patient." *Pediatr Neurosurg.* 2018;53(4):247-253.

Sasaki T, Asano T, Takakura K, Sano K, Kassell NF., 1984 "Nature of the vasoactive substance in CSF from patients with subarachnoid hemorrhage." *J Neurosurg.* Jun;60(6):1186-91.

Sasaki T, Wakai S, Asano T, Watanabe T, Kirino T, Sano K., 1981 "The effect of a lipid hydroperoxide of arachidonic acid on the canine basilar artery: an experimental study on cerebral vasospasm." *J Neurosurg.* 54:357-65.

Savvina, Irina A., Zabrodskaya Yu. M., et al. 2021. « Cerebral vasospasm: Mechanisms, Pathomorphology, Diagnostics, Treatment». In *Cerebrovascular Diseases – elucidating Key Principles,* Edited by Patricia Bozzetto Ambrosi. London: IntechOpen. doi: http://dx.doi.org/10.5772/intechopen.101229.

Schievink WI, van der Werf DJ, Hageman LM, Dreissen JJ., 1988 "Referral pattern of patients with aneurysmal subarachnoid hemorrhage." *Surg Neurol.* 29:367–71.

Schievink WI., 1997 "Intracranial aneurysms." *N Engl J Med* 336:28.

Schirmer CM, Hoit DA, Malek AM., 2007 "Decompressive hemicraniectomy for the treatment of intractable intracranial hypertension after aneurysmal subarachnoid hemorrhage." *Stroke.* Mar;38(3):987-992.

Shevelev, Oleg A., and Grechko A. V. 2019. *Therapeutic hypothermia.* Moscow: Publishing house of Russian University of Friendship of Peoples.

Shimoda M, Oda S, Mamata Y, Tsugane R, Sato O., 1997 "Surgical indications in patients with an intracerebral hemorrhage due to ruptured middle cerebral artery aneurysm." *J Neurosurg.* Aug;87(2):170-5.

Shuaifeng Yang, Tinghua Wang, Chao You, Wenke Liu, Ke Zhao, Hong Sun, Boyong Mao, Xuehua Li, Anqi Xiao, Xue Ye Mao&Heng Zhang. 2013 "Association of polymorphisms in the elastin gene with sporadic ruptured intracranial aneurysms and unruptured intracranial aneurysms in Chinese patients." *Int J Neurosci.* 123(7):454-8.

Smith ER, Carter BS, Ogilvy CS., 2002 "Proposed use of prophylactic decompressive craniectomy in poor-grade aneurysmal subarachnoid hemorrhage patients presenting with associated large sylvian hematomas." *Neurosurgery.* Jul;51(1):117-124: discussion 124.

Srivastava T, Sannegowda RB, Sharma B, Tejwani S., 2013 "Lenticulostriate artery aneurysm presenting as primary intraventricular haemorrhage." *BMJ Case Rep.* Jun 26;2013:bcr2013009968.

Steiner I, Gomori JM, Melamed E., 1984 "The prognostic value of the CT scan in conservatively treated patients with intracerebral hematoma." *Stroke.* 15: 279-282.

Suarez JI, Tarr RW, Selman WR., 2006 "Aneurysmal subarachnoid hemorrhage." *N Engl J Med* 354(4):387–96.

Suarez, Jose I. 2015. "Diagnosis and management of subarachnoid hemorrhage." *Neurocritical Care.* 21(5):1263–1287.

Suwatcharangkoon S, Meyers E, Falo C, Schmidt JM, Agarwal S, Claassen J, Mayer SA., 2015. "Loss of Consciousness at Onset of Subarachnoid Hemorrhage as an Important Marker of Early Brain Injury." *JAMA Neurol.* Jan;73(1):28-35.

Tam AK, Ilodigwe D, Mocco J, Mayer S, Kassell N, Ruefenacht D, Schmiedek P, Weidauer S, Pasqualin A, Macdonald RL., 2010 "Impact of systemic inflammatory response syndrome on vasospasm, cerebral infarction, and outcome after subarachnoid hemorrhage: exploratory analysis of CONSCIOUS-1 database." *Neurocrit Care.* Oct;13(2):182-9.

Templin C, Ghardi JR, Diekmann J, et al. 2015 "Clinical features and outcomes of Takotsubo (Stress) Cardiomyopathy." *N Eng J Med.* 373:929-38.

Theodore J, Robin ED, 1976 "Speculations on neurogenic pulmonary edema (NPE)." *Am Rev Respir Dis.* 113:405-411.

Tokuda Y, Inagawa T, Katoh Y, Kumano K, Ohbayashi N, Yoshioka H., 1995 "Intracerebral hematoma in patients with ruptured cerebral aneurysms." *Surg Neurol.* Mar;43(3):272-7.

Topkoru B, Egemen E, Solaroglu I, Zhang JH., 2017 "Early Brain Injury or Vasospasm? An Overview of Common Mechanisms." *Curr Drug Targets.* 18(12):1424-1429.

Trufanov, Gennadiy E. 2006. *Radio diagnostics of vascular malformations and arterial aneurysms of the brain.* Saint Petersburg: GEOTAR-Media.

Uozumi Y, Sakowitz O, Orakcioglu B, Santos E, Kentar M, Haux D, Unterberg A., 2014 "Decompressive craniectomy in patients with aneurysmal subarachnoid hemorrhage: a single-center matched-pair analysis." *Cerebrovasc Dis.* 37(2):109-115.

Vahedi K, Hofmeijer J, Juettler E, Vicaut E, George B, Algra A, Amelink GJ, Schmiedeck P, Schwab S, Rothwell PM, Bousser MG, van der Worp HB, Hacke W., 2007 "DECIMAL, DESTINY, and HAMLET investigators. Early decompressive surgery in malignant infarction of the middle cerebral artery: a pooled analysis of three randomized controlled trials." *Lancet Neurol.* Mar;6(3):215-22.

Vahedi K, Vicaut E, Mateo J, Kurtz A, Orabi M, Guichard JP, Boutron C, Couvreur G, Rouanet F, Touzé E, Guillon B, Carpentier A, Yelnik A, George B, Payen D, Bousser MG, 2007 "DECIMAL Investigators. Sequential-design, multicenter, randomized, controlled trial of early decompressive craniectomy in malignant middle cerebral artery infarction (DECIMAL Trial)." *Stroke.* Sep;38(9):2506-17.

Vale FL, Bradley EL, Fisher WS 3rd., 1997 "The relationship of subarachnoid hemorrhage and the need for postoperative shunting." *J Neurosurg.* 86:462–6.

van Asch CJ, van der Schaaf IC, Rinkel GJ., 2010 "Acute hydrocephalus and cerebral perfusion after aneurysmal subarachnoid hemorrhage." *AJNR Am J Neuroradiol.* Jan;31(1):67-70. doi: 10.3174/ajnr.A1748.

van der Schaaf IC, Brilstra EH, Buskens E, Rinkel GJ., 2002 "Endovascular treatment of aneurysms in the cavernous sinus: a systematic review on balloon occlusion of the parent vessel and embolization with coils." *Stroke.* Jan;33(1):313-8.

van Gijn J, Kerr RS, Rinkel GJ., 2007 "Subarachnoid haemorrhage." *Lancet* 369(9558):306–18.

van Gijn J, Rinkel GJ., 2001 "Subarachnoid haemorrhage: diagnosis, causes and management." *Brain* 124:249–78.

van Rooij WJ., 2012 "Endovascular treatment of cavernous sinus aneurysms." *Am J Neuroradiol.* 33:323–326.

Vanakker OM. 2011, "Hereditary Connective Tissue Diseases in Young Adult Stroke: A Comprehensive Synthesis" [Electronic resource]. *Stroke Res Treat.*,:1-18. https://doi.org/10.4061/2011/712903.

Vannemreddy P, Nanda A, Kelley R, Baskaya MK., 2001. "Delayed diagnosis of intracranial aneurysms: confounding factors in clinical presentation and the influence of misdiagnosis on the outcome." *South Med J.* 94:1108–11.

Vergouwen MD, Vermeulen M, van Gijn J, Rinkel GJ, Wijdicks EF, Muizelaar JP, Mendelow AD, Juvela S, Yonas H, Terbrugge KG, Macdonald RL, Diringer MN, Broderick JP, Dreier JP, Roos YB., 2010 "Definition of delayed cerebral ischemia after aneurysmal subarachnoid hemorrhage as an outcome event in clinical trials and observational studies: proposal of a multidisciplinary research group." *Stroke.* Oct;41(10):2391-5.

Verma A, Maheshwari MC, Bhargava S., 1987 "Spontaneous intraventricular haemorrhage." *J Neurol.* May;234(4):233-6.

Vermeij FH, Hasan D, Vermeulen M, Tanghe HL, van Gijn J., 1994 "Predictive factors for deterioration from hydrocephalus after subarachnoid hemorrhage." *Neurology.* Oct;44(10):1851-5.

Voth D., 1987. "Der zerebraleVasospasmusnachSubarachnoidalblutung. Neue Aspekte der Diagnostik und Therapie" [Cerebral vasospasm following subarachnoid hemorrhage. New aspects of diagnosis and therapy]. *ZentralblNeurochir.* 48(2):89-101. German.

Wan A, Jaja BN, Schweizer TA, Macdonald RL., 2016 "Clinical characteristics and outcome of aneurysmal subarachnoid hemorrhage with intracerebral hematoma." *J Neurosurg.* Dec;125(6):1344-1351.

Wang HJ, Ye YF, Shen Y, Zhu R, Yao DX, Zhao HY., 2014 "Surgical treatment of poor grade middle cerebral artery aneurysms associated with large sylvian hematomas following prophylactic hinged craniectomy." *J Huazhong Univ Sci Technolog Med Sci.* Oct;34(5):716-721.

Wheelock B, Weir B, Watts R, Mohr G, Khan M, Hunter M, Fewer D, Ferguson G, Durity F, Cochrane D, Benoit B., 1983 "Timing of surgery for intracerebral hematomas due to aneurysm rupture." *J Neurosurg.* Apr;58(4):476-81.

Wong GK, Poon WS, Wai S, Yu LM, Lyon D, Lam JM., 2002 "Failure of regular external ventricular drain exchange to reduce cerebrospinal fluid infection: a result of a randomized controlled trial." *J Neurol Neurosurg Psychiatry.* Dec;73(6):759-61.

Yasargil MG, Yonekawa Y, Zumstein B, Stah HJ., 1973 "Hydrocephalus following spontaneous subarachnoid hemorrhage." *J Neurosurg* 39:474-479.

Yasuno K, Bakırcıoğlu M, Low SK, Bilgüvar K, Gaál E, Ruigrok YM etal. A common variant near the endothelin receptor type A (EDNRA) gene is associated with intracranial aneurysm risk. *Proc Natl. Acad. Sci. USA.* 2011; 108 (49): 19707-19712.23.

Yoneoka Y, Ezuka I, Takai N, Oda T, Tamura T, Yamashita S., 1998 "Ruptured distal anterior choroidal artery aneurysm presenting with casting intraventricular haemorrhage." *Acta Neurochir (Wien).* 140(2):185-9.

Zubkov YN, Nikiforov BM, Shustin VA., 1984 "Balloon catheter technique for dilatation of constricted cerebral arteries after aneurysmal SAH." *Acta Neurochir (Wien).* 70(1-2):65-79.

Zubkov YuN, Khilko VA. 1982. *Intravascular neurosurgery*. Moscow : Medicine.

Zubkov YuN., 1989 "Treatment of patients with intracranial arterial aneurysms in the hemorrhagic period." Ph.D. diss. Moscow.

Zyablova EI, Tkachev VV, Porkhanov VA, 2021 "The contribution of CT angiography to the verification of the source of non-traumatic intracranial hemorrhage in the emergency department. " *Innovative medicine of Kuban*. 1(21): 34-38.

Zyablova, EI, Porkhanov VA, Sinitsyn VE, 2021 "Preoperative radio diagnostics of acute subarachnoid hemorrhages due to rupture of cerebral aneurysms." *Russian Electronic Journal of radiation diagnostics*. 11(2): 19-31 doi 10.21569/2222-7415-2021-11-1-125-136.

Chapter 4

Anesthetic Management of Cerebral Aneurysm Surgery

Irina A. Savvina[1,2,*], DScMed and Anna O. Petrova[1], PhD

[1]Department of Anesthesiology and Intensive Care, Almazov National Medical Research Centre of Ministry of Health Care of Russian Federation, Saint Petersburg, Russian Federation

[2]Department of Anesthesiology and Intensive Care named after Vladimir L. Vanevskii of the North-Western State Medical University named after Ilya I. Mechnikov of Ministry of Health Care of Russian Federation, Saint Petersburg, Russian Federation

Abstract

Subarachnoid hemorrhage (SAH) secondary to rupture cerebral aneurysm carries a poor outcome and high mortality. Preoperative grading scales, such as Hunt and Hess scale, are useful to estimate prognosis. Complications of SAH are not only intracranial but also extracranial (myocardial ischemia, arrhythmia, or neurological pulmonary edema). Preoperative management of cerebral vasospasm, arrhythmia, pulmonary edema, hypovolemia, and hyponatremia is required. Premedication differs according to the patient's grade. There are many invasive and noninvasive monitoring systems for the central nervous system during perioperative period. The induction of anesthesia and the hemodynamic response should be controlled adequately without compromising cerebral perfusion pressure (CPP). Total intravenous anesthesia (TIVA) is preferred particularly when motor evoked potential

*Corresponding Author's Email: irinasavvina@mail.ru.

In: Aneurysmal Subarachnoid Hemorrhage
Editor: Irina Savvina
ISBN: 979-8-88697-251-1

measurement is performed. BIS monitoring is required to control the depth of anesthesia. Artificial ventilation is controlled to prevent hypercapnia which may increase intracranial pressure (ICP). Induction and maintenance of anesthesia are carried out with opioids and α_2-adrenoagonists for neurovegetative stabilization supporting the optimal CPP level and neuroprotection. Anesthetic management of the both "open" neurosurgery and endovascular procedures is based on the general principles of neuroanesthesia.

Keywords: Subarachnoid hemorrhage (SAH) from a cerebral aneurysm, anesthetic management, α_2-adrenoagonists, total intravenous anesthesia (TIVA), intraoperative neuroprotection

Abbreviations

CNS -	central nervous system
CSWS -	cerebral salt-wasting syndrome
EEG -	electroencephalography
DI -	diabetes insipidus
ICP -	intracranial pressure
MAP -	mean arterial pressure
MDU -	microvascular Doppler ultrasonography
MEPs -	motor-evoked potentials
$P_{ET\ CO2}$ -	end-tidal CO2 concentration
SERs -	sensory-evoked responses
SIADH -	syndrome of inappropriate antidiuretic hormone secretion
SpO2 -	saturation
SSEPs -	somatosensory-evoked potentials
tcMEPs -	transcranial motor-evoked potentials

Introduction

Successful implementation of neurosurgical interventions for cerebral aneurysms is undoubtedly determined by the contribution of anesthetic management factors in managing intracranial volumes, maintaining a satisfactory intraoperative state of the brain, reliable hemostasis, and harmonious awakening of the patient. The quality of the anesthesia provided determines the conditions of surgical access, the possibility of comfortable exposure of the aneurysm neck during neurosurgery of cerebral aneurysm clipping, and effective intraoperative monitoring.

Patients with aneurysmal SAH often have either increased ICP or decreased intracranial compliance, secondary to the mass of SAH, parenchymal injury from ischemia or hydrocephalus. Complications of SAH are not only intracranial but also extracranial (myocardial ischemia, arrhythmia, or neurological pulmonary edema). So preoperative management of cerebral vasospasm, arrhythmia, pulmonary edema, hypovolemia, and hyponatremia is required. Successful anesthetic management of patients with cerebral aneurysms requires a thorough understanding of the natural history, pathophysiology, and surgical requirements of the procedures.

Anesthetic Management of "Open" Neurosurgical Operations of Clipping of Cerebral Aneurysm

Neuroanesthesiologists should make plans for the anesthetic management before surgery. The basic goals are as follows (Table 1).

α_2-adrenergic agonists are recommended for induction and maintenance of anesthesia for cerebral aneurysm surgery. Dexmedetomidine or clonidine as the component of neurovegetative stabilization reduces cerebral blood flow and cerebral metabolic requirement of oxygen, provides stable cerebral hemodynamics without sudden increase in ICP during intubation, extubating and head pin insertion. It exerts its neuroprotective effects through several mechanisms (activation of the central adrenergic structure - nucleus locus coeruleus in the rostral-ventrolateral region of the medulla oblongata) which make the usage of these drugs a promising tool during cerebral ischemia (Bekker et al., 2005; Kondratyev 1993). The pioneer of central α_2-adrenoagonists use in neuroanesthesia is Professor Anatoly N. Kondratyev. Dexmedetomidine modulates spatial working memory, enhancing cognitive performance besides having sedative, analgesic, and anxiolytic action through the α_2-adrenoreceptors (Franowicz et al., 1998).

Table 1. Anesthetic management of patients with intracranial aneurysms (Talke P., Flexman A., 2011)

Preoperative	Neurologic evaluation is performed to look for evidence of increased intracranial pressure and vasospasm Electrocardiogram changes frequently are present HHH therapy is indicated if vasospasm is present Calcium channel blockers
Induction	Avoid increases in systemic blood pressure Maintain cerebral perfusion pressure to avoid ischemia
Maintenance	Opioid plus propofol and/or volatile anesthetic is the recommended regimen Mannitol (0,25-1,0 g/kg IV) also can be given Maintain normal to increased systemic blood pressure to avoid ischemia during temporary clipping
Postoperative	Maintain normal to increased systemic blood pressure Early awakening is recommended to facilitate neurologic assessment HHH therapy is given as needed

HHH – hypervolemia, hypertension, hemodilution.

Preoperative Assessment and Premedication

To allow accurate assessment of the patient's immediate preoperative neurologic condition and clinical grade, preoperative medications are best omitted. The Hunt and Hess scale has been used as a preoperative neurological symptom grading scale (Table 2).

As the World Federation of Neurological Surgeons (WFNS) grading scale is based on the Glasgow coma scale (GCS), the scale is designed more simply and clinically estimates the prognosis by combining the GCS with major focal neurological deficits (aphasia, hemiparesis, or hemiplegia) (Table 3).

Preoperative evaluation includes a review of the patient's intracranial pathological condition, including the performing of computed tomography (CT) and angiograms; assessment of other systemic functions, premorbid as well as current condition, with emphasis on systems affected by SAH; discussion with neurosurgeon about positioning, anticipated difficulty and technique to clip and special monitoring requirements (Pong and Lam 2017).

Table 2. Hunt and Hess grading scale (Hunt WE, Hess RM, 1968)

Grade	
I	Asymptomatic or minimal headache and slight nuchal rigidity
II	Moderate to severe headache, nuchal rigidity, no neurological deficit other than cranial nerve palsy
III	Drowsiness, confusion, or mild focal deficit
IV	Stupor, moderate to severe hemiparesis, possibly early decerebrate rigidity, and vegetative disturbances
V	Deep coma, decerebrate rigidity, moribund appearance

Table 3. World Federation of Neurological Surgeons (WFNS) grading scale (Drake CG, 1988)

WFNS Grade	GCS score	Motor deficit
I	15	Absent
II	14-13	Absent
III	14-13	Present
IV	12-7	Present or absent
V	6-3	Present or absent

Preoperative medications such as anticonvulsants or steroids, are continued. Drugs for gastric conditions, either an H2 antagonist or metoclopramide, are given before the induction of anesthesia. Giving small doses of opioids or benzodiazepine, or both, may be effective in good-grade patients. Conversely, almost all poor-grade patients do not receive hypnotic premedication but receive blood pressure control. If the patient is intubated, medication for sedation and muscle relaxation may be given. Because of the hypovolemia after SAH, hydration with isotonic crystalloid solution is required before induction.

Induction of Anesthesia

The hemodynamic response evoked by direct laryngoscopy, tracheal intubation, and particularly the placement of head pins should be controlled adequately without compromising the CPP. After optimal head position is obtained, an opioid (fentanyl, 2-5 mcg/kg; morphine, 20-50 mcg/kg;

remifentanil, 0.5 mcg/kg/min), α_2-adrenoagonist (clonidine 1,45 mcg/kg; dexmedetomidine 0,7 – 1,0 mcg/kg) and a hypnotic agent (propofol, 2 mg/kg; thiopental, 3-5 mg/kg; midazolam, 0,1-0,2 mg/kg) are administrated intravenously, followed by a muscle relaxant (rocuronium, 0.6 mg/kg; vecuronium, 0.1 mg/kg) to facilitate insertion of an endotracheal tube. Lidocaine (1,5 mg/kg) is given before laryngoscopy and intubation, if needed. All procedures are carried out with a 100% oxygen mask and in some cases adding a low-dose inhalation anesthetic (0.5 MAC). Clonidine and dexmedetomidine attenuates hemodynamic stress response to intubation and extubating by sympatholysis (Guler et al., 2005).

Maintenance of Anesthesia

A volatile anesthetic (sevoflurane, desflurane) can be chosen under condition of normal intracranial pressure (ICP), but total intravenous anesthesia (TIVA) with propofol 4,0-7,0 mg/kg/h, fentanyl 5,0 mcg/kg/h and clonidine 0,45 mcg/kg/h or dexmedetomidine 0,2-0,4 mcg/kg/h is suitable for cerebral aneurysm surgery, particularly in a patient with a high ICP. BIS monitoring is useful to control the depth of anesthesia (target values BIS 30-40) (Savvina et al., 2022). Although lurching or other movement while the patient's head is fixed is very dangerous, no addition of muscle relaxant after intubation is required when MEP measurement is performed.

Artificial lung ventilation is carried out to maintain the PaCO2 between 30 and 35 mmHg, averting hypercapnia which may increase the ICP. Generally, the respiratory rate is raised to add minute volume, but simultaneously high airway pressure, which also may increase ICP, shoud be inhibited.

The systemic blood pressure before clipping is maintained within the patient's normal range or a mean arterial pressure (MAP) between 70 and 80 mmHg, thus optimizing the CPP ($\geq$ 50 mHg). During temporary proximal occlusion, MAP is maintained in the high-normal range to facilitate perfusion through the collateral circulation and to prevent distal cerebral ischemia or infarction caused by regional hypotension. At this time, a vasopressor (phenylephrine, 0,1-0,2 mg IV; dopamine, 3-5 mcg/kg/min; norepinephrine, 0,1-0,2 mcg/kg/min) can be used to raise the MAP gently (Ogihara 2015:303-319). After placement of a cerebrovascular clip, as the aneurysm is isolated from the systemic circulation, a MAP as high as 110 mmHg is acceptable, which may be of value in preventing postoperative vasospasm (Savvina et al., 2022).

Some type of lactated or acetated Ringer's solution is preferred to normal saline. The maintaining euvolemia is an important matter. Colloids (6% hetastarch or 4% succinylated gelatin or 5% albumin) are acceptable.

Hemodynamic Monitoring

Invasive arterial blood pressure measurement, performed before induction, is essential to strictly control systemic blood pressure and to prevent rupture of aneurysms and cerebral ischemia caused by violent fluctuations in blood pressure. Moreover, several blood samples via the arterial route may be obtained for analyzing blood gas, measuring blood sugar level, or other clinical factors.

Intermittent noninvasive blood pressure can be useful to indicate the risk of rebleeding.

Central venous pressure (CVP) for the monitoring of preload is of great importance for several indications, such as preoperative hypovolemia, severe heart disease, and excessive bleeding intraoperatively.

Transesophageal echocardiography (TEE) is performed to evaluate left cardiac system function and air embolism.

The V_5 lead of 12-lead ECG represents heart rate, rhythm, and cardiac ischemia.

Noninvasive Conventional Monitoring

Percutaneous oxygen saturation (S_pO_2) measurement via the pulse oximeter is helpful to prevent hypoxemia.

End-tidal CO_2 concentration ($P_{ET\,CO2}$) conveniently suggests the status of the cerebrovascular autoregulation of the brain, relaxed or tight. In addition, a sudden decrease in the $P_{ET\,CO2}$ may enable early detection of an air embolism.

Deep body temperature measured at the tympanic or nasopharyngeal region reflects brain temperature and is useful to help protect the brain from hyperthermia.

Urine output may be an estimate of the intravascular volume and renal function intraoperatively. When excessive urine output occurs, hypovolemia and electrolyte imbalances may exist, and diabetes insipidus (DI), SIADH, or CSWS needs to be considered.

BIS monitoring is required to control the depth of anesthesia (Savvina et al., 2022).

Neurophysiological Monitoring for Intracranial Neurovascular Surgery

EEG Monitoring

The surgical incision and brain retraction diminish the utility of placing EEG scalp or brain surface electrodes that could detect cerebral ischemia in at-risk cortex. Recording electrodes placed on the surface of the brain have been used successfully, but they are commonly considered "in the way" by neurosurgeons. Thus, EEG is typically used only to confirm metabolic suppression during temporary clip placement.

Motor-Evoked Potentials (MEPs)

Monitoring of MEPs outperforms other CNS monitoring such as SSEPs or microvascular Doppler ultrasonography (MDU), in detecting subcortical ischemia in the brain, which brings about motor dysfunction (Neuloh et al., 2004).

Somatosensory-Evoked Potentials (SSEPs)

SSEPs have been extensively studied during cerebral aneurysm surgery. For aneurysms involving the anterior cerebral circulation, SSEP monitoring has an excellent, but not perfect, record for predicting postoperative neurologic function. Most patients without surgically induced SSEP changes during the procedure awaken with an unchanged neurologic examination. Patients with significant SSEP changes that do not revert to normal awaken with a new neurologic deficit. Patients with significant intraoperative SSEP changes that return to normal may show at least a transient postoperative deficit, with the severity and duration of that deficit increasing as the severity of the SSEP change increases. Many authors have reported significant utility of SSEP monitoring in detecting improper aneurysm clip placement and in guiding intraoperative blood pressure management, particularly in patients already showing, or at significant risk for vasospasm after subarachnoid hemorrhage (Christoph et al., 2019).The same success cannot be reported, however, for posterior circulation aneurysms. In these cases, many areas of the cortex and subcortical structures are at risk for damage that cannot be monitored at all by somatosensory pathway function.

An important concern during aneurysm surgery is injury to perforating vessels near the aneurysm, which risks damage to subcortical pathways in the internal capsule and may account for half the new neurologic deficits immediately postoperatively. Anatomically, the motor pathway runs anterior to the sensory pathway in the internal capsule and is at greater risk if the anterior choroidal artery, lenticulostriate perforator vessels, or even perforating branches of the anterior cerebral artery are injured during dissection and clip placement. Two concerns need to be addressed if tcMEP is to be incorporated successfully in these cases. First, motion caused by stimulation needs to be minimized to not interfere with the surgery. Second and more importantly, stimulus parameters need to be set to limit deep current spread that would activate the corticospinal tract distal to the internal capsule and obscure ischemia of the proximal pathway. The use of longer stimulus trains at intensities close to the motor threshold addresses both concerns and have made tcMEP monitoring a useful adjunct during aneurysm surgery in many centers (Christoph et al., 2019).

Transient Cardiac Pause (Cardioplegia Using Adenosine)

To facilitate clipping of a large aneurysm with a broad neck and reduce the risk of rupture, transient cardiac arrest can be induced with a bolus of adenosine (Pong and Lam 2017). After a dose response has been established with the use of two to three incremental doses of adenosine between 6 and 18 mg (Hashimoto et al., 2000), a duration of approximately 30 seconds of asystole can be induced with an average dose of 30 to 36 mg of adenosine. Recovery of cardiac rhythm is spontaneous and may be followed by rebound tachycardia and hypertension. This technique is contraindicated in patients with preexisting cardiac conduction abnormalities or severe asthma.

Intraoperative Cerebroprotection

Because experimental studies in cerebral ischemia have demonstrated that even mild hypothermia can exert significant cerebroprotective effects by suppressing release of excitotoxic amino acids (Busto et al., 1989; Minamisawa et al., 1990), the practice of maintaining the body temperature between 33° and 35° C during the periods when the patient is considered to be at risk for cerebral ischemia was quite routine. The Intraoperative Hypothermia for Aneurysm Surgery Trial (IHAST) evaluated the effects of mild hypothermia (33,5^{O}C) and found no effect on neurologic outcome in patients with favorable clinical grade aneurysm (Todd et al., 2005).

Pharmacological metabolic suppression or use of mannitol (total 2 g/kg) just before the proximal vessel occlusion appears to provide some brain protection without the complications of moderate hypothermia. When temporary occlusion is necessary, propofol is recommended to induce burst suppression in addition to the use of mannitol (Pong and Lam 2017). Prophylaxis of local cerebral ischemia and cerebral vasospasm following temporary occlusion of the afferent artery during surgical clipping cerebral aneurysm was proposed with short intervals of vessels occlusion in combination with intraoperative intravenous administration of Inosine+Nicotinamide+Riboflavin+Succinic Acid (20,0 ml). Such tactics expands the tolerability to artery occlusion in patients operated in the "cold" period, reduces the possibility of neurological deficit, reduces the recovery period and resuscitation bed-day after neurosurgery (Savvina et al., 2019).

Studies suggest the likelihood of neuroprotective action of dexmedetomidine as a component of general anesthesia by reducing the levels of circulating and brain catecholamines and thus balancing the ratio between cerebral oxygen supplies, reducing excitotoxicity, and improving the perfusion in the ischemic penumbra. It reduces the levels of the glutamate responsible for cellular brain injury, especially in subarachnoid hemorrhage (Bekker et al., 2005).

Anesthesia Management of Endovascular Neurosurgical Procedures for Cerebral Aneurysm

The anesthetic concerns of particular importance for endovascular neurosurgical procedures as the field of interventional neuroradiology are maintaining the patient's immobility during the procedure to facilitate imaging and to prevent intervention-related complications; either enabling rapid recovery from anesthesia at the end of operation to facilitate neurological examination and monitoring or providing for intermittent evaluation of neurologic function during the procedure; managing anticoagulation; treating and managing sudden unexpected procedure-specific complications during the procedure, such as hemorrhage or vascular occlusion, which may involve manipulating systemic blood pressure; guiding the medical management of critical care patients during transport to and from radiology suites; and recognizing self-protection issues related to radiation safety (Young and Pile-Spellman 1994; 80; Young et al., 1997).

Preoperative Patient Assessment and Premedication

Patient with aneurysmal SAH is the emergency and critically ill, with possibility of cerebral vasospasm development, so it is necessary to evaluate the level of neurological deficit and prognosis (Table 2, Table 3). Because the incidence and severity of vasospasm is related to the amount of subarachnoid blood present, computed tomography (CT) findings are often graded according to the Fisher's grading system (Table 4) (Fisher et al., 1980). Despite criticisms of Fisher grading (Smith et al., 2005) and proposed modifications (Frontera et al., 2006), it remains the primary method of describing the CT findings with regard to clot burden and the risk of vasospasm in aneurysmal SAH (Pong and Lam 2017).

Table 4. Fisher grades for computed tomography findings in subarachnoid hemorrhage

Grade	CT Finding(s)
1	No blood detected
2	Diffuse thin layer of subarachnoid blood (vertical layers <1 mm thick)
3	Localization clot or thick layer of subarachnoid blood (vertical layers ≥1 mm thick)
4	Intracerebral or intraventricular blood with diffuse or no subarachnoid blood)

CT, computed tomography.

Patients who have a history of significant contrast agent reactions are needed in premedication with steroids, antihistamines and H2 blockers prior to the procedure. The patient's renal function should be evaluated before the procedure due to nephrotoxicity of the contrast agents.

General anesthesia is used for endovascular emergency neurosurgical procedures in patients with ruptured cerebral aneurysm and SAH. According to general neuroanesthesia principles, the best option is TIVA (propofol 4,0-6,0 mg/kg/h; fentanyl 2,5 - 5,0 mcg/kg/h and clonidine 0,45 mcg/kg/h or dexmedetomidine 0,2-0,4 mcg/kg/h) with intubation and artificial lung ventilation. Of course, the specific choice of anesthetics may be guided primarily by cardiovascular and cerebrovascular considerations. Normocapnia or modest hypocapnia consistent with the safe conduct of positive-pressure ventilation should be maintained.

Hemodynamic monitoring during endovascular neurosurgery includes beat-to-beat arterial pressure monitoring and blood sampling can be facilitated by the placement of an intra-arterial catheter. The systemic blood pressure before coiling is maintained within the patient's normal range or a mean arterial pressure (MAP) between 70 and 80 mmHg, thus optimizing the CPP ($\geq$ 50 mmHg). The MAP after embolization with coiling need not change from the normal range (Ogihara 2015: 303-319).

The anesthesiologist should be prepared for aneurysmal rupture and acute SAH at all times, from spontaneous rupture of a leaky sac to direct injury of the aneurysm wall by the vascular manipulation, perianeurysmal thrombus formation, or arterial branch occlusion. The morbidity and mortality of intraprocedural rupture is high. One report found that, in the 5% of the studied coiling cases, 63% of patients with intraprocedural rupture had periprocedural death (Elijovich et al., 2008). If a rupture occurs, anticoagulation must be immediately reversed (1 mg protamine for each 100 units of heparin given) and low normal mean arterial pressure. There are also increasingly more reports on the use of specific clotting factors, such as recombinant factor VIIa and factor IX complex, to rescue severe life-threatening bleeding, including intracranial hemorrhage uncontrolled by standard transfusion therapy.

Conclusion

The contribution of neuroanesthesia to the improved results of the surgical treatment of cerebral aneurysms is indisputable. There are specific features of anesthesia during cerebral aneurysm clipping operations and endovascular treatment of cerebral aneurysms. The risk of complications and death increases with aneurysm rupture. The anesthesiologist should be ready for this dramatic plot. Perioperative neuroprotection includes general anesthesia (TIVA) with neurovegetative stabilization with opioids and α_2-adrenoagonists, mild hypothermia, mannitol. BIS monitoring is recommended to control the depth of anesthesia. Neurophysiological monitoring (EEG, MEPs, SSEPs) is necessary to predict the cerebral damage due to neurosurgical manipulations and delayed ischemia. Anesthetic management of cerebral aneurysm surgery is based on the basic principles of neuroanesthesiology.

References

Bekker A, Sturaitis MK. 2005. Dexmedetomidine for neurological surgery. *Neurosurgery.* 57:1-10.

Busto R, Dietrich WD, Globus MY, Ginsberg MD. 1989. The importance of brain temperature in cerebral ischemic injury. *Stroke.* 20:1113-1114.

Christoph N. Seubert, John J. Mcauliffe III, and Michael Mahla. 2019."Neurologic Monitoring." In *Anesthesia,* edited by R. Miller, 1243-1276. NewYork: Elsevier.

Drake CG. 1988. Report of world federation of neurological surgeons committee on a universal subarachnoid hemorrhage scale. *J Neurosurg.* 68: 985-986.

Elijovich, Lucas, Randall T. Higashida, Michael T. Lawton, Gary Duckwiler, Steven Giannotta, and S. Claiborne Johnston. 2008. Predictors and outcomes of intraprocedural rupture in patients treated for ruptured intracranial aneurysms: The CARAT study. *Stroke.* 39:1501-1506.

Fisher CM, Kistler JP, Davis JM. 1980. Relation of cerebral vasospasm to arachnoid hemorrhage visualized by computerize tomographic scanning. *Neurosurgery.* 6:1-9.

Frontera, Jennifer A., Jan Claassen, J. Michael Schmidt, Katja E. Wartenberg, Richard Temes, E. Sander Connolly, R. Loch Macdonald, and Stephan A. Mayer. 2006. Predicton of symptomatic vasospasm after subarachnoid hemorrhage: The modified Fisher scale. *Neurosurgery.* 59:21-27.

Franowicz JS, Arnsten AF. 1998. The alpha-2a noradrenergic agonist, guanfaciane, improves delayed response performance in young adult rhesus monkeys. *Psychopharmacology (Berl).* 136:8-14.

Guler G, Akin A, Tosun E, Eskitafloglu E, Mizrak A, Boyaci A. 2005. Single-dose dexmedetomidine attenuates airway and circulatory reflexes during extubating. *Acta Anaesthesiol Scand.* 49:1088-91.

Hashimoto T, Young WL, Aagaard BD, Joshi S, Ostapkovich ND, and John Pile-Spellman J. 2000. Adenosine-induced ventricular asystole to induce transient profound systemic hypotension in patients undergoing endovascular therapy: Dose-response characteristics. *Anesthesiology.* 93: 998-1001.

Hunt WE, Hess RM. 1968. Surgical risk as related to time of intervention in the repair of intracranial aneurysms. *J Neurosurg.* 28: 14-20.

Kondratyev, Anatoly N. 1993. "Combined effects on the opioid and adrenergic antinociceptive systems in the anesthetic provision of neurooncological operations." PhD diss. St.Petersburg Medical Academy of Postgraduate Education.

Minamisaws H, Nordstrom CH, Smith ML, Siesjo BK. 1990. The influence of mild body and brain hypothermia on ischemic brain damage. *J Cereb Blood Flow Metab.* 10:365-374.

Neuloh G, Schramm J. 2004. Monitoring of motor evoked potentials compared with somatosensory evoked potentials and microvascular Doppler ultrasonography in cerebral aneurysm surgery. *J Neurosurg.* 100:389-399.

Pong RP, Lam AM. 2017. "Anesthetic Management of Cerebral Aneurysm Surgery." In *Neuroanesthesia,* edited by Cottrell J. and Patel P., 223-247. New York: Elsevier.

Savvina IA, Cherebillo VY, Zabrodskaya YM, Petrova AO, Sergeev AV, Paltsev AA, et al. 2019. The intraoperative prophylaxis of local ischemical brain damage in neurosurgical patients with cerebral aneurysm. *Pirogov Journal of Surgery.* 5:65-71.

Savvina IA, Zabrodskaya YuM, Petrova AO. 2022. "General anesthesia and autonomic nervous system: control and management in neurosurgery." In *Autonomic Nervous System –Special Interest Topics*, edited by TheodorosAslanidis and Christos Nouris, 53-76. London: IntechOpen.

Savvina IA, Zabrodskaya YuM, Petrova AO, Samochernykh KA. 2022. "Cerebral vasospasm: Mechanisms, Pathomorphology, Diagnostics, Treatment." In *Cerebrovascular Diseases - elucidating Key Principles*, edited by Dr. Patricia Bozzetto Ambrosi. London: IntechOpen. doi: http://dx.doi.org/10.5772/intechopen.101229.

Smith, Michael L., John M. Abrahams, Sid Chandela, Michelle J. Smith, Robert W. Hurst, and Peter D. Le Roux. 2005. Subarachnoid hemorrhage on computed tomography scanning and the development of cerebral vasospasm: The Fisher grade revisited. *Surg Neurol.* 63:229-234; discussion 234-235.

Talke P, Flexman A. 2011. "Central nervous system disease." In *Basics of anesthesia*, edited by Miller RD, Pardo MC Jr, 476-485. Philadelphia: Elsevier.

Todd MM, Hindman BJ, Clarke WR, Torner JC. 2005. Mild intraoperative hypothermia during surgery for intracranial aneurysm. *N Engl J Med.* 352:135-145.

Yukihiko Ogihara. 2015. "Anesthesia for Intracranial Vascular Surgery." In *Neuroanesthesia and Cerebrospinal Protection*, edited by Hiroyuki Uchino, Kazuo Ushijima, Yukio Ikeda, 303-319. Tokyo: Springer.

Young WL, Pile-Spellman J. 1994. Anesthetic considerations for interventional neuroradiology. *Anesthesiology.* 80: 427-456.

Young WL, Pile-Spellman J, Hacein-Bay L, Joshi S. 1997. Invasive neuroradiologic procedures for cerebrovascular abnormalities: Anesthetic considerations. *Anesthesiol Clin N Am.* 15:631-653.

Chapter 5

Hemostasiological Disorders in Patients with Aneurysmal Subarachnoid and Intracranial Hemorrhage

Natalia V. Dryagina,* PhD

Department of Laboratory Diagnostics, Russian Polenov Scientific Research Neurosurgical Institute – branch of the Almazov National Medical Research Centre of Ministry of Health Care of Russian Federation, Saint Petersburg, Russian Federation

Abstract

The chapter summarizes the basics of the functioning of the coagulation and fibrinolytic systems and the role of coagulation factors in maintaining hemostatic balance. Most components of hemostasis have a wide range of concurrent functions that are not directly related to the processes of coagulation and fibrinolysis in the systemic bloodstream. Factors of coagulation and fibrinolytic systems are expressed on the cell membranes of various organs, including the tissues of the brain and meninges. These components of hemostasis, acting outside of plasma hemostasis, mediate many cellular processes, such as adhesion, migration, proliferation, apoptosis, angiogenesis, inflammation and tissue healing. There is an increasing understanding of the involvement of these factors both in the physiology of the central nervous system and in the pathogenesis of diseases of the nervous system. With intracranial hemorrhages, the ingress of thromboplastically active substances from the damaged brain into the CSF and then into the systemic bloodstream tissue leads to hypercoagulation and increases the risk of thrombotic

*Corresponding Author's Email: nvdryagina@mail.ru.

In: Aneurysmal Subarachnoid Hemorrhage
Editor: Irina Savvina
ISBN: 979-8-88697-251-1

complications. In subarachnoid hemorrhages, the ingress of a large number of plasma coagulation factors into the subarachnoid space changes the procoagulant and fibrinolytic properties of the cerebrospinal fluid, affecting the sanitation of the cerebrospinal fluid pathways from the blood. Prognostic significance in the development of a number of posthemorrhagic complications has been established for liquor levels of D-dimers and PAI-1.

Keywords: aneurysmal subarachnoid hemorrhage (SAH), cerebrospinal fluid (CSF), coagulation, fibrinolysis, intraventricular hemorrhage, cerebral-subarachnoid hemorrhage, CSF pathways

Abbrevations

BBB –	Blood–brain barrier
CSF –	Cerebrospinal fluid
IVH –	Intraventricular hemorrhage
PAI-1 –	Plasminogen activator inhibitor of type 1
SAH –	Aneurysmal subarachnoid hemorrhage
TF –	Tissue factor
tPA –	Tissue type plasminogen activator

Introduction

Getting of blood into the subarachnoid space and brain tissue as a result of aneurysmal hemorrhage causes pronounced changes in the composition of cerebrospinal fluid (CSF). The content of coagulation and fibrinolytic system factors increases, which significantly affect the rate of rehabilitation of the cerebrospinal fluid pathways. The entry of thromboplastically active substances of cerebral origin from the resorbed cerebrospinal fluid into the bloodstream can lead to violations of systemic hemostasis. The absence of unidirectional changes and correlations between the markers of coagulation and fibrinolysis in CSF and peripheral blood indicates the autonomy of hemostatic processes in the blood poured into the intracranial space. Meanwhile, there is a connection between the cerebrospinal fluid level of many markers of the coagulation and fibrinolytic systems and the development of complications such as posthemorrhagic hydrocephalus, cerebral vasospasm, fibrin deposition on the membranes and hemispheres of the brain. Thus, a detailed study of the processes occurring in the subarachnoid space after an aneurysmal hemorrhage can provide additional objective information to the attending physician, and the determination of individual markers of coagulation and fibrinolysis in CSF can have not only prognostic value, but also become a target for therapeutic decisions.

General Ideas about the Hemostasis System

According to modern concepts, the hemostasis system is a complex biological system, the main functions of which are the preservation of blood in the bloodstream in a liquid state and the prevention of blood loss in case of vascular damage. Its main structural and functional components are the vascular wall, blood cell elements, mainly platelets, and plasma factors. All components are in dynamic equilibrium, providing a hemostatic balance. Conditionally, plasma proteins of hemostasis are divided into two enzymatic systems – the coagulation system and the fibrinolysis system.

Basic Principles of Functioning of the Coagulation and Fibrinolytic Systems

Normally, almost all proteins of the coagulation system are in a latent state. The exception is factor VII, 1-2% of which normally circulates in active form (Dolgov, Vavilova and Svirin 2019). Activation of plasma proteins in both systems occurs due to a multi-stage (cascade) enzymatic process involving non-enzymatic cofactors, during which the initial signal is amplified (Sang et al. 2021). Each system has a number of activators and inhibitors. Inhibitors of the coagulation system are often isolated into a separate anticoagulation system (Dolgov and Svirin 2005). The presence of coagulation inhibitors allows you to keep the blood in a liquid state and limit thrombosis to the site of damage. The most significant physiological anticoagulants include antithrombin, protein C system, tissue factor pathway inhibitor and α2-macroglobulin (Versteeg et al. 2013).

The fibrinolysis system provides restriction of clot growth, gradual dissolution of the thrombus and restoration of normal blood flow. Its main components are the plasminogen proenzyme, its activators – tissue type plasminogen activator tPA, urokinase plasminogen activator (urokinase) uPA, and their inhibitors – plasminogen activator inhibitor of type 1 PAI-1 and type 2 PAI-2 (Yildiz 2014).

As a result of activation, one key enzyme is formed in each system. In the coagulation system, it is thrombin, which ensures the formation of a fibrin clot. In the fibrinolysis system, this is plasmin, under the action of which fibrin is destroyed (Hoffman and Monroe 2006).

At all stages of hemostasis, the presence of calcium ions is necessary, which is involved in the binding of tenase and prothrombinase complexes with platelet anionic phospholipids, the formation of bonds between clotting factors, platelet activation, fibrin clot stabilization and many other reactions (Sang et al. 2021).

According to the currently accepted cellular theory of coagulation, all coagulation processes take place on the cell membranes of subendothelial cells and shaped blood elements, mainly platelets (Swieringa et al. 2018; Hoffman and Monroe 2001). After damage to the vessel, blood contacts subendothelially located smooth muscle cells and fibroblasts expressing tissue factor (TF), as a result of binding TF to circulating VIIa, their complex is formed, activating factors IX and X, which means the beginning of the initiation phase.

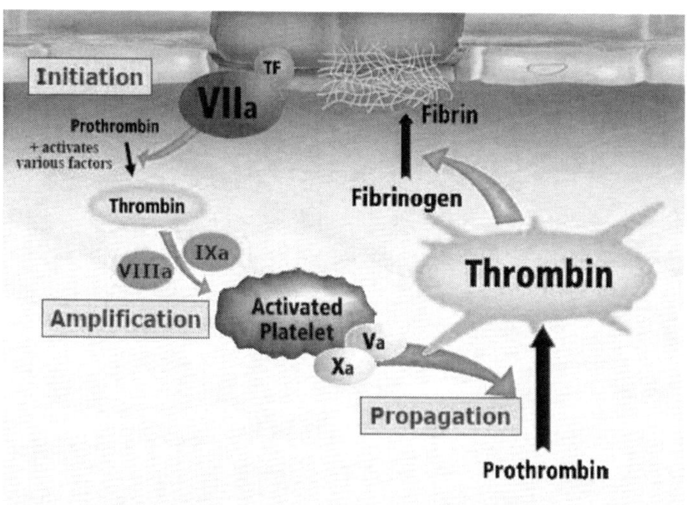

Source: M. Hoffman, D. M. Monroe. A cell-based model of hemostasis. Thromb Haemost. 2001;85(6):958-65.

Figure 1. Diagram of the cascade of the blood coagulation system.

Activated factor X is capable of producing trace amounts of thrombin in the absence of its cofactor Va, i.e., without the formation of the prothrombinase complex Xa-Va. Under the influence of this initial amount of thrombin, the second phase of coagulation is triggered – amplification, in which factor VIII is released from its complex with Willebrand factor, activation of factor V and other plasma coagulation factors, as well as activation of platelets, at this stage already tightly adhered to the subendothelial structures of the vascular wall (Hoffman and Monroe 2007). With the formation of tenase IXa-VIIIa and prothrombinase Xa-Va complexes on the platelet surface, the third phase of coagulation begins –propagation (Versteeg et al. 2013; Sang et al. 2021). The thrombin produced in this phase is sufficient to form a fibrin clot. While the reactions of the first phase occur mainly on subendothelial surfaces, by the beginning of the third phase, the main processes are localized on platelet membranes. As a final stage, the formation of transverse covalent bonds between adjacent fibrin chains with the formation of a dense fibrin thrombus occurs under the action of XIIIa (Versteeg et al. 2013; Hoffman and Monroe 2006).

Thus, due to the expression of TF on the cell membrane, the localization of the coagulation cascade is ensured where it is necessary to stop bleeding. As we move away from the site of injury, the coagulation potential weakens, intact endothelial cells have anticoagulation properties, which allows us to limit the growth of the clot (Ivanciu and Stalker 2015).

Extravascular Functions of Hemostasis Components

Currently, it is obvious that many components of the coagulation and fibrinolytic systems, in addition to performing the main task, have a number of other functions that can be conditionally designated as "part-time" or "extravascular". Thus, thrombin participates in the regulation of various cellular functions, such as signaling in the cell, proliferation, migration and growth of cells; in the processes of embryogenesis, angiogenesis and tissue repair; affects the permeability of the endothelium, increasing the migration of leukocytes into the extravascular space, which is an important component of inflammation and edema; stimulates chemotaxis and cytokine production (Crawley et al. 2007; Maragoudakis 2009; Lal, Dittus and Holmes 2013). Its expression is widespread in tissues, which is consistent with numerous functions of thrombin (Maragoudakis 2009). Similar extravascular effects have been found for another key component of the coagulation system – tissue factor (Cimmino and Cirillo 2018; Hoffman and Monroe 2012).

For the factors of the fibrinolytic system involved in the regulation of cellular functions, the name "plasminogen activation system" is used. It includes urokinase, which plays a key role, since it is the main activator of plasminogen in tissues, tPA, their inhibitors, primarily PAI-1, uPAR receptor, plasminogen and plasmin itself (Adcock and Ramanathan 2004; McRae and Porter 2012). These factors, through their proteolytic activity, can destroy extracellular proteins, in addition, activating other proteolytic enzymes, for example, matrix metalloproteinases, can have indirect effects on the state of the extracellular matrix (Cesari, Pahor and Incalzi 2010). The plasminogen activation system is involved in various processes based on the degradation of the extracellular matrix – angiogenesis, apoptosis, bacterial invasion, migration of various cell types (leukocytes, endothelial cells, etc.) (Sillen and Declerck 2021; Ismail, Shaker and Bajou 2022; Schuliga 2015).

The Role of Hemostasis Components in the Pathogenesis of CNS Diseases

The fact that the brain tissue is rich in thromboplastic substances, and the meninges contain fibrinolysis activators, has been known for a long time. The widely used to date prothrombin Quick test was proposed in 1935; the reagent for it was thromboplastin (an obsolete name for tissue factor) obtained from the brain of laboratory animals (Quick 1935). In the human body, the brain is the most thromboplastin-rich organ. In 1950, it was shown that the meninges of dogs have fibrinolytic activity due to the presence of a plasminogen activator. Subsequently, these data were confirmed for human brain membranes (Takashima, Koga and Tanaka 1969; Fantl and Fitzpatrick 1950; Albrechtsen 1957). J. M. Porter (1969), who observed a high frequency of dissolution of subarachnoid and subdural clots without the development of obstructive hydrocephalus, suggested that meningeal membranes and cerebrospinal fluid have pronounced fibrinolytic activity (Porter et al. 1969).

The presence of fibrinolysis factors in normal CSF was indirectly confirmed by the fact that it has lytic properties. Clinical observations have shown that CSF, even containing a large number of cellular elements or dead nerve tissue, is gradually freed from them by dissolving the cells and removing them in dissolved form outside the subarachnoid space (Moltke 1958; Shamburov 1954).

The development of immunohistochemical methods made it possible to detect the expression of many factors of the hemostasis system in nerve and glial cells of various parts of the central nervous system – prothrombin, factor X, tissue factor, thrombin, antithrombin, thrombomodulin, plasminogen, PAI-1, tPA (Arai et al. 2006; Eddleston et al. 1993; Salles and Strickland 2002). The presence of these factors in brain tissue together with receptors indicates their importance in the work of the central nervous system, especially in the embryonic period and in children, when the processes of cell proliferation, differentiation and migration are most intense. The expression of coagulation factors in the brain is regulated by proinflammatory cytokines and growth factors (Maragoudakis 2009; Paugh et al. 2008; Yepes, Woo and Martin-Jimene 2021).

Thrombin, among other proteinases, under normal conditions regulates the morphology of astrocytes, their migration and proliferation, retraction of the processes of neurons, proliferation of glia, synaptic activity of the brain. The effects of thrombin on nerve tissue in brain damage depend on its expression – in low concentrations it promotes the survival of neurons and astrocytes and the preservation of their functions, in high concentrations it causes their apoptosis (Maragoudakis 2009; Yarovaya, Blokhina and Neshkova 2009). A similar involvement in the processes of cellular regulation was also found for tissue factor, the main sources of which in the brain are astrocytes and arachnoendothelial cells. It participates in embryonic development and inflammatory reactions, promotes tissue healing, angiogenesis, cell adhesion and migration (Cimmino and Cirillo 2018; Hoffman and Monroe 2012; Chu 2011; Zelaya, Rothmeier and Ruf 2018).

The physiological significance of the plasminogen activation system in the brain is due to its participation in the growth, migration and differentiation of neurons, as well as in cognitive functions (Salles and Strickland 2002; Benchenane et al. 2005). High expression of tPA was found in the brain regions responsible for motor skills (cerebellum), endocrine regulation (hypothalamus), fear and anxiety (amygdala), learning and memory (hippocampus), which indirectly indicates the role of the plasminogen activation system in these processes (Salles and Strickland 2002; Strickland 2001). The expression of plasminogen and PAI-1 is detected in a much smaller amount in the brain, which increases in the case of excitotoxic or ischemic damage (Salles and Strickland 2002; Xin et al. 2010).

The plasminogen activation system is capable of having both protective and damaging effects on nerve tissue, depending on the substrate that destroys plasmin (Strickland 2001).

In strokes, tPA is able to potentiate excitotoxic damage to the cerebral parenchyma, activating microglia and leading to degradation of extracellular matrix components and neurons (Benchenane 2005; Xin et al. 2010; Jeon et al. 2012). Plasmin, through its proteolytic function, can participate in the demyelination underlying neurodegenerative diseases (Strickland 2001). Activated tPA plasmin, destroying the connection of neurons with the components of the extracellular matrix, contributes to the death of neurons and the restructuring of synaptic connections in the hippocampus, which are typical morphological signs of temporal lobe epilepsy (McRae and Porter 2012). On the other hand, tPA and plasmin can perform a protective function by splitting fibrin deposits on damaged nerve tissue (Strickland 2001).

PAI-1 in cerebral ischemia prevents apoptosis, reduces brain edema and axonal degeneration. With excitotoxic damage, PAI-1 by inactivation of tPA prevents degradation of the extracellular matrix, protects neurons and promotes axonal regeneration (Xin et al. 2010; Jeon et al. 2012). In inflammatory processes in the brain, PAI-1 suppresses phagocytosis and migration of microglial cells (Jeon et al. 2012). However, in Alzheimer's disease, PAI-1, due to inhibition of tPA, blocks the cleavage of β-amyloid, leading to the progression of the disease.

Factors of Coagulation and Fibrinolytic Systems in the Cerebrospinal Fluid

Hemostasis factors with a small molecular weight are present in small amounts in normal CSF. In people without neurological diseases, plasminogen, its activators, PAI-1, D-dimers, fragments of prothrombin F1+2 were found in the cerebrospinal fluid, and the CSF concentration of TF is 5 times higher than its concentration in the blood (Suzuki et al. 1999; Feng, Guibin and Wenzhou 2003; Weisfelt et al. 2007; Van Dreden et al. 2014). Determination of factors of the coagulation and fibrinolytic systems in the cerebrospinal fluid in CNS diseases revealed their connection with the occurrence of complications and prognosis. In this regard, D-dimers and PAI-1 are the most interesting.

D-dimers in the cerebrospinal fluid under physiological conditions are most likely of plasma origin. The liquor concentration of D-dimers in a healthy person is, according to various authors, from 14 to 500 ng/ml (Feng, Guibin and Wenzhou 2003; Weisfelt et al. 2007; Van Dreden et al. 2014). In CNS diseases, the content of D-dimers in the cerebrospinal fluid increases both due to increased permeability of the blood–brain barrier (BBB), and as a result of lysis of a blood clot or fibrin deposits directly in the subarachnoid space.

PAI-1 in normal CSF is present in a low concentration, from 0.58 to 2.0 ng/ml. The source of PAI-1 in CSF can be the endothelium of small cerebral vessels and glial cells. An increase in the concentration of PAI-1 in the cerebrospinal fluid is observed in subarachnoid hemorrhage (SAH) and intraventricular hemorrhage (IVH) (Feng, Guibin and Wenzhou 2003; Weisfelt et al. 2007; Ikeda et al. 1997). The cerebrospinal fluid concentration of PAI-1 after intracranial hemorrhages correlates with the outcome (Hansen, Lapp and Brugnara 2000; Zoair, Abd El-Aziz and Awny 2008; Dryagina et al. 2013). Higher levels of PAI-1 in the cerebrospinal fluid of patients with vasospasm indicate that this complication of SAH occurs against the background of suppression of fibrinolysis in the subarachnoid space (Ikeda et al. 1997).

Blood, shaped elements, endothelium of small vessels of the meninges and choroidal plexus, as well as glial cells can serve as sources of components of the coagulation and fibrinolytic systems in the cerebrospinal fluid (Suzuki et al. 1999; Ikeda et al. 1997; Anderson, Matthews and Stuart 1978; Hansen 1998). The penetration of coagulation factors from the vascular bed through a damaged or intact BBB does not explain the presence of coagulation factors in the cerebrospinal fluid in quantities, in some cases tens of times higher than their blood levels, as well as the distinct dynamics of cerebrospinal fluid levels with their unchanged plasma content (Suzuki et al. 1999; Ikeda et al. 1997; Kasuya et al. 1988).

Hemostasiological Disorders in Patients with Aneurysmal SAH and Intracranial Hemorrhage

Activation of coagulation and fibrinolysis processes in the cerebrospinal space occurs:

1) in the case of SAH by contact activation via Hageman factor XII after blood contact with collagen trabeculae (internal pathway) (Kasuya et al. 1988);
2) in the case of intracranial hematomas and intraventricular hemorrhages due to the release of TF (external pathway) from damaged brain tissue (Hansen 1998; Kasuya et al. 1988).

The result is the formation and persistence of clots in the cerebrospinal fluid pathways. Following the activation of the coagulation system in the subarachnoid space, the fibrinolytic, kinin and complement systems associated with it are activated (Kasuya et al. 1988). Biologically active compounds formed during the launch of these systems, as well as the breakdown products of erythrocytes in the cerebrospinal fluid, can cause damage to the BBB, trigger inflammatory processes in the subarachnoid space and lead to delayed cerebral ischemia after aneurysmal SAH (Kasuya et al. 1988; Bagley 2000; Dreier et al. 2000). Pronounced activation of coagulation or suppression of fibrinolysis in the subarachnoid space after hemorrhage contributes to secondary ischemic changes due to vasospasm, deterioration of the sanitation of the cerebrospinal fluid pathways from the blood, the occurrence of meningeal fibrosis and hydrocephalus (Hansen 1998; Beuth et al. 1997).

In intracranial hemorrhages, an increase in the concentration of D-dimers in the cerebrospinal fluid is observed, significantly exceeding their plasma levels, which reflects the high intensity of local lysis of blood coagulated in the cerebrospinal fluid pathways. A decrease in the liquor concentration of D-dimers in the first days indicates a slowdown in fibrinolysis in the subarachnoid space, which contributes to the persistence of a blood clot and the occurrence of vasospasm (Hirashima et al. 1997). A high concentration of D-dimers in the blood is a predictor of early neurological deterioration of patients and death in the first week after intracranial hemorrhage (Delgado et al. 2006). In patients who died after suffering severe subarachnoid hemorrhage, there is a negative correlation between the cerebrospinal fluid concentration of D-dimers and the time of death, which may indicate that this indicator reflects more the massiveness of hemorrhage, rather than the intensity of fibrinolysis (Dryagina 2016). The determination of D-dimers can be used to differentiate SAH and traumatic lumbar puncture, in which the cerebrospinal fluid contains an admixture of travel blood (Juliá-Sanchis et al. 2007).

The revealed negative correlation between the time of death and the concentration of PAI-1 in the cerebrospinal fluid after SAH confirms the unfavorable role of inhibition of local fibrinolysis in the cerebrospinal space on the purification of the cerebrospinal tract from blood (Dryagina 2016; Dryagina and Nazarov 2017). According to the results of our studies, in children with intraventricular hemorrhage, the concentration of PAI-1 in the cerebrospinal fluid below 150 ng/ml is a criterion for a favorable prognosis, i.e., recovery without progressive posthemorrhagic hydrocephalus (Dryagina

2016). A more pronounced increase in PAI-1 leads to a significant inhibition of fibrinolysis, which worsens the sanitation of the cerebrospinal fluid pathways from the blood and contributes to the progression of posthemorrhagic hydrocephalus (Hansen, Lapp and Brugnara 2000; Zoair, Abd El-Aziz and Awny 2008; Dryagina et al. 2013). In addition, a link has been established between the high level of PAI-1 in CSF and the ineffectiveness of prescribing fibrinolysis activators to children with IVH (Hansen, Lapp and Brugnara 2000; Zoair, Abd El-Aziz and Awny 2008).

An increase in the levels of coagulation factors and fibrinolysis in the cerebrospinal fluid was found not only after intracranial hemorrhages, but also in other neurological diseases in which damage occurs to the BBB – CNS infections, ischemic stroke, multiple sclerosis, Alzheimer's disease, lymph and myeloblastic leukemia, occurring with the involvement of the central nervous system (Feng, Guibin and Wenzhou 2003; Weisfelt et al. 2006; Kwieciński et al. 2009). The deposition of fibrin on the membranes and brain matter in bacterial infections of the central nervous system is a consequence of the penetration of fibrinogen through the BBB and simultaneous activation of coagulation in the subarachnoid space. The detection of higher concentrations of PAI-1 in the cerebrospinal fluid of patients with bacterial meningitis with subsequent cerebral infarction than in patients without infarction indicates the importance of suppressing fibrinolysis in the pathogenesis of this complication (Weisfelt et al. 2007). A strong correlation of the liquor concentration of PAI-1, D-dimers, and markers of neuronal and astrocyte damage in patients with systemic lupus erythematosus involving the central nervous system may mean that the deposition of fibrin on brain tissue against the background of suppression of fibrinolysis leads to subsequent tissue damage (Kwieciński et al. 2009).

In our opinion, the physiological meaning of the presence of a tissue factor both in the cerebrospinal fluid and in brain tissues is due to the need to quickly stop bleeding, since even a relatively small hemorrhage in the closed cranial space is deadly. Large amounts of thromboplastically active substances coming from the brain tissue into the cerebrospinal fluid during intracranial hemorrhage, traumatic brain injury or as a result of neurosurgical intervention serve as a mechanism for triggering the coagulation of blood trapped in the cerebrospinal space. This activates a cascade of reactions of the coagulation system aimed at the implementation of the main function – stopping bleeding from the cerebral vessels. Just as in the blood, the signal to start the coagulation system is the appearance of TF on the surface of the vascular wall, in the cerebrospinal fluid pathways, the trigger mechanism is the ingress of blood and missing coagulation factors into the cerebrospinal fluid, where TF is contained in physiological conditions.

The high fibrinolytic activity of the cerebrospinal fluid after hemorrhage is explained by the need to quickly sanitize the subarachnoid space, because the persistence of blood clots in the cerebrospinal fluid pathways, leading to a violation of the balance between the production and resorption of the cerebrospinal fluid, can be fatal. The activation of fibrinolysis, necessary for the dissolution of the formed fibrin clot, in the cerebrospinal fluid, as well as in the blood, occurs secondary to the clotting processes and is aimed at sanitizing the cerebrospinal space from clotting products, similar to restoring the patency of the vascular bed after stopping bleeding.

Thus, the coagulation factors contained in the cerebrospinal fluid are involved in the processes of inflammation, make it possible to stop bleeding from cerebral vessels, clear the cerebrospinal fluid pathways from coagulation products or fibrin deposits. Under the influence of these components, the intensity of local processes of coagulation and fibrinolysis of blood entering the cerebrospinal space during neurosurgical intervention or as a result of intracranial hemorrhage is regulated. However, changes in the composition of the cerebrospinal fluid that occur as a result of the receipt of hemostatically active substances from damaged brain tissues can contribute to the systemic activation of the coagulation system and lead to the development of hemostatic complications (Gerlach et al. 2009; Adueva 1996; Kondratiev 1986; Novikov 2004).

Systemic Hemostasis during Neurosurgical Interventions

Any surgical intervention causes activation of coagulation and fibrinolysis processes not only at the site of the surgical wound, but also in the systemic blood flow. These changes are caused by damage to the endothelium and subsequent contact of TF with plasma proteins of hemostasis; the release of plasminogen activators from endotheliocytes and shaped elements; the realization of stress reactions associated with an increase in the concentration of a number of hormones, including adrenaline in the blood; blood loss exceeding 10% of the volume of circulating blood (Kondratiev 1986; Tanaka, Key and Levy 2009). Activation of the hemostasis system during neurosurgical operations is associated, in addition to the listed reasons, with the influence of thromboplastic and fibrinolytic factors of cerebral origin, which is associated with the risk of hemostatic complications (Gerlach et al.

2009; Adueva 1996; Kondratiev 1986; Novikov 2004). However, at present, the problem of hemorrhagic disorders in neurosurgery is not so acute compared to the recent past, since the improvement of surgical intervention technologies has reduced the traumatism and duration of surgery, which has ensured a reduction in intraoperative blood loss and a decrease in the frequency of postoperative hematomas (Gerlach et al. 2009; Gvozdev 2006). Another important component of this issue is the emergence of new methods of general anesthesia, which lead to a decrease in stress activation of the blood coagulation system (Kondratiev 2014). At the same time, the frequency of thromboembolic complications in the systemic bloodstream remains quite high (the frequency of deep vein thrombosis is about 25% of the total number of neurosurgical patients, pulmonary embolism is from 1.5 to 3.5%) and does not tend to decrease (Lubnin 2011; Smith et al. 2015), and the occurrence of postoperative hematomas, despite the low frequency (from 0.7 to 8%), leads to a fatal or unfavorable outcome in 55% of cases (Gerlach et al. 2009).

The powerful buffering properties of the coagulation and fibrinolytic systems in most cases make it possible to avoid significant hemostasis disorders during brain surgery, when the output of coagulation factors into the vascular pool is maximal. With the development of hemorrhagic complications in neurosurgical patients, 2 strategies are used – either to compensate for the deficiency of coagulation factors by transfusion of donor plasma or prothrombin complex preparations, or the introduction of fibrinolysis inhibitors (tranexam). Prevention of thromboembolic complications is carried out taking into account age-adjusted levels of D-dimers, risk assessment of thromboembolic complications according to one of the existing scales, the results of ultrasound examination of the lower extremities. Prevention includes both mechanical measures (compression knitwear) and pharmacological methods (administration of low molecular weight heparins in the postoperative period) (De Hert et al. 2018).

The activation of fibrinolysis occurring during surgery may be secondary to the activation of the coagulation system, and also occur due to the entry into the blood of fibrinolysis activators contained in the endothelium of cerebral vessels in large quantities. Nevertheless, despite the severity of changes in the state of systemic hemostasis, the reliability of blood buffer systems avoids critical disorders in the form of thromboembolic or hemorrhagic complications in most cases of surgical interventions.

Conclusion

Violation of the natural balance between the components of the coagulation and fibrinolytic systems in the cerebrospinal fluid occurs as a result of both the underlying disease and neurosurgical intervention. The severity of the imbalance depends on the severity of the pathological process (disease) and the traumatic nature of the operation.

Further study of biomarkers has great prospects. The search for highly specific markers and their panels, easily detectable in available fluids, with diagnostic and prognostic value, will simplify and speed up diagnosis, determine the severity and mechanism of damage, clarify indications for additional examination methods, evaluate the effectiveness of treatment, predict the outcomes of the disease.

Acknowledgments

The author expresses gratitude to Professor Kozlov A.V., North -Western State Medical University named after I.I. Mechnikov of the Ministry of Health of the Russian Federation, for valuable advice when writing the text, Professor Savvina I.A., Almazov National Medical Research Center, for assistance in preparing and editing the chapter and Dr. Petrova A.O. for translating the text.

References

Adcock, D. M. Ramanathan, R. 2004. "The fluid and tissue phases of the plasminogen system". *Laboratory medicine.* 6(35): 364-367. Published June 1, 2004. doi:10.1309/JKPHN8YUN297P1NE.

Adueva, S. A. 1996. "*Changes in hemocoagulation in patients after removal of brain tumors and ways of their correction*". PhD diss., St. Petersburg. [Russian].

Albrechtsen, O. K. 1957. "The fibrinolytic activity of human tissues". *British journal of haematology.* 3(3):284-291. doi: 10.1111/j.1365-2141.1957.tb05798.x.

Anderson, M., Matthews, K. B., Stuart, J. 1978. "Coagulation and fibrinolytic activity of cerebrospinal fluid". *Journal of clinical pathology.* Published May, 1978. 31(5): 488-492. doi: 10.1136/jcp.31.5.488.

Arai, T., Miklossy, J., Klegeris, A., Guo, J. P., McGeer, P. L. 2006. "Thrombin and prothrombin are expressed by neurons and glial cells and accumulate in neurofibrillary tangles in Alzheimer disease brain". *Journal of neuropathology and experimental neurology.* 65(1):19-25. Published Jan 2006. doi: 10.1097/01.jnen.0000196133.74087.cb.

Bagley, R. S. 2000. "Bleeding into the central nervous system". *Materials of the 18th Ann. Meet. Ved. Med. Forum.* 2000: 334-336.

Benchenane, K., Berezowski, V., Ali, C., Fernández-Monreal, M., López-Atalaya, J. P., Brillault, J., Chuquet, J., Nouvelot, A., MacKenzie, E. T., Bu, G., Cecchelli, R., Touzani, O., and Vivien, D. 2005. "Tissue-type plasminogen activator crosses the intact blood-brain barrier by low-density lipoprotein receptor-related protein-mediated transcytosis". *Circulation.* 111(17):2241-9. Epub Apr 25, 2005. doi: 10.1161/01.CIR.0000163542.48611.A2.

Beuth, W., Kasprzak, H. A., Rość, D., Kotschy, M., Osinski, P., and Śniegocki, M. 1997. "Fibrinolysis disorders in some conditions of neurosurgical practice. Our experiences". *Clinical Neurology and Neurosurgery.* 99(Supplement 1): S43.

Cesari, M., Pahor, M., Incalzi, R. A. 2010. "Plasminogen activator inhibitor-1 (PAI-1): a key factor linking fibrinolysis and age-related subclinical and clinical conditions". *Cardiovascular therapeutics.* 28(5):e72-91. Epub Jul 7, 2010. doi: 10.1111/j.1755-5922.2010.00171.x.

Chu, A. J. 2011. "Tissue factor, blood coagulation, and beyond: an overview". *International journal of inflammation.* 2011:367284. Epub Sep 20, 2011. doi: 10.4061/2011/367284.

Cimmino, G., Cirillo, P. 2018. "Tissue factor: newer concepts in thrombosis and its role beyond thrombosis and hemostasis". *Cardiovascular diagnosis and therapy.* 8(5):581-593. Accessed Oct, 2018. doi: 10.21037/cdt.2018.10.14.

Crawley, J. T. B., Zanardelli, S., Chion, C. K. N. K., Lane. D. A. 2007. "The central role of thrombin in hemostasis". *Journal of thrombosis and haemostasis.* 5 Supplement 1:95-101. Accessed 2007 Jul. doi: 10.1111/j.1538-7836.2007.02500.x.

De Hert, S., Staender, S., Fritsch, G., Hinkelbein, J., Afshari, A., Bettelli, G., Bock, M., Chew, M. S., Coburn, M., De Robertis, E., Drinhaus, H., Feldheiser, A., Geldner, G., Lahner, D., Macas, A., Neuhaus, C., Rauch, S., Santos-Ampuero, M. A., Solca, M., Wappler, F. 2018. "Pre-operative evaluation of adults undergoing elective noncardiac surgery: Updated guideline from the European Society of Anaesthesiology". *European journal of anaesthesiology.* 35(6):407-465. Published Jun, 2018. doi: 10.1097/EJA.0000000000000817.

Delgado, P., Alvarez-Sabin, J., Abilleira, S., Santamarina, E., Purroy, F., Arenillas, J. F., Molina, C. A., Fernandez-Cadenas, I., Rosell, A., and Montaner, J. 2006. "Plasma d-dimer predicts poor outcome after acute intracerebral hemorrhage". *Neurology.* 11;67(1):94-8. Published Jul, 2006. doi: 10.1212/01.wnl.0000223349.97278.e0.

Dolgov, V. V, and Svirin, P. V. 2005. *Laboratory Diagnostics of Hemostasis Disorders.* M.; Tver: Triad. [Russian].

Dolgov, V. V., Vavilova, T. V., and Svirin, P. V. 2019. *Laboratory Diagnostics of Hemostasis Disorders: an Educational and Methodical Manual.* M. Tver: LLC "Publishing House "Triada". [Russian].

Dreier, J. P., Ebert, N., Priller, J., Megow, D., Lindauer, U., Klee, R., Reuter, U., Imai, Y., Einhäupl, K. M., Victorov, I., and Dirnagl, U. 2000. "Products of hemolysis in the subarachnoid space inducing spreading ischemia in the cortex and focal necrosis in rats: a model for delayed ischemic neurological deficits after subarachnoid hemorrhage?" *Journal of neurosurgery.* 93(4):658-66. Published Oct, 2000. doi: 10.3171/jns.2000.
93.4.0658.

Dryagina, N. V., Kozlov, A. V., Lashko, E., Iova A. S., Kryukov E. 2013. "The state of the coagulation and fibrinolytic systems in the cerebrospinal fluid of children with intraventricular hemorrhage". *Neurosurgery and neurology of childhood.* 2(36):92-97. [Russian].

Dryagina, N. V. 2016. "Procoagulant and fibrinolytic properties of cerebrospinal fluid in patients with neurosurgical profile". PhD diss. St. Petersburg. [Russian].

Dryagina N., Nazarov R. 2017. "Components of coagulation and fibrinolysis in the assessment of cerebrospinal fluid clearance after cerebral subarachnoid hemorrhage". *Emergency medical care.* 6(1):49-55. [Russian].

Eddleston, M., de la Torre, J. C., Oldstone, M. B., Loskutoff, D. J., Edgington, T. S., and Mackman, N. 1993. "Astrocytes are the primary source of tissue factor in the murine central nervous system. A role for astrocytes in cerebral hemostasis". *The Journal of clinical investigation.* 92(1):349-58. Published Jul, 1993. doi: 10.1172/JCI116573.

Fantl, P., Fitzpatrick M. 1950. "Fibrinolysis induced by brain extracts". *The British Journal of Experimental Pathology.* 31(2):131-137.

Feng, L., Guibin, Z., Wenzhou, Z. 2003. "Coagulation and fibrinolytic activity in patients with acute cerebral infarction". *Chinese medical journal.* 116(3): 475-477.

Gerlach, R., Krause, M., Seifert, V., Goerlinger, K. 2009. "Hemostatic and hemorrhagic problems in neurosurgical patients". *Acta neurochirurgica (Wien).* 151(8):873-900. Epub Jun 26, 2009. doi: 10.1007/s00701-009-0409-z.

Gvozdev, P. B. 2006. "Reducing the risk of neurological complications in the surgical treatment of deep-localized brain formations using the stereotactic method": PhD diss., Yekaterinburg. [Russian].

Hansen, A. 1998. "CNS fibrinolysis: a review of the literature with a pediatric emphasis". *Pediatric neurology.* 18(1):15-21. Published Jan, 1998. doi: 10.1016/s0887-8994(97)00127-6.

Hansen, A. R., Lapp, S., Brugnara, S. 2000. "Plasminogen activator inhibitor-1: defining characteristics in the cerebrospinal fluid of newborns". *The Journal of pediatrics.* 137(1):132-4. Published Jul, 2000. doi: 10.1067/mpd.2000.106229.

Hirashima, Y., Nakamura, S., Suzuki, M., Kurimoto, M., Endo, S., Ogawa, A., and Takaku, A.1997. "Cerebrospinal fluid tissue factor and thrombin-antithrombin III complex as indicators of tissue injury after subarachnoid hemorrhage". *Stroke.* 28(9): 1666-1670. Published Sep, 1997. doi: 10.1161/01.str.28.9.1666.

Hoffman, M., Monroe 3rd, D. M. 2001. "A cell-based model of hemostasis". *Thrombosis and haemostasis.* 85(6):958-65.

Hoffman, M., Monroe, D. M. 2007. "*Coagulation 2006: a modern view of hemostasis*". Hematology/oncology clinics of North America. 21(1):1-11. Published Feb, 2007. doi: 10.1016/j.hoc.2006.11.004.

Hoffman, M., Monroe, D. M. 2012. "The multiple role of tissue factor in wound healing". *Frontiers in bioscience (Scholar edition).* 4(2):713-21. Accessed Jan 1, 2012. doi: 10.2741/s295.

Ikeda, K., Asakura, H., Futami, K., Yamashita, J. 1997. "Coagulative and fibrinolytic activation in cerebrospinal fluid and plasma after subarachnoid hemorrhage". *Neurosurgery.* 41(2):344-9. Published Aug, 1997. doi: 10.1097/00006123-199708000-00002.

Ismail, A. A., Shaker, B. T., Bajou, K. 2022. "The Plasminogen-Activator Plasmin System in Physiological and Pathophysiological Angiogenesis". *International journal of molecular sciences.* 23(1): 337. Published Dec 29, 2021. doi: 10.3390/ijms23010337.

Ivanciu, L., Stalker, T. J. 2015. "Spatiotemporal regulation of coagulation and platelet activation during the hemostatic response in vivo". *Journal of thrombosis and haemostasis.* 13(11): 1949-1959. Published online 2015 Oct 23. doi: 10.1111/jth.13145.

Jeon, H., Kim, J.-H., Kim, J.-H., Lee, W.-H., Lee, M.-S., and Suk, K. 2012. "Plasminogen activator inhibitor type 1 regulates microglial motility and phagocytic activity". *Journal of neuroinflammation.* 29;9:149. Epub Jun 29, 2012. doi: 10.1186/1742-2094-9-149.

Juliá-Sanchis, M. L., Estela-Burriel, P. L., Lirón-Hernández, F. J., and Guerrero-Espejo, A. 2007. "Rapid differential diagnosis between subarachnoid hemorrhage and traumatic lumbar puncture by D-dimer assay". *Clinical chemistry.* 53(5):993. Published May, 2007. doi: 10.1373/clinchem.2007.085613.

Kasuya, H., Shimizu, T., Okada, T., Takahashi, K., Summerville, T., and Kitamura, K.1988. "Activation of the coagulation system in the subarachnoid space after subarachnoid haemorrhage: serial measurement of fibrinopeptide A and bradykinin of cerebrospinal fluid and plasma in patients with subarachnoid haemorrhage". *Acta neurochirurgica (Wien).* 91(3-4):120-125. doi: 10.1007/BF01424566.

Kondratiev, A. N. 1986. "Changes in hemocoagulation and principles of its correction during removal of brain tumors in conditions of neuroleptanalgesia". PhD diss., Leningrad. [Russian].

Kondratiev, A. N. 2014. *Neurotrauma through the eyes of an anesthesiologist-resuscitator.* Moscow: Medicine. [Russian].

Kwieciński, J., Kłak, M., Trysberg, E., Blennow, K., Tarkowski, A., and Jin, T. 2009. "Relationship between elevated cerebrospinal fluid levels of plasminogen activator inhibitor 1 and neuronal destruction in patients with neuropsychiatric systemic lupus erythematosus". *Arthritis and rheumatism.* 60(7):2094-101. Published Jul, 2009. doi: 10.1002/art.24603.

Lal, I., Dittus, K. Holmes, C. E. 2013. "Platelets, coagulation and fibrinolysis in breast cancer progression". *Breast cancer research.* 15(4):207. doi: 10.1186/bcr3425.

Lubnin, A. Yu. 2011. "*Practical problems of contemporary neuroanesthesiology*". Zhurnal Voprosy Neirokhirurgii Imeni N.N. Burdenko. 2011;75(1):47-56. [Russian].

Maragoudakis, M. E. 2009. *Thrombin: Physiology and Disease.* New York: Springer.

McRae, P. A., Porter, B. E. 2012. "The perineuronal net component of the extracellular matrix in plasticity and epilepsy". *Neurochemistry international.* 61(7):963-72. Epub Aug 29, 2012. doi: 10.1016/j.neuint.2012.08.007.

Moltke, P. 1958. "Plasminogen activator in animal meninges". Proceedings of the *Society for Experimental Biology and Medicine.* 98(2):377-379. doi: 10.3181/00379727-98-24049.

Novikov, V. Yu. 2004. "*Local and systemic changes in hemostasis in children during neurosurgical operations*". PhD diss., St. Petersburg. [Russian].

Paugh, B. S., Paugh, S. W., Bryan, L., Kapitonov, D., Wilczynska, K. V., Gopalan, S. M., Rokita, H., Milstein, S., Spiegel, S. and Kordula, T. 2008. "EGF regulates plasminogen activator inhibitor-1 (PAI-1) by a pathway involving c-Src, PKCdelta, and sphingosine kinase 1 in glioblastoma cells". *FASEB journal.* 22(2):455-65. Epub Sep 12, 2007.doi: 10.1096/fj.07-8276com.

Porter, J. M., Acinapura, A. J., Kapp J. P., Silver, D. 1969. "Fibrinolysis in the central nervous system". *Neurology.* 19(1):47-52.

Quick, A. J. 1935. "The prothrombin in hemophilia and in obstructive jaundice". *Proc. Am. Soc. Biol. Chem., J. Biol. Chemistry.* 109(2): lxxiii-lxxiv.

Salles, F. J., Strickland, S. 2002. "Localization and regulation of the tissue plasminogen activator-plasmin system in the hippocampus". *The Journal of neuroscience.* 22(6):2125-34. Published Mar 15, 2002. doi: 10.1523/JNEUROSCI.22-06-02125.2002.

Sang, Y., Roest, M., de Laat, B., de Groot, P. G., Huskens, D. 2021. "Interplay between platelets and coagulation". *Blood Reviews.* 46: 100733. Published online 2020 Jul 12. doi: 10.1016/J.blre.2020.100733.

Smith, T. R., Nanney 3rd, A. D., Lall, R. R., Graham, R. B., McClendon Jr, J., Lall, R. R., Adel J. G., Zakarija, A., Cote, D. J. and Chandler, J. P. 2015. "Development of venous thromboembolism (VTE) in patients undergoing surgery for brain tumors: results from a single center over a 10 year period". *Journal of clinical neuroscience.* 22(3):519-25. Epub Dec 18, 2014. doi: 10.1016/j.jocn.2014.10.003.

Schuliga, M. 2015. "The inflammatory actions of coagulant and fibrinolytic proteases in disease". *Mediators of inflammation.* 2015:437695. Epub Mar 24, 2015. doi: 10.1155/2015/437695.

Shamburov, D. A. 1954. *Cerebrospinal fluid.* M.: Medgiz. [Russian].

Sillen, M., Declerck, P. J. 2021. "A Narrative Review on Plasminogen Activator Inhibitor-1 and Its (Patho) Physiological Role: To Target or Not to Target?" *International journal of molecular sciences.* 22(5):2721. Published Mar 8, 2021. doi: 10.3390/ijms22052721.

Strickland, S. 2001. "Tissue plasminogen activator in nervous system function and dysfunction". *Thrombosis and haemostasis.* 86(1): 138-43.

Suzuki, M., Kudo, A., Otawara, Ya., Hirashima, Yu, Takaku, A. and Ogawa, A. 1999. "Extrinsic pathway of blood coagulation and thrombin in the cerebrospinal fluid after subarachnoid hemorrhage". *Neurosurgery.* 44(3):487-494. doi: 10.1097/ 00006123-199903000-00029.

Swieringa, F., Spronk, H. M. H., Heemskerk, J. W. M., van der Meijden, P. E. J. 2018. "Integrating platelet and coagulation activation in fibrin clot formation". *Research and practice in thrombosis and haemostasis.* 2(3): 450-460. Accessed 2018 May 20. doi: 10.1002/rth2.12107.

Takashima, S., Koga, M., Tanaka, K. 1969. "Fibrinolytic activity of human brain and cerebrospinal fluid". *British journal of experimental pathology.* 50: 533-539.

Tanaka, K. A., Key, N. S., Levy, J. H. 2009. "Blood coagulation: hemostasis and thrombin regulation". *Anesthesia and Analgesia.* 108(5):1433-46. Published Jun, 2009. doi: 10.1213/ane.0b013e31819bcc9c.

Van Dreden, P. V., Hue, G., Dreyfus, J. F. Woodhams, B. and Vasse, M. 2014. "Procoagulant phospholipids and tissue factor activity in cerebrospinal fluid from patients with intracerebral haemorrhage". *Advances in hematology.* 2014:576750. Epub Feb 17m 2014. doi: 10.1155/2014/576750.

Versteeg, H. H., Heemskerk, J. W., Levy, M., Reitsma, P. H. 2013. "New fundamentals in hemostasis". *Physiological Reviews.* 93(1):327-58. Published Jan, 2013. doi: 10.1152/physrev.00016.2011.

Weisfelt, M., Determann, R. M., de Gans, J., van der Enda, A., Levi, M., van de Beek, D. and Schultz, M. J. 2007. "Procoagulant and fibrinolytic activity in cerebrospinal fluid from adults with bacterial meningitis". *The Journal of infection.* 54(6):545-50. Epub Jan 4, 2007. doi: 10.1016/J.jinf.2006.11.016.

Xin, H., Li, Y., Shen, L. H., Liu, X., Wang, X., Zhang, J., Pourabdollah-Nejad D, S., Zhang, C., Zhang, L., Jiang, H., Zhang, Z. G., and Chopp, M. 2010. "Increasing tPA activity in astrocytes induced by multipotent mesenchymal stromal cells facilitate neurite outgrowth after stroke in the mouse". *PloS One.* 3;5(2):e9027. Epub Feb 3, 2010. doi: 10.1371/journal.pone.0009027.

Yarovaya, G. A., Blokhina, T. B., Neshkova, E. A. 2009. "Proteinase-activated receptors (PARs) are a signaling pathway initiated by limited proteolysis". *Laboratory medicine.* 10:23-34. [Russian].

Yepes, M., Woo, Y., Martin-Jimene, C. 2021. "Plasminogen Activators in Neurovascular and Neurodegenerative Disorders". *International journal of molecular sciences.* 22(9): 4380. Published Apr 22, 2021. doi: 10.3390/ijms22094380.

Yildiz, S. Y., Kuru, P., Oner, E. T., Agirbasli, M. 2014. "Functional stability of plasminogen activator inhibitor-1". *Scientific World Journal.* 2014: 858293. Epub Oct 15. 2014. doi: 10.1155/2014/858293.

Zelaya, H., Rothmeier, A. S., Ruf, V. 2018. "Tissue factor at the crossroad of coagulation and cell signaling". *Journal of thrombosis and haemostasis.* 16(10):1941-1952. Epub Oct, 2018. doi: 10.1111/jth.14246.

Zoair, A. M., Abd El-Aziz S. A., Awny, M. M. 2008. "Neonatal CSF plasminogen and plasminogen activator inhibitor-1 assay as predictors of posthemorrhagic hydrocephalus". *Journal of Pediatric Neurology.* 6(3): 237-242.

Chapter 6

Subarachnoid Haemorrhage in Pregnancy

Aynagul Zh. Bayalieva*, Munir Mohsin, Veronika R. Davydova and Roman Ya. Shpaner
Department of Anesthesiology and Resuscitation, Disaster Medicine, Kazan State Medical University, Kazan, Russian Federation

Abstract

In this chapter, we describe the clinical, diagnostic, and tactical features of the treatment of subarachnoid haemorrhages (SAH) in pregnant women. SAH in this category of patients is not so rare and accounts for 5 to 13% of all causes of maternal death. Surgical treatment for SAH is carried out at any stage of pregnancy if there is a threatening haemorrhage clinic. In the absence of signs of haemorrhage, pregnant women should be observed throughout the pregnancy. In such cases, it is possible to perform operative delivery and neurosurgical surgery. The chapter will present physiological changes in the body of pregnant women, which are important to consider in the treatment of SAH. Based on the pharmacological effects of drugs used to treat patients of this category, their effect on the fetus, and options for safe methods of pain relief during surgical treatment will be presented. A characteristic will be given to the drugs used during the neurosurgical intervention in terms of safety for the fetus at various stages of pregnancy. In the chapter, we will consider the postoperative management of pregnant women with SAH. The chapter will address the issues of the prevention of pulmonary embolism in pregnant women with SAH.

*Corresponding Author's Email: bayalieva1@yandex.ru.

In: Aneurysmal Subarachnoid Hemorrhage
Editor: Irina Savvina
ISBN: 979-8-88697-251-1

Keywords: stroke, subarachnoid haemorrhage, pregnancy, eclampsia, preeclampsia

Introduction

Subarachnoid haemorrhage (SAH) is a type of stroke, which occur when there is bleeding in the subarachnoid space around the brain. SAH during pregnancy and postpartum period results in catastrophic maternal outcomes. There are few demographic estimates of pregnancy-related SAH, however, pregnancy including the postpartum period may increase the risk of SAH. SAH increases maternal mortality and significant morbidity; the risk of the unborn child is also significant in this population group. Urgent neurosurgical conditions usually override obstetrics considerations and the treatment of SAH is similar in both pregnant and non-pregnant women. Effective management of such patients demands a thorough knowledge of the physiology of pregnancy and the pathophysiology of different obstetric conditions.

Epidemiology

It is difficult to obtain a precise epidemiological perspective on SAH in pregnancy. Studies on SAH in pregnancy are scant. There are some studies on intracranial haemorrhage which show the cases of SAH during pregnancy and the postpartum period. One cohort-crossover design study by Jennifer et al., (2020) which were based on the data obtained from all hospital admissions for New York, California, and Florida for a 7-10 year period. Participants included all women (of a different race) admitted for labor and delivery who were older than 12 years and did not have a prior diagnosis of ICH and data were reported as rate ratios and 95% Cls. This study showed that 3 314 945 pregnancies found an increase of ICH during the 3rd trimester (2.9 vs 0.7 cases/100 000 pregnancies) and the first 6-12 post-partum weeks (4.4 vs 0.5 cases/100 000 pregnancies). Pregnancy-related ICH was associated with a higher risk of maternal (relative risk difference, 792.6; absolute risk difference, 0.18) and fetal (relative risk difference, 5.3; absolute risk difference, 0.03) death, compared with pregnancies without ICH. These studies suggest that the risk of ICH is significantly higher during the 3rd trimester of pregnancy and the 1st 12 weeks post-partum (Jennifer et al., 2020;

Jacob and Marcus, 2009; Brian et al., 2012). There are age and race disparities in ICH risk that are associated with devastating maternal and fetal outcomes. These data illustrate the critical need for continuous monitoring and aggressive management of ICH-associated risk factors (Jennifer et al. 2020; Jacob and Marcus, 2009).

Another study by Jacob and Marcus (2009) suggests the overall frequency of pregnancy-related SAH during pregnancy is thought to be 0.01–0.03%. Up to 90% of these SAHs occur during pregnancy, 2% during delivery, and 8% during the puerperium (Jennifer et al., 2020). The tendency for a higher frequency of SAH with advancing gestation suggests that hemodynamic or other physiological changes in pregnancy do influence the rate of aneurysmal growth or rupture (Jacob and Marcus, 2009).

In another study by Brian et al. (2012) in which about 639 cases (5.8 per 100,000 deliveries) of pregnancy were observed in age 15-44 years during the period 1995-2008. During the study period, SAH was associated with 4.1% of all pregnancy-related in-hospital deaths. More than half of the SAH cases occurred postpartum. Advancing age, African-American race, Hispanic ethnicity, hypertensive disorders, coagulopathy, tobacco, drug or alcohol abuse, intracranial venous thrombosis, sickle cell disease, and hypercoagulability were independent risk factors for pregnancy-related SAH. Compared with SAH in non pregnant controls, pregnancy-related SAH had lower clipping/coiling rates (12.7% vs. 44.5%, $P < 0.001$) (Brian et al., 2012).

The risk of SAH was previously believed to be increased during pregnancy (Dias and Sekhar, 1990; Salonen Ros et al., 2001), which can be caused by pregnancy-induced increased circulating blood volume, cardiac output, and the hormonally-induced changes in the arterial wall (Meyers et al., 2000). Recent studies (Kim et al. 2013; Tiel Groenestege et al., 2009) however do not find an increased association between pregnancy or delivery and the risk of rupture of cerebral aneurysms (1.4% and 0.05%, respectively, comparable to the rates of aneurysm rupture in the general population). Parity may confer a moderate long-term protective effect on the risk of SAH (Gaist et al., 2004). Once ruptured, prompt aneurysmal obliteration (either surgical clipping or endovascular coiling) should be undertaken to decrease the rate of poor outcomes.

Vascular Physiology in Pregnancy

It is well appreciated that pregnancy and labour are hyperdynamic states. Blood volume increases in early pregnancy and reaches a plateau at 32 weeks, by which time (during the third trimester) blood volume has increased by 50-60%. Plasma volume increases disproportionately during this time leading to a reduction in haematocrit. Although cardiac output increases by 30–50% over the first 24 weeks of pregnancy, systemic vascular tone falls and blood pressure decreases. During the first stage of labour, cardiac output increases by 50% from the pregnancy baseline. The mean arterial pressure also increases by up to 20% during uterine contractions. By 24 h after delivery, all hemodynamic variables are returned to the prelabour baseline (Robson et al., 1987; Bayalieva et al., 2013).

Normally, the blood-brain barrier (BBB) prevents the extravasation of proteins, sodium, and potassium into the extracellular space of the brain. This uniquely alters local Starling's forces so that the osmotic pressure exerted by ions retained in the vascular compartment opposes the transit of water into the brain. This feature prevents vasogenic edema under usual conditions. Several studies have shown that pregnancy increases BBB permeability in the presence of hypertension, with some regional variation (Euser and Cipolla, 2007).

Cerebral blood flow (CBF) and perfusion pressure have been measured indirectly in pregnancy with transcranial Doppler middle cerebral artery (MCA) flow measurements and velocity-encoded magnetic resonance imaging (MRI). As gestation progresses, MCA flow decreases, and CBF decreases (Cipolla, 2007). Some authors have found that CBF decreases by 20% in the latter stages of pregnancy and posit that vascular resistance falls to minimize the change in perfusion (Zeeman et al., 2003). Probably, the range of cerebral blood flow autoregulation changes during pregnancy, and the relative hypertension of preeclampsia, and eclampsia may lead to rupture of vessels at a lower pressure than in non-pregnant women.

Pregnancy is also a state where changes occur in the haemostatic system. Typically, there is hypercoagulability with alterations in both mechanisms of coagulation and fibrinolysis. Procoagulant factors including factors VII, VIII, and X, von Willebrand's factor, and fibrinogen are increased. Protein S decreases and fibrinolytic activity is also decreased (Brenner, 2004). In the puerperium, physiological intravascular volume changes in the context of this haemostatic milieu may predispose further to thrombotic events.

Preeclampsia and Eclampsia as Risk Factors for SAH

Preeclampsia presents with hypertension blood pressure (BP) greater than 140/90 mmHg and proteinuria >300 mg/day. The clinical flow of preeclampsia is often silent but may cause neurological symptoms like headache, vision disorder, and impairment of consciousness. Eclampsia occurs with seizures but may not have the above neurological symptoms. Some patients also have stroke-like episodes of focal neurological deficit. Systemic vascular resistance increases in preeclampsia with resultant hypertension and reduction in cardiac output and plasma volume (Ganzevoort et al., 2004; Walker, 2000). Major cerebrovascular changes in eclampsia are thought to be similar to those of hypertensive encephalopathy with edema (Mas and Lamy, 1998) and a state of cerebral hyperperfusion. Generally, the imaging features are reversible with neuroimaging characteristics of cerebral edema and a predilection for the posterior parietal and occipital lobes (Cipolla, 2007).

In the same above-mentioned cohort by Jennifer et al., (2020), nearly one-third (35.29%) of pregnant women who experience ICH had eclampsia or preeclampsia. This report showed that ICH during pregnancy or the postpartum period was independently associated with hypertension, gestational hypertension, coagulopathy, and tobacco use. Eclampsia, preeclampsia tends to produce hypertensive encephalopathy like cerebrovascular changes, which leads to cerebral hyperperfusion and edema (Cipolla, 2007). Eclampsia is one of the important causes of serious and often fatal ICH. This study also showed that the ICH during pregnancy and postpartum period has been ascribed to eclampsia-related causes, coagulopathies, and other vascular abnormalities. Pregnancy is generally described as a state of hypercoagulation, which is considered an adaptive physiological response to reduce haemorrhagic risk. However, systematic activation of the coagulation cascade by circulating thromboplastin factors followed by depletion of procoagulants and secondary activation of the fibrinolytic system results in disseminated intravascular coagulation. Disseminated intravascular coagulation manifests as life-threatening haemorrhage and is a major contributor to maternal mortality. In the same data, 9.20% of patients with ICH also had a diagnosis of nonspecific coagulopathy, among whom one-half had disseminated intravascular coagulation (Creanga et al., 2014). These factors were independently associated with ICH risk during pregnancy. Nonspecific coagulopathies may be due to the other rare yet life-threatening complications of pregnancy and eclampsia, such as HELLP (hemolysis, elevated liver enzymes, and low platelet count) syndrome (Haram et al., 2009). Thrombocytopenia, although significantly associated with ICH risk in some analyses, was not independently associated with ICH risk.

Etiologies

SAH during pregnancy is due to a range of etiologies and is less likely to be because by a cerebral aneurysm, than SAH occurring in the non-pregnant patient. SAH in pregnancy frequently occurs in the setting of hypertensive disorders.

SAH is the part of intracranial haemorrhagic syndromes that include bleeding inside of the skull, but outside of the brain like subdural haemorrhage, epidural haemorrhage, and parenchymal bleeding like intracerebral haemorrhage (ICH), contusions, petechial haemorrhage, dural haemorrhages. SAH and ICH are the two most common forms of haemorrhagic stroke. In the general population, SAH is most often associated with an intracerebral aneurysm. SAH and ICH in most pregnancies occur due to ruptured saccular and mycotic aneurysms (Kanani et al., 2007; Jaigobin and Silver, 2000; Powell and Rijhsinghani, 1997) (almost all of the time cause of SAH), ruptured arteriovenous malformations ("

Dias and Sekhar, 1990; Jaigobin and Silver, 2000) (mostly causing ICH), intracranial venous thrombosis (Ko et al., 2007), pregnancy-induced hypertension leading to vessel rupture (Shah, 2003), intracranial vertebral artery dissection (Tuluc et al., 2006), Moyamoya disease (Matsumoto et al., 2009), posterior reversible encephalopathy syndrome, and postpartum angiopathy, which is a form of the reversible cerebral vasoconstriction syndrome (Servillo et al., 2003; Singhal, 2004).

Population-based data by Brian et al., (2012) suggest that the incidence of SAH is increased in the period around delivery (most of the cases were observed in the 3rd trimester). However, a recent study from the Netherlands using a case-crossover study design demonstrated that the risk of aneurysmal SAH is not increased during pregnancy, labour, or the puerperium. This suggests the need for further study, SAH was shown to be a leading cause of indirect maternal mortality in the triennial, Confidential Enquiry into Maternal and Child Health in the United Kingdom; it was second only to cardiac disease and accounted for indirect maternal deaths in 2003–2005 (Lewis, 2007).

Clinical Presentation

Pregnancy does not alter the clinical presentation of SAH. About one-third of patients present with a poor neurological grade, and with impaired consciousness. The other patients who present with a preserved consciousness complaint of sudden onset of severe headache (Jennifer et al., 2020; Jacob and Marcus, 2009; Brian al., 2012) which may be associated with nausea, vomiting, photo- and phonophobia. The headache can be aggravated by physical work, emotional stress, and increased blood pressure (ANSRF, 2015). Sudden and severe headache is accounted for by the sudden rise in ICP which occurs at rupture. Meningism - meningeal irritation caused by blood in subarachnoid space, seizures, and confusion/agitation is mostly seen with SAH and focal neurological deficits due to focal ischemia and/or cranial nerve involvement may be associated with intracerebralhaemorrhage. The initial symptoms may be similar to eclampsia or preeclampsia. At the time of admission, two-thirds of patients have a depressed level of consciousness with a GCS score of less than 8 is usually associated with increased ICP. Systemic dysfunction is common in the acute phase and may include cardiac ischemia, and neurogenic pulmonary edema (WFSA, 2009).

Clinical assessment and investigations can be performed by several grading systems. The World Federation of Neurosurgeons (WFNS) clinical grading system is used world widely (Table 1).

Table 1. WFNS Grading scale for SAH. GCS, Glasgow Coma Score (WFSA, 2009)

Grade	GCS score	Motor deficit
I	15	Absent
II	13-14	Absent
III	13-14	Present
IV	7-12	Present or absent
V	3-6	Present or absent

Diagnosis

Immediate unenhanced (non-contrast) computed tomography (CT) is the investigation of choice for diagnosing SAH. Cranial CT is indicated in all patients complaining of sudden onset severe headache lasting for longer than one hour and with no alternative explanation. There may be a temptation to use MRI rather than CT in pregnant patients, But MRI is not sensitive in the detection of acute SAH. CT should perform as soon as possible after the patient presents, since SAH may not be evident on delayed CT if blood reabsorption has begun. However, if the presentation is delayed, the sensitivity of CT is reduced and the change in haemoglobin and red cell breakdown makes MRI a more sensitive method of detecting the presence of SAH. CT can miss 2-7% of subtle SAH and in the case of negative CT and MRI, a lumbar puncture with the spectrophotometric examination of CSF for bilirubin will provide definitive evidence of the presence or absence of SAH. Once a diagnosis of SAH has been made, further investigations are performed to identify the cause of SAH, which may be an aneurysm or other pathological process. Differentiation of aneurysm may be performed by contrast CT angiography, MRA, and catheter angiography. Angiography not only identifies the aneurysm but also gives detailed anatomical configuration to optimally manage the SAH. These all investigations should be performed with appropriate shielding of the fetus from ionizing radiation (Jennifer et al., 2020; Jacob and Marcus, 2009; Brian et al., 2012; Dias and Sekhar, 1990; ANSRF, 2015; WFSA, 2009).

Management

There are no separate dedicated guidelines for pregnant patients with SAH. In all patients with SAH after the early making of diagnosis, the interventional occlusion therapy method should be chosen whether endovascular coiling should be done or open Clipping. Early occlusion prevents rebleeding. Early clipping and coiling, within 72 hours, is now the goal for all grades of SAH (WFNS I-V), replacing the previous approach of delayed aneurysm occlusion (until after the period of vasospasm) for poor grade SAH. Early evacuation of subarachnoid blood by clipping may also reduce the incidence of vasospasm (WFSA, 2009).

SAH aneurysm clipping requires a craniotomy, which is performed under general anesthesia (GA). It takes about 4-8h and is better to perform in patients having large (>50 ml) intraparenchymalhaematomas and middle cerebral artery (MCA) aneurysms. It has a mortality rate of 1-3% (Indu et al., 2018).

On the other hand, coiling is a minimally invasive percutaneous endovascular intervention, which is a safe alternative to traditional surgical clipping of the aneurysm, and may be associated with a better outcome in some selected patients. Coiling may be preferred in elderly patients, patients with basilar apex aneurysms, and those presenting with a poor grade SAH. Coiling is a technique in which the packing of an aneurysm is performed with detachable coils, and is performed under general anesthesia. In some low-grade SAH (WFNS I-II) with relatively preserved consciousness coiling is performed without GA. Coiling avoids craniotomy which speeds up the recovery. It is not indicated in about 5-15% of cases, due to the morphology and position of the aneurysm (Indu et al., 2018).

There is a largest randomized controlled trial comparing the two treatments is the International Subarachnoid trial (ISAT). This multicenter randomized trial compared the efficacy and safety of endovascular coiling with surgical clipping in a patient with aneurysmal SAH. This trial enrolled 2143 patients, between 1994-2002 which showed that the poor outcome (death and dependency) for the coiled group was 24% compared with 31% for the clipped group. This trial shows that coiling has 7% survival benefits (Indu et al., 2018).

Time and Method of Delivery

If the gestational age is < 24 weeks, neurosurgical intervention should proceed, and all care should be taken to optimize maternal hemodynamics to preserve fetal well-being. Fetal management following surgery then proceeds as guidelines by obstetric indications.

At gestational age > 24 weeks, one of the following three decisions should be made:

1. The Cesarean delivery followed by neurosurgery as sequential procedures
2. The neurosurgical intervention is followed by the continued support of the pregnancy for as long as possible to ensure fetal maturity.
3. An undesirable but temporary decision to postpone neurosurgical intervention due to the lack of the possibility of specialized neurosurgical care, to perform delivery with subsequent intervention at later date.

The Cesarean section most certainly should be the priority if the gestational age of the fetus is more than 32 weeks. Regardless of the timing of delivery, the fundamentals of avoiding maternal hypoxemia, hypotension, and acid-base changes remain the top priority (Indu et al., 2018).

Radiation Exposure

According to the recommendation of the International Commission on Radiation Protection (ICRP) on Radiological Protection, the radiation threshold above which abortion should be considered is 100 mGy (ICRP, 2000). As well as the report by Kuon et al., with optimized lead shielding the coiling-related fetal radiation is negligible (ICRP, 2000; Kuon et al., 2002). An experiment was performed by Marshman et al. (2005) that utilized a standard body phantom conducted in a digital subtraction angiography (DSA) suite, in a general endovascular procedure the absorbed fetal dose was measured to be 2.8 mGy (which is a magnitude below the risk threshold as mentioned above) (Marshman et al., 2005). Therefore the radiation risk associated with the endovascular procedure is minimal. This might be reassuring to the pregnant patient, especially because abdominal shielding is also employed.

The risk of radiation exposure depends on the time of gestation and the amount of absorbed radiation dose. The most sensitive period is the prenatal period and time of fetal organogenesis (10-12 weeks of gestation). The risks of radiation to the fetus include prenatal death, growth retardation, impaired mental ability, low intelligence quotient, and childhood cancer. Various precautions should be employed, including keeping the radiation dose as low as reasonably achievable levels, minimizing the total time of the procedure, and using decreased magnification and lead shielding of the abdomen. During the third trimester (the period in which most of the SAH occurs) fetal organogenesis has been completed; therefore the above-mentioned risks of radiation to the fetus are negligible (Guidelines, 2018).

Contrast Agent Hazards

The most commonly used contrast agent in endovascular coiling is Omnipaque (iohexol). This contrast is injected through a proximally inserted catheter, which creates a fluoroscopic image of the vascular anatomy of the brain. Reproduction studies have been performed in animals with the maximum recommended human dose. Which demonstrates no evidence of impaired fertility or harm to the fetus by Omnipaque. There is no study has been conducted on humans. Therefore animal reproductive studies are not always predictive of human response; this drug should be used during pregnancy only if the expected benefits overweigh the risks (Drug.com).

Anticoagulants Hazards

The anticoagulant of choice during pregnancy is heparin, as it does not cross the placenta due to its highly ionized polysaccharide structure. Warfarin, on the other hand, is contraindicated in pregnancy, as it readily crosses the placental membrane and has a potential teratogenic effect on the fetus. If fetal distress is detected by FHR monitoring, the heparin should be immediately reversed and the procedure canceled (Indu et al., 2018).

Goals to Maintain Perioperative Condition of the Patients

1. To prevent a rise in intracranial pressure or the development of brain edema.
2. To maintain cerebral homeostasis with adequate cerebral perfusion pressure.
3. To maintain uteroplacental perfusion and fetal oxygenation by avoiding hypoxia, hypotension, hypocapnia, acidosis, and hypothermia
4. To maintain hemodynamic stability, particularly at the induction and maintenance phases until the aneurysm is secured.

General anesthesia (GA) may be performed for clipping and coiling (for coiling; WFNS grade III-IV, grade I-II can be performed without GA depending on conditions of consciousness); and the principles are the same for both. Give a good neuroanesthesia understanding of neurophysiology is very essential. The cerebral perfusion pressure (CPP) should be maintained, sudden swings in intracranial pressure (ICP) should be avoided, transmural pressure gradient of an aneurysm (TMPG) should be controlled, optimal brain relaxation for surgery should be provided and enable rapid awakening for assessment in good clinical grade patients (WFSA, 2009).

The CPP=MAP-ICP thus an adequate MAP for brain perfusion and oxygenation is very essential, especially in the presence of impaired autoregulation and elevated ICP (normal ICP-5-15 mmHg; more than 20 mmHg shows intracranial hypertension). The MAP should be 90-110 mmHg for an adequate CPP. TMPG=MAP-ICP, therefore maintenance of the MAP, maintains the TMPG to avoid the sudden aneurysm rupture. Patients with good clinical grade I-II or with no neurological deficit and normal ICP may tolerate a lower MAP which also avoids the risk of aneurysm rupture. However, the patients with poor clinical grade III-IV depend on the high MAP for cerebral perfusion (WFSA, 2009).

Monitoring

Along with basic monitoring electrocardiography (ECG), non-invasive blood pressure (NIBP), pulse oximetry (SpO_2), and end-tidal carbon dioxide concentration ($ETCO_2$). Invasive blood pressure monitoring is indicated like arterial blood pressure and CVP before the induction to have close control of blood pressure in this crucial time, if available. IBP is also required to have close control of uteroplacental perfusion and oxygenation. Fetal heart rate (FHR) monitoring may be useful to guide and maintain adequate uterine perfusion and oxygenation. All patients should have urinary output and core temperature measured. Some patients can have ICP monitoring which may be useful during induction.

Some neurophysiological monitoring like evoked potentials and jugular venous bulb monitoring has not been shown to improve the outcome and is not routinely used (ANSRF, 2015; Thorsten et al., 2013). The bispectral index scale (BIS) is a simple, noninvasive, and continuous electroencephalographic monitor that could reflect the level of consciousness. Can be used as a predictor of neurologic outcomes in patients with SAH during GA or sedation (Wang et al., 2015). The BIS value should be ranged from 80-70 for sedation and 60-50 during GA (Yousefi-Banaem et al., 2020).

Brain Relaxation

Optimal brain relaxation increases surgical exposure and facilitates the clipping of aneurysms. Brain relaxation can be achieved by maneuvers, brain ventricular drains, and pharmacological agents.

Positioning

Proper positioning of the neurosurgical patient is very important to decrease the ICP. 15-30° head up position is optimal to decrease the ICP. Excessive neck flexion or rotation should be avoided. The endotracheal tube should be taped instead of typing around the neck (ANSRF, 2015; Thorsten et al., 2013). Also, the pregnant women should be placed in the left lateral tilt position at 30° to avoid vena cava compression and return of the blood (Frédérique and Pascale, 2006).

Hyperventilation

Temporary hyperventilation to produce mild hypocapnia (aiming for $PaCO_2$ of 30 mmHg) causes cerebral vasoconstriction and can reduce the bulk in poor grade patients. However, excessive hyperventilation carries the risk of inducing cerebral ischemia, especially in poor-grade patients. Thus the use of hyperventilation should be individualized according to the operating conditions. A reasonable approach is to institute mild hypocapnia (30-35 mmHg) before the dura is open, moderate hypocapnia (25-30 mmHg) after the dura is open and normocapnia during induced hypotension and after the aneurysm is clipped (ANSRF, 2015; Thorsten et al., 2013; Pong and Lam, 2010).

Mannitol

Use of mannitol in pregnancy is limited. Mannitol has been assigned to pregnancy category C by the FDA. Animal studies have not been reported. There are no controlled data on human pregnancy. Mannitol is only recommended for use during pregnancy when the benefit outweighs the risk.

It is an osmotic diuretic, is usually the first choice of drug to decrease the brain water content, and is often administered post induction of anesthesia for surgical clipping. If the BBB is damaged as occurs with brain damage, then mannitol may follow its pressure gradient and worsen cerebral edema. Its mechanism of action is complex and can cause electrolyte dysbalance and metabolic acidosis. Mannitol is usually given as a 20% solution, at a dose of 0.5-1.0g/kg over 20 minutes. Quick administration of mannitol can cause an abrupt decrease in ICP, which may increase the risk of aneurysm rupture (ANSRF, 2015; WFSA, 2009; Thorsten et al., 2013). Mannitol worsens the condition in patients with renal impairment. It can also worsen the electrolyte abnormalities, including hyponatremia (increasing the intravascular water in the first phase). In the second phase of action, mannitol gets excreted in the urine with excess free water, potentially causing hypernatremia due to the induced diuresis. Electrolytes should be monitored carefully with mannitol use (Steven et al., 2022).

Hypertonic Saline

NaCl 3% is equally effective with 20% mannitol in the extent of brain relaxation. However, mannitol remains the agent of choice for intraoperative brain relaxation. Hypertonic saline can also impair the electrolyte balance of the blood (Indu et al., 2018).

Furosemide

A meta-analysis of almost 7000 neonates that were exposed to diuretics during pregnancy, did not find an increased risk of adverse effects, such as birth defects, fetal growth restriction, thrombocytopenia, or diabetes, among neonates exposed to diuretics in utero (Mosa et al., 2009). It reduces the CSF formation and water and ion movement across the BBB. The usual dose of 5-20 mg is sometimes given in combination with mannitol (or used alone at higher doses) to enhance its effect, but caution should be employed to avoid over dieresis and hypervolemia (WFSA, 2009).

CSF Drainage

Provide an effective means of reducing brain bulk by decreasing the volume of CSF. Using of lumber subarachnoidal or ventriculostomy catheter is an effective method to achieve satisfactory brain relaxation. During the insertion of drain CSF loss should be minimized, sudden decrease in ICP, as to avoid an abrupt change in TMPG and rebleed of an aneurysm (Indu et al., 2018; Thorsten et al., 2013).

Anesthetic Conduct

The principles of administering smooth anesthetic care are discussed above. It is very important to maintain normal uteroplacental circulation for the development of a healthy fetus, therefore about this, an adequate depth of anesthesia should be achieved to maintain an arterial pressure within 20% of baseline, and avoid sudden increases which may increase the TMPG and thus cause aneurysm rupture. At the same time, maintenance of arterial pressure within 20% of baseline, maintaining adequate uterine blood flow and normal placental function. Transfer of drug through the placenta occurs by simple diffusion, the rate of which depends on the physicochemical characteristics of the drug, such as molecular size, protein binding, lipid solubility, and degree of ionization. Inhalational agents cross the placenta freely due to their low molecular weight and high lipid solubility and may be able to cause fetal depression if administered for a long duration (WFSA, 2009; Indu et al., 2018).

Induction of anesthesia is usually intravenous. Induction agents can be used as Propofol (most commonly used due to its rapid redistribution and metabolism), Thiopental sodium, and Etomidate (which are good alternatives to Propofol). Ketamine has been avoided in the past due to its effect on ICP; however recent evidence of its safe use in head injury is emerging. It has been demonstrated that a 1-1.5 mg/kg dose of Ketamine can reduce the ICP and increase the CPP (Eric and Michele, 2013). Although Ketamine crosses the placenta rapidly, it does not produce neonatal depression unless used in doses above 1-1.5 mg/kg (Demet Dogan and Ismail, 2018). All these above-mentioned induction agents have limited effect on the fetus due to their rapid redistribution and metabolism.

Neuraxial anesthesia is recommended for obstetrical procedures but is contraindicated in acute neurological conditions that can raise ICP (NYSORA).

Muscle relaxants preferably should be used as non-depolarizing muscle relaxants (NDMR) (like Rocuronium, and Vecuronium, as these are recommended and have a relatively short time of onset and rapid elimination (Demet Dogan and Ismail, 2018) are less lipophilic and predominantly ionized at physiological pH and their rate of transfer therefore limited. The depolarizing muscle relaxant (DMR) succinylcholine can also be used with caution as it may cause a slight increase in cerebral blood flow and ICP in some patients. However there exist some controversial studies on the use of succinylcholine in C-sections and neurosurgeries) (Abu-Halaweh et al., 2007; Carlos et al., 2017).

The reversal agents used like Atropine is a lipid-soluble tertiary amine and would be expected to cross the placenta in the form of the free base therefore may cause tachycardia in the fetus and can be used if the benefit outweighs the risk to the fetus. Neostigmine can cross the placenta and should be used with atropine to avoid fetal bradycardia (Grant et al., 2021). Glycopyrrolate is a beta-agonist that may potentially interfere with uterine contractility. Animal studies with Glycopyrrolate do not indicate direct or indirect harmful effects concerning reproductive toxicity at clinically relevant exposures (Kuczkowski, 2004). Regarding Sugammadex, no safety studies had been conducted in humans, and therefore, unless it is a case of vital necessity, it is discouraged to use because of potential harm (Nicolas and Félix, 2015).

Remifentanil given as an infusion can be titrated against the blood pressure and used to obtund the pressor response at intubation. Opioids have a relatively low degree of ionization and considerable lipid solubility. They cross the placenta readily and because pH is lower in the fetus, will be subject to ion trapping (WFSA, 2009; Indu et al., 2018).

Maintenance of anesthesia is the same for both pregnant and non-pregnant patients. Anesthesia can be maintained with either volatile or total intravenous anesthesia. Sevoflurane is the first choice volatile agent, as it causes the least change in cerebral blood flow (and thus ICP) at concentrations of 1 MAC. At deeper levels of anesthesia, cerebral vasodilatation will occur (WFSA, 2009; Indu et al., 2018). Intravenous agents (propofol, thiopental, remifentanil, fentanyl, etc.) have the advantage of reducing cerebral blood flow and metabolic rate, thus conferring some cerebral protective effect, which may be of significance in patients with raised ICP. However large and prolonged doses of the above-mentioned drugs should be avoided as they may increase the risk of toxic and teratogenic effects (Bayalieva et al., 2013).

Mechanical ventilation should be maintained as normoventilation. Positive end-expiratory pressure (PEEP) can impair cerebral venous drainage and can increase the ICP.

There are several critical stimulating points, including insertion of a head pin and raising of a bone flap which may require boluses of remifentanil to overcome the pressor response. Similarly, there will be stages of minimal surgical stimulation, especially after opening the dura. This is preferable to reducing the depth of anesthesia, but awakening and coughing of the patient should be avoided. When it may be necessary to administer a vasopressor such as phenylephrine or noradrenaline to maintain the MAP.

A randomized prospective International Hypothermia Aneurysm Trial (IHAST), which include 1001 patients, with WFNS grade I-III showed that induced mild hypothermia (33°C) has not been shown to improve neurological outcomes after craniotomy for aneurysm clipping and lead to a higher incidence of bacteremia. Normovolaemia should be the goal until the aneurysm is clipped, the careful volume loading may help to reduce the incidence of postoperative cerebral vasospasm (WFSA, 2009).

The use of short-acting analgesics, such as remifentanilperioperatively is ideal, to wake up all good clinical grade patients postoperatively to assess their neurological status.

Postoperatively in the recovery phase, all patients should be admitted to ICU. The emergence should be rapid and smooth, to allow early neurological assessment. The pregnant patient is at a high risk of aspiration following extubation and therefore extubated only after the patient is fully awake and airway reflexes are intact. If emergence is delayed, or there is some new neurological deficit, then CT or angiography should be performed.

Postoperative Concerns

The patient is closely monitored in ICU. Correction of hypertension by antihypertensive drugs should be performed. Adequate postoperative analgesia should be achieved for maternal comfort and morbidity and to reduce undesirable hemodynamic changes. Multimodal analgesia using local infiltration of the incision site/scalp blocks, intravenous paracetamol or acetaminophen, and opioids such as morphine 2-5 mg should be administered. Tramadol is discouraged in neurosurgical patients because it lowers the seizure threshold. The non-steroidal anti-inflammatory drugs can also be used if there are no contraindications.

Deep Vein Thrombosis Prophylaxis

Pregnant women have a 4-5 fold increased risk of thromboembolism compared to the non-pregnant population, which is due to a hypercoagulation state. European Stroke Organization Guidelines forThe Management of Intracranial Aneurysms and Subarachnoid Haemorrhage show the combination of stockings and intermittent pneumatic compression may be the preferred strategy for prophylaxis of DVT. Pharmacological prophylaxis with heparin and low molecular weight heparin like enoxaparin 40 mg subcutaneous after surgery may increase the risk of bleeding (Indu et al., 2018; Annika et al., 2021).

Statins are not recommended in pregnancy due to their teratogenic effect. The recently published placebo-controlled randomized trial results and meta-analysis did not show any effect of statins on the development of clinical outcome SAH (Dean and Alethea, 2016).

Antifibrinolytic drugs such as tranexamic acid or antiplatelet drugs can improve outcomes. The potential protection offered against re-bleeding is offset by the increased risk of thromboembolism and cerebral ischemia (Roos et al., 2003; Clinical trail, 2018).

Cerebral Vasospasm/Ischemia

In about two third of SAH patients, cerebral vasospasm is most likely to develop 3-12 days, lasting approximately 2 weeks. Half of the patients develop symptomatic cerebral ischemia, increasing the neurological deficit. It may also lead to increased ICP, secondary to infarction. It can be diagnosed both clinically and radiologically, using angiography, CT angiography, and transcranial Doppler (TCD). A large amount of subarachnoid blood on CT is a predictor of the development of vasospasm.

Prophylaxis of vasospasm includes oral nimodipine 60 mg orally every 4 hours, for 21 days. The oral or NG route is as effective as IV administration but is associated with less hypotension (WFSA, 2009; Frédérique and Pascale, 2006). However, animal studies have demonstrated that nimodipine might increase the risk of intrauterine growth retardation and congenital abnormalities; however, in a given situation risk and benefit should be weighed against the overall maternal and fetal outcome. The usual practice is still to administer nimodipine in all cases having SAH (Magee et al., 1996).

Although, the pregnant patients are somewhat protected from cerebral artery vasospasm in their relatively hemodiluted and hypervolemic state. However, hypertension, hypervolemia, and hemodilution (triple-H) should be maintained as the cerebral blood flow depends on the blood pressure once autoregulation is impaired, therefore an increase in blood pressure, and a decrease in blood viscosity, may reverse vasospasm. To achieve good cerebral blood flow systolic blood pressure should be 120-150 mmHg in untreated aneurysms and up to 200 mmHg in aneurysms that have been clipped or coiled. Regarding triple-H therapy, serious complications, including pulmonary edema, respiratory insufficiency, and myocardial ischemia should be recognized and managed (WFSA, 2009).

The patients who have deteriorating neurological function are unresponsive to medical treatment. Angiography with balloon angioplasty with or without concomitant intra-arterial administration of papaverine can be done, which can dilate the dependent artery. The complications including arterial dissection rupture and thrombosis can increase morbidity and mortality (WFSA, 2009; Indu et al., 2018).

Magnesium sulfate the drug of choice for preventing and treating eclampsia has been shown to reduce the severity of vasospasm after SAH. However, according to MASH-2 (Magnesium for Aneurysmal Subarachnoid Haemorrhage), randomized placebo-controlled trials revealed that magnesium treatment is not superior to placebo in the reduction of poor outcomes (Indu et al., 2018; Thorsten et al., 2013).

Complications of SAH

Cardiac Dysfunction

The sympathetic nervous system is affected by the SAH, which causes the excessive release of catecholamines and cardiac dysfunction. This leads to systematic and pulmonary hypertension, neurogenic pulmonary edema, cardiac dysrhythmias, myocardial infarction, and cardiogenic shock. ECG and cardiac troponin may be abnormal in this regard. Management is mainly supportive of the administration of inotropes and mechanical ventilation (WFSA, 2009; Thorsten et al., 2013).

Electrolyte Dysbalance

Electrolyte dysbalance occurs in both pregnant and non-pregnant patients with SAH, secondary to either cerebral salt wasting syndrome (CSWS) or inappropriate secretion of antidiuretic hormone (SIADH). Hyponatremia with volume depletion is the commonest electrolyte abnormality which is caused by the secretion of the brain and arterial natriuretic peptide, which is managed by the IV administration of normal saline and hydrocortisone. SIADH is associated with excessive free water loss, which is managed with normal or hypertonic saline instead of water restriction. Potassium, calcium, and magnesium should be controlled and corrected with appropriate supplementation. Hyperglycemia may occur secondary to sympathetic stimulation should be correct and can improve the outcome. Recommendation for Blood Glucose Management-Hyperglycemia over 10 mmol/l should be treated (WFSA, 2009; Thorsten et al., 2013).

Antiepileptic Treatment

The development of seizures in pregnant with SAH has not been studied yet. But the pregnant patients with SAH are 2-3 fold more prone to develop seizures due to their altered physiology. Seizures have been seen in patients 7-10% with SAH, this incident may increase in pregnant. Intermittent or continued EEG monitoring does not improve the outcome. There are prospective, randomized, double-blind, placebo-controlled trials that suggested that the outcome was worse in the 65% of patients receiving prophylactic antiepileptic drugs than in the other 35% of patients who did not receive prophylactic antiepileptic medication. Given the lack of evidence in favor of prophylactic treatment with antiepileptic drugs and the possible disadvantage of serious adverse drug reactions, the current advice should be not to start antiepileptic drugs as prophylactic treatment until seizures are clinically apparent (Thorsten et al., 2013).

However, despite it, phenytoin is commonly used in neurosurgical patients, yet its deleterious effect in pregnancy like fetal hydantoin syndrome (includes microcephaly, craniofacial abnormalities, distal phalangeal hypoplasia, and developmental delay) (Hanson and Smith, 1975). Similar abnormalities have been seen with barbiturate use. Neural tube defects have been observed with sodium valproate. Carbamazepine may have the least risk of teratogenicity, but it is not commonly used in acute neurosurgical practice because of the lack of an intravenous preparation (WFSA, 2009).

Steroids

A Cochrane review placebo-controlled trial on hydrocortisone in patients with SAH showed that it does not improve the clinical outcome (class IV, level C). This drug should be used during pregnancy only if the potential benefit justifies the potential risk to the fetus (Thorsten et al., 2013; Drug.com, 2021).

Clinical Case

We present in this chapter of the book a clinical case in which the patient after a cesarean section developed: subdural hematoma with the displacement of the median structures of the brain and the development of ischemia of the brainstem, subarachnoid haemorrhage with severe vasospasm and the formation of 3 ischemic foci. The etiology of this pathology is difficult to establish.

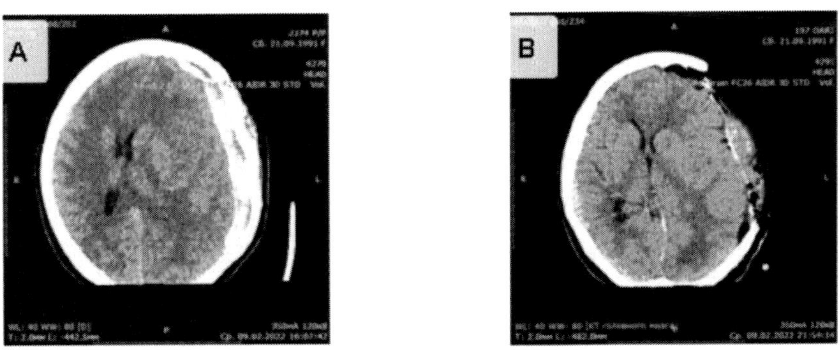

Figure 1. Patient O., 31 years old. CT scan of the brain, axial view. Acute subdural hematoma of the left fronto-parietal-temporal region, about 120 cm3 in volume. Lateral dislocation of the brain (A). Condition after decompressive craniotomy in the left fronto-parietal-temporal region, removal of an acute subdural hematoma (B).

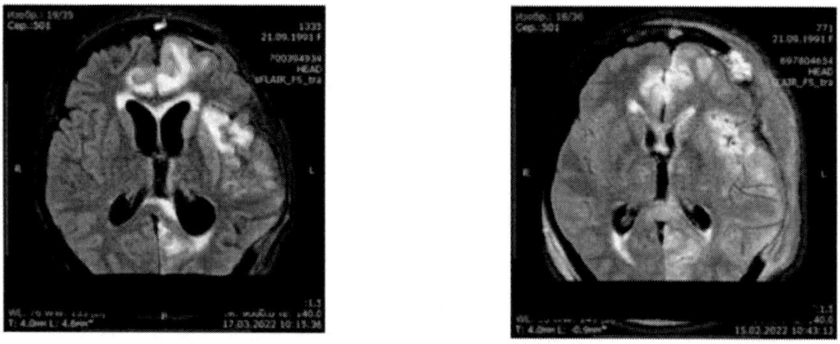

Figure 2. Patient O., 31 years old. Brain MRI, axial view, Flair IP. 7th day after decompressive craniotomy in the left fronto-parietal-temporal region, removal of an acute subdural hematoma. A fragment of a subdural hematoma with a volume of about 5 cm3 in the region of the left frontal lobe. Regression of lateral dislocation. In the medial sections of both frontal lobes, the insula of the left temporal lobe and the medial sections of the left occipital lobe, zones of ischemic changes are determined. The ventricular system of the brain is expanded. The medulla prolapses into the bone defect.

A 31-year-old woman was admitted to the maternity hospital with the diagnosis: Pregnancy at 33 weeks. Underweight fetus with Frank Breech presentation. Mild anemia. Vaginitis. Subclinical hypothyroidism. Patient later laser correction of vision.

In the hospital, the woman was taken under observation and given general supportive therapy for two weeks. After that, it was decided to perform a cesarian section (CS) at 35 weeks of pregnancy due to the severe fetal growth retardation (FGR), chronic decompensated placental insufficiency, and pelvic breech presentation of the fetus.

CS was performed under spinal anesthesia (SA) with Bupivacaine 0.5% 12.5 mg. The course of the CS and SA was without any significance. An alive female, low weight (1990 g) neonate was delivered with Apgar score-5-6. After CS woman was shifted to the ICU with normal consciousness and stable hemodynamics, from where after recovering from anesthesia, shifted to the after-birth observation department. She was prescribed pain killers Tramadol 100 mg IM once and Paracetamol 1 g PO three a day but the patient refused to take Paracetamol as her Visual analog scale score was 0-1.

The next day afternoon she complained of a sudden severe headache, and soon after lost consciousness. GCS was 6-5 (moderate coma). To protect the airway and to confirm adequate oxygenation patient was shifted to MV with slight hyperventilation. After taking emergency labs and performing a CT scan without contrast, it was diagnosed as subdural hematoma and SAH with dislocation of middle structures (Figure 1A).

It was decided to perform emergency left-sided decompression trepanation of the skull and evacuated 120 ml of blood (histological examination of hematoma showed, no malformation found) (Figure 1B). This life-saving surgery was performed under GA. During anesthesia, MAP was kept at 90-110 mmHg. The neurological status of the patient after surgery was a coma, GCS- 5.

During anesthesia, MAP was kept at 90-110 mmHg. The neurological status of the patient after surgery was a coma, GCS- 5. MRI of the brain of the patient on the 7th day after neurosurgical intervention is shown in Figure 2. Tracheostomy was performed on the 10th day after surgery and mechanical ventilation (MV) continued sedation for MV was performed by Dexmedetomidine IV infusion. The effectiveness of MV was controlled by ABGs. Treatment of vasospasm is performed with nimodipine 60 mg PO every 6h under control of BP. Control of electrolytes, blood glucose level, and fluid balance was observed. Anticonvulsant therapy was performed with Valproic acid infusion 0.8 - 1.35 мг/кг/час. Nutritional support was observed on a daily calories bases. DVT prophylaxis was started soon after surgery, an elastic bandage was applied, and on the 3rd day after surgery, Enoxaparin had been started due to the large hematoma and risk of rebleeding. Hemodynamics was stable, breathing was adequately through tracheostomy, and oxygenation was normal. The patient was shifted to the neurological department with a chronic persisting neurological deficit with low rehabilitation potential, for further management.

In summary, the algorithm for diagnostics and treatment of pregnancy patients with SAH is shown in Figure 3.

Conclusion

Although SAH is rare, it is an important cause of morbidity and mortality during pregnancy. Subarachnoid haemorrhage occupies a special place in the pathologies of the nervous system in pregnant women. It can be a complication of pathologies of pregnancy, such as hypertension, preeclampsia, HELLP-syndrome, DIC, and other coagulopathies; the background may be cerebral vascular pathologies like cerebral aneurysms and vascular malformations. Any obstetric pathology with hypertension should be under the supervision of specialists (therapists and cardiologists) and blood pressure should be corrected. In this way, the development of complications can be prevented. In several cases, pregnancy proceeds without complications during the whole course of pregnancy. Subarachnoid haemorrhage develops due to the rupture of an aneurysm, which had previously been asymptomatic. Treatment should be based on the same principles as those for non-pregnant patients with awareness of the influence that pregnancy has on certain conditions.

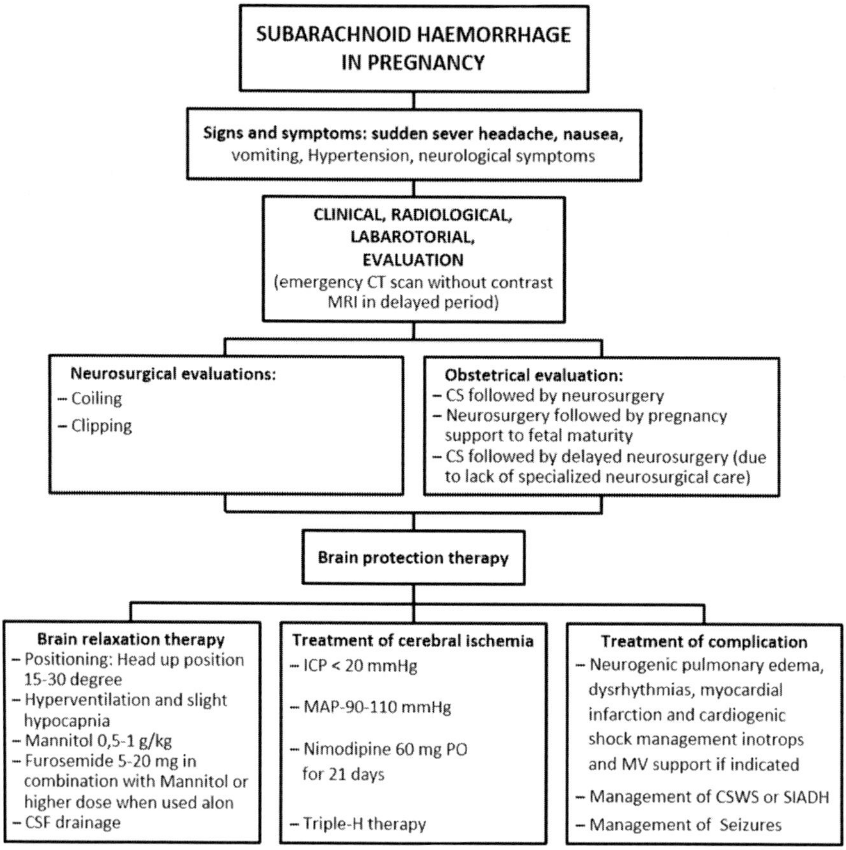

Figure 3. The algorithm of diagnostics and treatment of pregnancy patients with SAH.

The clinical case, which is presented in this chapter, demonstrates that in addition to subarachnoid haemorrhage, subdural haematoma, pronounced dislocation syndrome, vasospasm, secondary ischemia, and cerebral edema have been developed. Despite the severity of brain damage and the development of a deep stupor in a short period, the neurosurgical decompression within an hour gave positive results and saved the patient's life. It is rare in obstetric practice when obstetric and neurosurgical services are present in the same hospital, and decisions about surgery are quickly made. At present, necessary investigations, and effective treatment of subarachnoid haemorrhage and intracranial haematomas in obstetrics, as a multidisciplinary problem in medicine, there are few clinical guidelines and treatment protocols in both obstetrics and neurosurgery.

References

Bateman B. T., Olbrecht V. A., Berman M. F., Minehart R. D., Schwamm L. H., &Leffert, L. R. 2012. Peripartum Subarachnoid Hemorrhage: Nationwide Data and Institutional Experience. *Anesthesiology*. 116:324–333. doi:10.1097/ALN.0b013e3182410b22.

Bayalieva A. Z., Shpaner R. Y., Bogdanova E. I., Ganeeva I. R. 2013. Features of anesthesia in pregnant women with subarachnoid haemorrhages. *Kazan medical journal*. 9(1): 89-95. doi: 10.17816/KMJ1778.

Bayalieva A. Z., Shpaner R. Y., Bogdanova E. I., Ganeeva I. R. 2013. Conducting anesthesia in pregnant women with subarachnoid hemorrhages. *Vestnik sovremennoi klinicheskoi medicine*. 6(5): 85-90. doi: 10.20969/VSKM.2013.6(5).1-170.

Bowles Eric D., Michele E-Gold. 2013. Rethinking the paradigm: evaluation of ketamine as a neurosurgical anesthetic. 81(1):18.

Brenner B. 2004. Hemostatic changes in pregnancy. *Thromb Res*. 114:409 –14.

Carlos Marcelo, Luis Abramides, Torres Hans, Donald de Boer. 2017. Is there still an indication for the use of succinylcholine in cesarean section? *Brazilian Journal of anesthesiology*. 67(5).

Cipolla M. J. 2003. Cerebrovascular function in pregnancy and eclampsia. *Hypertension*. 50:14– 24.

Clinical recommendations. 2015. Surgical treatment of non-traumatic ICH in pregnancy. Association of Neurosurgery of Russian Federation.

Clinical trial. gov. 2018. "Tranexamic acid in pregnancies with vaginal bleeding." Last update: 01.22.2020. https://clinicaltrials.gov/ct2/show/NCT03632824.

Committee Opinion No. 723. 2018. Guidelines for Diagnostic Imaging During Pregnancy and Lactation. *Obstet Gynecol*. 132(3):786. doi: 10.1097/AOG.0000000000002858.

Creanga A. A., Berg C. J., Ko J. Y., et al. 2014. Maternal mortality and morbidity in the United States: where are we now? *J Women's Health*. 23(1):3-9. doi:10.1089/jwh. 2013.4617.

Dean G. Karalis, Alethea N Hill. 2016. *The risks of statin use in pregnancy: a systematic review*. doi.1016/j.jacl.2016.07.002.

Demet Dogan Erol and Ismail Aytac. 2018. Current anesthesia for Cesarean Section. *Clinical journal of obstetrics and gynecology*. 1:061-066. doi: 10.29328/journal. jog.1001011.

Dias M. S., Sekhar L. N. 1990. Intracranial hemorrhage from aneurysms and arteriovenous malformations during pregnancy and the puerperium. *Neurosurgery*. 27:855–866.

Drug.com. *Iohexol Pregnancy and Breastfeeding Warnings*. https://www.drugs.com/pregnancy/iohexol.html.

Drug.com. 2021. *Hydrocortisone topical pregnancy and breastfeeding warning*. Last update Apr 21, 2021. www.drugs.com/pregnancy/hydrocortisone.html.

Euser A. G., Cipolla M. J. 2007. Cerebral blood flow autoregulation and edema formation during pregnancy in anesthetized rats. *J Hypertension*. 49:334 –40.

Fairhall Jacob M., Marcus A. Stoodley. 2009. Intracranial hemorrhage in pregnancy. Published online 2009 Nov 30. doi: 10.1258/om.2009.090030.

Frédérique Henry, Pascale Quatresooz. 2006. Blood vessel changes during pregnancy: areview. *American journal of clinical dermatology*. 7(1):65-9. doi: 10.2165/00128071-200607010-00006.

Gaist D., Pedersen L., Cnattingius S., Sorensen H. T. 2004. Parity and risk of subarachnoid hemorrhage in women. *Stroke*. 35:28–33.

Ganzevoort W., Rep A., Bonsel G. J., de Vries J. I., Wolf H. 2004. Plasma volume and blood pressure regulation in hypertensive pregnancy. *J Hypertension*. 22:1235–42.

Grant A. Neely, Sarah Sabir, Arpan Kohli. 2021. Neostigmine. Last update: 22.08.2021. https://www.ncbi.nlm.nih.gov/books/NBK470596/.

Hanson J. W., Smith D. W. 1975. "The fetal hydantoin syndrome." *J Pediatric*. 87:285–90.

Hantsche A., Wilhelmy F., Kasper J., Wende T., Hamerla G., Rasche S., Meixensberger J., Lindner D. 2021. Early prophylactic anticoagulation after subarachnoid hemorrhage decreases systemic ischemia and improves outcome. *Clinical Neurology and Neurosurgery*. 207:106809. doi: 10.1016/j.clineuro.21.106809.

Haram K., Svendsen E., Abildgaard U. 2009. The HELLP syndrome: clinical issues and management. *BMC Pregnancy Child birth*. 9(1):8. doi:10.1186/1471-2393-9-8.

International Commission on Radiological protection. 2000. Pregnancy and medical radiation. *Ann ICRP*. 30:1-43.

Jaigobin C., Silver F. L. 2000. Stroke and pregnancy. *Stroke*. 31:2948–51.

Kanani N., Goldszmidt E. 2007. Postpartum rupture of an intracranial aneurysm. *Obstet Gynecol*. 109:572–4.

Kapoor Indu, Charuma Hajan, Heman Shuprabhakar. 2018. *Pregnancy with subarachnoid hemorrhage*. http://www.snacc.org/wp-content/uploads/2018/06/SAH-with-pregnancy-FINAL.pdf.

Kim Y. W., Neal D., Hoh B. L. 2013. Cerebral aneurysms in pregnancy and delivery: pregnancy and delivery do not increase the risk of aneurysm rupture. *Neurosurgery*. 72:143–150.

Ko Y. P., Hsu C. Y., Yang C. L, Cheng S. J., Tsai H. J., Chen C. P., Hsu Y. W. 2007. Postcesarean subarachnoid hemorrhage as the initial presentation of cerebral venous thrombosis. *Taiwan J Obstet Gynecol*. 46:317–9.

Kuczkowski K. M. 2004. Nonobstetric surgery during pregnancy: what are the risks of anesthesia? *Obstet Gynecol Surv*. 59:52 –6.

Kuon E., Schmitt M., Dahm J. B. 2002. Significant reduction of radiation exposure to operator and staff during cardiac interventions by analysis of radiation leakage and improved lead shielding. *Am J Cardiol.* 89:44–49.

Lewis G. 2007. The Confidential Enquiry into Maternal and Child Health. Saving mothers' lives: Reviewing maternal deaths to make motherhood safer – 2003–2005. The 7th report of the Confidential Enquiries into Maternal Deaths in the UK. London, CEMACH, 2007.

Magee L. A., Schick B., Donnenfeld A. E., Sage S. R., Conover B., Cook L., McElhatton P. R., Schmidt M. A., Koren G. 1996. "The safety of calcium channel blockers in human pregnancy: a prospective, multicenter cohort study. *Am J Obstet Gynecol.* 174:823 –8.

Marshman L. A., Rai M. S., Aspoas A. R. 2005. Comment to "endovascular treatment to ruptured intracranial aneurysms during pregnancy: report of three cases." *Arch Gynecol Obstet.* 272:93.

Mas J. L., Lamy C. 1998. Stroke in pregnancy and the puerperium. *J Neurol.* 245:305 –13.

Matsumoto Y., Asada M., Mukubou M. 2009. Postpartum subarachnoid hemorrhage due to Moyamoya disease associated with renal artery stenosis. *J Obstet Gynaecol.* 35:787–9.

Meeks J. R., Bambhroliya A. B., Alex K. M., Sheth S. A., Savitz S. I., Miller E. C., McCullough L. D., Vahidy F. S. 2020. Association of primary intracerebral hemorrhage with pregnancy and the postpartum period. Jama network open. *Neurology.* April 14, 2020. doi:10.1001/jamanetworkopen.2020.2769.

Meyers P. M., Halbach V. V., Malek A. M., Phatouros C. C., Dowd C. F., Lawton M. T., Lempert T. E., Higashida R. T. 2000. Endovascular treatment of cerebral artery aneurysms during pregnancy: report of three cases. *Am J Neuroradiol.* 21:1306–1311.

Mosa'b Al-Balas, Pina Bozzo, Adrienne Einarson. 2009. Use of diuretics during pregnancy. *Canadian Family Physician.* 55(1): 44–45.

NYSORA. Neuroaxial anesthesia. https://www.nysora.com/techniques/neuraxial-and-perineuraxial-techniques/spinal-anesthesia/.

Pong R. P., Lam A. M., 2010. "Anesthetic management of cerebral aneurysm surgery." In: *Cottrell's and Young's Neuroanesthesia,* ed. Cottrell J. E., Oung W. L. 218-46. 5th ed. Philadelphia: Mosby Elsevier.

Powell S., Rijhsinghani A. 1997. Ruptured bacterial intracranial aneurysm in pregnancy. A case report. *J Reprod Med.* 42:455–8.

Robson S. C., Dunlop W., Boys R. J., Hunter S. 1987. Cardiac output during labour. *Br Med J.* 295:1169 –72.

Roos Y. B., Rinkel G. J., Vermeulen M., Algra A., van Gijn J. 2003. Antifibrinolytic therapy for aneurysmal subarachnoid haemorrhage. *Cochrane Database Syst Rev.* CD001245.

Salonen Ros H., Lichtenstein P., Bellocco R., Petersson G., Cnattingius S. 2001. Increase drisks of circulatory diseases in late pregnancy and puerperium. *Epidemiology.* 12:456–460.

Sami Abu-Halaweh, Islam Massad, Hamdi M. Abu-Ali, Izdiad Z. Badran, Bassam A. Barazangi, Michael A. Ramsay. 2007. Rapid sequence induction and intubation with 1 mg/kg rocuronium bromide in cesarean section, comparison with suxamethonium. *Saudi Medical Journal*. 28(9):1393-6.

Servillo G., Striano P., Striano S., Tortora F., Boccella P., De Robertis E., Rossano F., Briganti F., Tufano R. 2003. Posterior reversible encephalopathy syndrome (PRES) in critically ill obstetric patients. *Intensive Care Med*. 29:2323–6.

Shah A. K. 2003. Non-aneurysmal primary subarachnoid hemorrhage in pregnancy-induced hypertension and eclampsia. *Neurology*. 61:117–20.

Singhal A. B. 2004. Postpartum angiopathy with reversible posterior leukoencephalopathy. *Arch Neurol*. 61:411–6.

Steiner T., Juvela S., Unterberg A., Jung C., Forsting M., Rinkel G. 2013. European stroke organization guidelines for the management of intracranial aneurysms and subarachnoid haemorrhage. *Journal of cardiovascular diseases*. 35(2):93-112. doi: 10.1159/000346087.

Steven Tenny, Roshan Patel, William Thorell. 2022. "Mannitol" Last Update: February 21, 2022. https:// www.ncbi.nlm.nih.gov/books/NBK470392/.

Task Group on Control of Radiation Dose in Computed Tomography. 2000. Managing patient dose in computed tomography. A report of the International Commission on Radiological Protection. *Ann ICRP*. 30:7–45.

Tiel Groenestege A. T., Rinkel G. J., van der Bom J. G., Algra A., Klijn C. J. 2009. The risk of aneurysmal subarachnoid hemorrhage during pregnancy, delivery, and the puerperium in the Utrecht population: case-crossover study and standardized incidence ratio estimation. *Stroke*. 40:1148–1151.

Tuluc M., Brown D., Goldman B. 2006. Lethal vertebral artery dissection in pregnancy: A case report and review of the literature. *Arch Pathol Lab Med*. 130:533–5.

Varela Nicolas., Félix Lobato. 2015. Sugammadex and pregnancy, is it safe? *Journal of Clinical Anesthesia*. 27(2):183-184.

Walker J. J. 2000. Pre-eclampsia. *Lancet*. 356:1260– 5.

Wang A. Y., Huang C. H., Chang W. T., Chen W. J. 2016. Bispectral index monitoring in subarachnoid hemorrhage–associated out-of-hospital cardiac arrest. *American journal of emergency medicine*. 34(5):934.e1-3. doi: 10.1016/j.ajem.2015.09.025.

WFSA. Management of subarachnoid haemorrhage. Anaesthesia tutorial of the week 163. 7th December 2009. https://resources.wfsahq.org/atotw/managememt-of-subarachnoid-haemorrhage-anaesthesia-tutorial-of-the-week-163/.

Yousefi-Banaem H., Goharani R., Hajiesmaeili M., Tafrishinejad A., Zangi M., Amirdosara M., Nashibi M. 2020. A Review of Bispectral Index Utility in Neurocritical Care Patients. *Arch Neurosci*. 7(3):e96490. doi: 10.5812/ans.96490.

Zeeman G. G., Hatab M., Twickler D. M. 2003. Maternal cerebral blood flow changes in pregnancy. *Am J Obstet Gynecol*. 189:968– 72.

Chapter 7

Differential Diagnosis and Treatment Tactics for Subarachnoid Hemorrhage in Children

Eleonora T. Nazaralieva[1,2,*], PhD and William A. Khachatryan[1], PhD

[1]Department of Pediatric Neurosurgery, Almazov National Medical Research Centre of Ministry of Health Care of Russian Federation, Saint Petersburg, Russian Federation

[2]National Hospital of Ministry of Health of Kyrgyz Republic, Bishkek, Kyrgyzstan

Abstract

In this chapter, we will focus on the etiological factors in the development of SAH in children, and the features of SAH in young children. According to statistical studies, the symptoms of SAH in children in the first year of life occur with approximately the same frequency as in adult patients. The frequency of SAH in children can vary from 1.9% to 4.6%. Timely differential diagnosis of SAH and assessment of the severity of the condition of a small patient is extremely important since SAH in children is one of the ten most common causes of death. The overall mortality of children with aneurysm rupture and SAH ranges from 13 to 34% in observations. Currently, earlier verification of SAH in children is the result of improved diagnostic capabilities and increased clinical awareness. SAH in childhood belongs to the group of heterogeneous conditions with a variable clinical picture and various etiological factors; therefore, the improvement of diagnostic methods and management tactics is a priority task of modern pediatric neurosurgery. In this chapter,

---

*Corresponding Author's Email: neleonora@yandex.com.

In: Aneurysmal Subarachnoid Hemorrhage
Editor: Irina Savvina
ISBN: 979-8-88697-251-1

we outline the principles of surgical and conservative treatment of children with SAH, depending on the etiological factor in the development of hemorrhage.

Keywords: subarachnoid hemorrhages, cerebral aneurysm, arteriovenous malformation of the brain, treatment of subarachnoid hemorrhages

Introduction

Although subarachnoid hemorrhages (SAH) relate to a rather rare pathology of childhood, there has been an increase in the number of SAH in recent years, including in children. According to statistical studies, symptoms of SAH in children in the first year of life occur with approximately the same frequency as in adult patients. The frequency of SAH in children can vary from 1.9% to 4.6%. Wider detection of SAH in children is probably the result of improved diagnostic capabilities and increased clinical awareness (Levy et al. 2022).

SAH in children is one of the top ten most common causes of death. The estimated mortality after the first bleeding in children is from 11 to 20% in comparison to 20-30% in adults. According to observations, the total mortality of children by ruptured aneurysm and SAH ranges from 13 to 34% (Levy et al. 2022; Shinkawa et al. 2018, 461-463; Skoch et al. 2017, 2153-2157).

This disease in childhood relates to a group of heterogeneous conditions with a variable clinical picture and etiological factors, therefore, the improvement of diagnostic methods and management tactics is a priority issue in modern pediatric neurosurgery.

The Main Causes of Subarachnoid Bleeding in Children and the Mechanisms of Disease Progress

SAH is a hemorrhage in the subarachnoid space (between the arachnoid membrane of the brain and soft tissues). SAH is diagnosed at any age, including in children from 0 to 18 years. Two main groups of SAH in childhood are neurosurgical and pediatric diseases.

The neurosurgical pathologies are arterial aneurysm, arteriovenous malformation of the brain arteries and spinal cord, Moyamoya disease, and brain tumors.

The main pediatric causes are blood diseases (haemoblastosis), chemotherapy treatment, severe infectious diseases with sepsis, v itamin K deficiency, connective tissue diseases, a cardiovascular pathology (heart defects, aortic coarctation).

Further, we will consider the main diseases that could cause SAH in children.

Aneurysms of Cerebral Arterial Vessels in Children

The aneurysm of cerebral arterial vessels is an abnormal dilation of the vessel wall. In this case, the most serious and formidable complication is the ruptured aneurysm. Cerebral arterial aneurysms are extremely rare in children in comparison to in adults, they are 4% of all intracranial aneurysms (Amelot et al. 2019).

Currently, there is no convincing evidence of the presence of any provoking factor for the aneurysm progress. Because the aneurysms are mostly located in the area of artery bifurcation, it is assumed that changes in hemodynamic indicators could cause the progress of the aneurysm (da Cunha and da Cunha Correia 2018, 219-221).

Congenital fenestration of the brain artery can also causeaneurysm formation. The arterial vessel fenestration is the split of the artery lumen into two channels, meanwhile, each channel will have its endothelium. Adventitia can be common or also separate, creating additional connecting "bridges." The fenestration of the brain vessels is a consequence of a dysfunction of the primitive vessels (embryonic arteries) formation or incomplete artery obliteration. Mostly, the vascular fenestration is in the anterior communicating artery and the middle cerebral artery during the research of the brain arteries (Krystkiewicz et al. 2021, 85-92).

The cerebral aneurysms are divided into single and multiple (10%). They can be small (<5 mm), large (6-24 mm) or giant (>25 mm) in size. There are histological characteristics such as sac-fusiform or delaminating during morphological research. Most often, the brain aneurysms are localized in the internal carotid artery, the middle cerebral artery, and the anterior cerebral artery (75%), in the main artery (25%). The location and size of the brain aneurysms are the same in children and adult patients (Krings et al. 2010, 1309-1318). It was impossible to find information in the literature on the detection of aneurysms duringroutine autopsy examinations in children. This may be due to the symptomatic nature of the aneurysmal dilations in children (Krings et al. 2010, 1309-1318).

The main causes of aneurysms in adults are aging of the body, hypertension, smoking, and alcohol and drug abuse. These factors do not matter in children, mostly the aneurysms are formed as "defective defense mechanisms" (Lasjaunias 2000, 160-165). Examples, abnormal self-repair of the vascular wall, systemic or genetic diseases with defects in the genes of the vascular wall or connective tissue (Marfan Syndrome, Ehlers-Danlos Syndrome), brain injuries, and inflammatory and infectious diseases. According to the literature, the causes of aneurysms in childhood can be detected in about 50% of cases, traumatic aneurysms are 5-10% of cases, and infection is 15% (Lasjaunias et al. 2006, 789-850). The saccular (classical) aneurysms occurred in 30% of cases, the dissection occurred more often in the first five years of the child's life.

Traumatic aneurysms are diagnosed in 5-10% of pediatric patients. The aneurysms localization in the distal part of the anterior cerebral artery is 40%, 35% of cases are in large vessels along the skull base, and 25% of cases are in distal cortical vessels (Hahn et al. 1990, 360-364; Ventureyra and Higgins 1994, 361-379; Yazbak et al. 1995, 15-19). The classic clinical picture after the injury is the progress of the hemorrhagic bleeding approximately 2-4 weeks after the first injury. At the same time, most of the children had a closed head injury. The traumatic brain injury causes the formation of a false sac (pseudoaneurysm). An extravascular hematoma is formed due to the destruction of the arterial wall throughout, which connects to the lumen of the artery. The fibrin complexes at the same time form the wall of the false aneurysm (Krings et al. 2008, 315-329).

Also, children may have aneurysms that have been caused by previous or current infectious diseases. For the first time, such aneurysms were described more than 100 years ago. In 1901 patients had bacterial endocarditis, and previously such aneurysms were called "mycotic arterial aneurysms" (Lasjaunias 2000, 160-165). This term is not used now, because most often such aneurysms have bacterial etiology. The term "infectious arterial aneurysm" is found in the literature (Barrow et al. 1990, 572-563; Bohmfalk et al. 1978, 369-382). According to the literature, approximately 15% ofintracranial aneurysms are caused by an infectious process. It is possible to detect Staphylococcus aureus, streptococci, and other gram-negative bacteria during detecting bacteria. The cerebrospinal fluid is seeded in compliance with all the rules for detecting microorganisms (Choux 1992, 123-131). Most often, the infectious aneurysms are localized in the distal arteries of the brain or near the skull base and cavernous sinuses. One of the mechanisms of aneurysm formation in case of infection is the direct action of infectious emboli on small-diameter vessels. If the aneurysm is located in the large vessels of the skull base, then this is a consequence of a long-term infection (osteomyelitis of the wedge-shaped sinus, thrombophlebitis of the cavernous sinus, infection with carotid artery damage). In this case, the infection spreads from the outside toward the vessels (Krings et al. 2008; Marsot-Dupuch et al. 2000, 891-898). Patients with infectious aneurysms have multiple characteristics. During angiography, they look likesmall aneurysms that can turn into hematoma. They can be fusiform without a neck, or they can be the false aneurysm, where the "neck" is the remainder of a ruptured vessel, and the "aneurysm" is the cavity of a hematoma.

The saccular aneurysms (often referred to as "classic" in the literature) are rarely found in newborns and children under 8 years of age. According to statistics, the number of saccular aneurysms increases in direct proportion with age (Lasjaunias et al. 2005, 437-450). Most often they are located in the bifurcation zone.

The aneurysm dissection is the most common pathogenetic mechanism of SAH formation due to the aneurysms in children. According to foreign sources, newborns and children in the first years of life have aneurysm dissection in 50% of cases. The dissection of the aneurysm can have a different clinical picture. We will consider the variants of SAH as a result of the aneurysm dissection. SAH often has a high tendency to repeated hemorrhages in the first 24 hours in 70% of cases, in the first week in 80% of cases, and only 10% of cases have it after 1 month due to the aneurysm dissection (Mizutani and Kojima 2000, 91-97).

Vascular Malformations in Children as a Cause of the Subarachnoid Hemorrhage

Vascular malformations are another cause of SAH in children, it ranks third in the frequency of detection (Fernando et al. 2021). Vascular malformations are a group of vascular lesions with various hemodynamic or structural properties. They can be caused by the following reasons. Moyamoya disease is a chronic occlusive cerebrovascular disease that causes progressive stenosis of the internal carotid artery and its branches. The exact causes of the progress of Moyamoya disease are not fully known. A certain role is given to genetic factors, specifically defects in the genes of class I and class II human leukocyte antigen (HLA) (Krings et al. 2008; Clatterbuck et al. 2001, 1246-12504; Can et al. 2017, 15-24; Google 2022). However, different races have the lesion of different gene loci, which may be the cause of the genetic characteristics of different racial groups. Immunological mechanisms also have an important role. Thus, the content of a large amount of IgG and IgM b C3 complement fraction was detected on the vascular wall in patients with the Moyamoya disease. Some authors observe the connection of autoimmune diseases (systemic lupus erythematosus, Graves' disease, antiphospholipidsyndrome) with vascular hyperplasia and the formation of Moyamoya syndrome (Huang et al. 2017, 246-253).

The capillary telangiectasia consists of capillaries, which have no elastic or smooth muscle fibers; they are thin-walled, but variably expanded structures. These channels with lined endothelium, as a rule, differ from normal capillaries only in caliber (Clatterbuck et al. 2001, 1246-1250).

The arteriovenous malformations are clusters of abnormal arteries and veins with an increased risk of intracranial bleeding, more common in young people. Vascular malformations are an innate feature of vessel development. In the histological description, they are ecstatic, fibrous growths of capillary vessels, which have a thin wall and are capable of spontaneous ruptures. Mortality in the case of vascular malformation rapture with late diagnosis and absence of surgical intervention is up to 30%, disability in 50% of cases (Can et al. 2017, 15-24; Google 2022).

Venous angioma (venous-medullary malformation (VMM)) is the most common malformation involving the intracranial venous system. VMM is characterized by a cluster of radially located medullary venous channels that converge and merge into a collecting vein. It causes the typical appearance of an umbrella or "jellyfish" on cerebral angiography. They are considered congenital anomalies of the brain venous system. The most widely described etiology of the VMM progress is atresia. The atresia is abnormal development or ischemia during intrauterine life with the secondary development of the abnormal venous structure. Considering the angioarchitecture of the medullary venous system, VMM is connected with the absence of superficial or deep venous collectors, which causes a hemodynamic imbalance. This leads to compensatory drainage in the direction of the deep venous system or the pial venous system through the collector's vein. It can be considered an anatomical change in the localized pathway of the venous drainage system of the brain (Nabavizadeh et al. 2016, 463-472). It is detected hyalinization and fibrous thickening, the absence of an elastic plate with poorly located layers of smooth muscles in morphological description (Ruiz et al. 2009, 271-283).

A mixed vascular malformation is vascular spaces of various sizes that are lined with a single layer of endothelin without distinct signs of arteries or veins (Chakravarthy et al. 2016, 458-464).

About 70-80% of the vascular malformations in the brain are located supratentorial and are usually solitary (Dalyai et al. 2011). About 25% of them are located in the brain stem (Abla et. al. 2011, 403-415). Most often, the rupture attacks the spinal cord, dura mater, cranial nerves, skin, and rarely the retina. Patients with vascular malformations should do genetic research for the exclusion of genetically mediated diseases (Abla et al. 2011, 403-415).

Frequent progress of the vascular malformations of the brain with genetic diseases and syndromes was also noted. Randu-Osler syndrome is a genetically determined disease with an autosomal dominant type of inheritance in the ENG gene. It encodes the synthesis of englin or a mutation in the ACVRL1 gene, encoding a receptor-like activin kinase. These mutations cause the dysregulation of angiogenesis with the progress of the mucocutaneous telangiectasia and visceral arteriovenous shunt (spinal, pulmonary, and hepatic) (Kikuchi et al. 1994, 374-80). The vascular malformations in this syndrome are most often located superficially and belong to the capillary type of malformations.

More rare genetic pathologies are capillary malformation type 1. It is a dominant autosomal disease caused by mutations of the RASA1 gene. These patients have multifocal capillary malformations (Josephson et al. 2012, 500-507). Capillary Malformation-Type 2 AVM syndrome is the dominant autosomal disease caused by an EPHB4 mutation. These patients have intra- and extracranial malformations, multifocal capillary malformations, andtelangiectasias (Lawton et al. 1997, 267-274).

Traumatic Subarachnoid Hemorrhages in Children

The traumatic SAH usually occurs near the site of a skull fracture and intracerebral contusion. Radiological signs of traumatic origin are localized bleeding in the superficial furrow, adjacent skull fracture, and brain contusion with external signs of traumatic injury (Shipman et al. 2019, 88-89).

Spontaneous Subarachnoid Hemorrhages in Children Due to Other Causes

The cause of the spontaneous subarachnoid hemorrhage in newborns may be the progress of hemorrhagic disease newborns. The main reason for this condition is a lack of vitamin K.

Vitamin K deficiency can easily develop in infants due to poor vitamin transfer through the placenta, the low vitamin K content in breast milk, and poor intestinal absorption due to immature intestinal flora and malabsorption in premature infants. Bleeding with vitamin K deficiency in infancy is classified by the time interval from the moment of delivery: early bleeding is within 24 hours after delivery, classic is within 1 week after birth, and later is at the age of 2 weeks to 6 months. The hemorrhagic disease in infancy can be life-threatening, especially with a late onset. Therefore, all children, including newborns, should have vitamin K prophylaxis. Exclusively breastfeeding and cholestasis are closely related to this deficiency and cause the late appearance of the hemorrhagic disease symptoms. The hemorrhagic manifestations mainly attack the gastrointestinal tract, skin, and central nervous system and are represented by intracranial and subarachnoid hemorrhages. According to a Japanese study of hemorrhagic nodes, intracranial hemorrhage was reported in 82.7% of infants with the idiopathic hemorrhagic syndrome (Araki et al. 2020).

Analyzing these results, we can conclude, that the causes of SAH in children are diverse, often due to genetic factors or the natural course of certain diseases. SAH in children still has a rare pathology, but it is necessary to identify the risk groups of the possible SAH progress and to do closer monitoring and diagnosis for preventive treatment or prevention.

The Clinical Picture of Subarachnoid Hemorrhages in Children

The onset of SAH is usually sudden and can be accompanied by headache, vomiting, deterioration of consciousness, convulsions, coma, paresis, paralysis of cranial nerves, fever, and meningism. Warning signs that point to large bleeding are sometimes observed in the form of "sentinel bleeding" with headache in 10-15% of patients. Patients may also have focal neurological deficits associated with the aneurysm dilatation, or symptoms of mass effect and cerebrospinal fluid obstruction (CSF) in the giant aneurysm rupture. One of the SAH characteristics is the appearance of symptoms in relative well-being. For example, a child's behavior may change (lethargy, drowsiness, anxiety, excitement). Children under one year old have a "brain cry," vomiting, swelling of the fontanel, decreased appetite, convulsions, focal symptoms, hemorrhagic shock, and retinal hemorrhages.

The symptoms of SAH in children under 5 years old are often accompanied by an increase in intracranial pressure (ICP) and symptoms of volumetric brain damage (Fung et al. 2019). Thus, the leading symptoms in SAH will be nausea, vomiting, swelling of the anterior fontanel, edema of the optic disc, paresis, and plegia.

Methods of Diagnosis of Subarachnoid Hemorrhages in Children

If SAH is suspected, all patients are examined by a neurologist, if it is necessary by a neurosurgeon. According to clinical recommendations, a child with neurological symptoms has a general "routine" neurological examination. If focal or meningeal symptoms are detected, a child has an additional examination, including various diagnostic methods, a general blood test, biochemical blood analysis, electrocardiography, CT of the brain, MRI of the brain, angiography of cerebral vessels, and other necessary examinations.

One of the primary methods of examination in children with focal neurological symptoms is a lumbar puncture. According to modern data from the medical literature, cerebrospinal fluid (CSF) is a dynamic, metabolically active body fluid that has many important functions. This keeps the "buoyancy" of the brain, helps to reduce the functional weight of the brain by 75%, and protects brain tissue from traumatic damage. Since the central nervous system has no lymph nodes, the cerebrospinal fluid also provides an immunological and protective function for the brain. CSF also has a certain antibacterial function and it can inhibit the growth and reproduction of bacteria (Bonadio 2014, 141-150). The cerebrospinal fluid is located in the subarachnoid space. The average volume of CSF ranges from 65 to 150 ml in children 4-13 years old. About 70% of the CSF is formed in the vascular plexuses of the ventricles, a structure of microvilli with a layer of epithelial cells, that are connected by dense connections forming a blood-brain barrier (Bonadio 2014, 141-150).

Normally, the cerebrospinal fluid is an ultrafiltrate of plasma, which consists of 99% water, and also contains protein, electrolytes, enzymes, and antibacterial factors. The presence of certain neurological diseases can be assumed by the change in the main parameters of the cerebrospinal fluid and its density. Therefore, sometimes a lumbar puncture (LP) is required with SAH. LP is contraindicated with increased intracranial pressure. In this case, a sharp pressure decrease in the cerebrospinal fluid can cause a resumption of bleeding from a damaged vessel, due to a decrease in the effectiveness of a thrombotic clot. Characteristic changes of SAH in LP are increased number of erythrocytes ("serrated erythrocytes"), increased fluid pressure, and xanthochromia.

It should be noted that the lumbar puncture is an auxiliary method for the diagnostics of SAH. The main importance in this disease is instrumental diagnostic methods (CT, MRI, angiography of cerebral vessels).

The gold standard for SAH diagnostics is CT of the brain without a contrast agent in the first 4-6 hours from the onset of the disease (Abraham and Chang 2016, 901-916). MRI is done less often due to the frequent lack of equipment in the medical institution. Both of these methods are reliable and highly sensitive for the detection of SAH. False-negative results may be with a small amount of hemorrhage and severe anemia, while the blood will have the same density as the brain tissue. Figure 1 shows the CT of the patient with subarachnoid hemorrhage (Figure 1 A, B, C).

Also, during a CT of the brain, it is possible to detect a lesion of the ventricular brain system, which is one of the prognostic unfavorable signs (Figure 2 A, B, C).

Also, patients with SAH undergo CT angiography with an examination of all four arteries and their branches (2 carotid and 2 vertebral).

The angiographic studies have a particular value during the diagnostics ofvascular malformations since they are often difficult to differentiate according to CT. Not specific signs in CT are bleeding from the vascular malformations that may be manifested by foci of increased density surrounded by an edematous mantle of the "frosted glass" type (Hegde et al. 2012, 380-388). According to MRI of the brain, SAH from the vascular malformations is visualized as a cluster of vessels shaped as "popcorn" or "mulberry" with a rim of signal attenuation on the periphery (Rigamonti et al. 1987, 18-24). MRI diagnostic is preferable since it is not always possible to find hidden bleeding from the malformations in angiography. Considering that CT is associated with a certain radiation strain, it is proposed to use the method of rapid magnetic resonance imaging of the brain (fbMRI) for rapid visualization of hydrocephalus in pediatric patients. The authors of this study emphasize that this MRI protocol can be considered as an alternative to CT diagnostics due to a decrease in radiation strain and an increase in diagnostic value (Shope et al. 2021, 475-481).

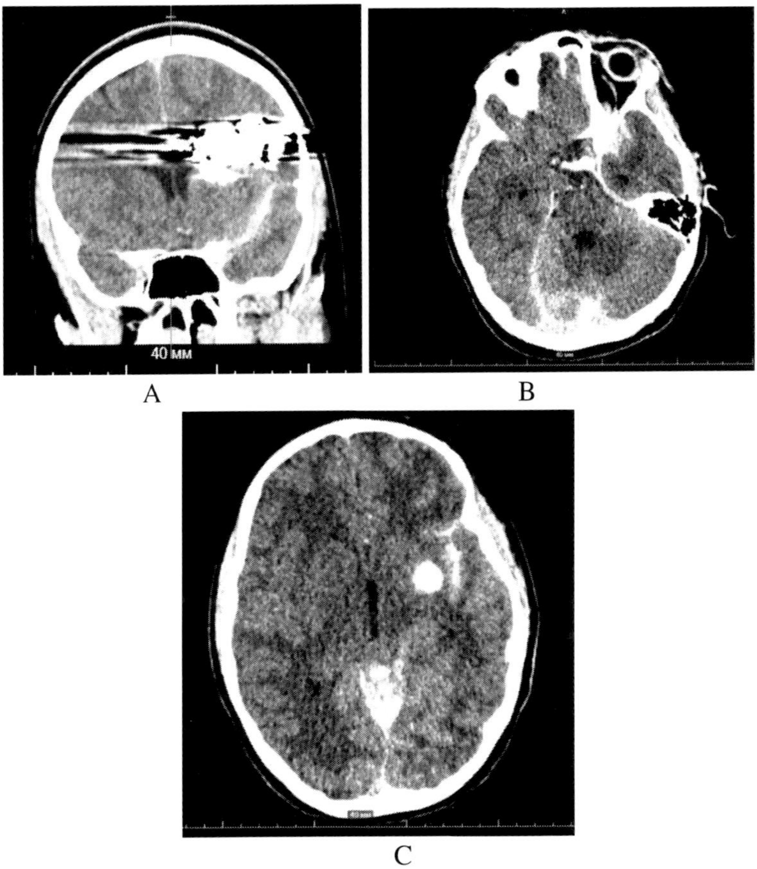

Figure 1. Patient Sh., 16 years old. SAH III. Condition after intravascular embolization of AVM of the left frontal lobe. On the CT scan of the brain, an intracerebral hematoma is determined in the left frontal lobe, against which a cast of embolizate is visualized. A significant amount of blood in the left lateral fissure of the brain, blood along the outline of the cerebellum. MPR in the coronary projection (A), axial projection (B, C).

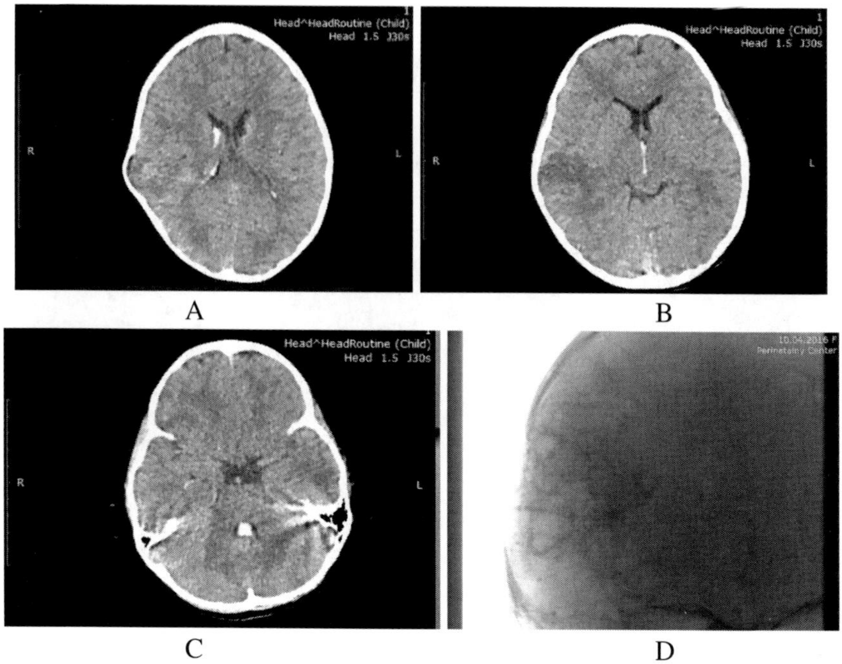

Figure 2. Patient G., 4 years old. AVM of the right temporal and parietal lobes. Intraventricular hemorrhage. On the CT scan of the brain in the axial projection, blood is determined in the right lateral (A), third (B) and fourth (C) ventricles. The ventricular system of the brain is not expanded. Cerebral angiography, direct projection (D). Filling of the AVM in the right temporal and parietal lobes from the hypertrophied branches of the right SMA is revealed, with the discharge of blood into the deep vein of the brain.

Also, the main laboratory tests are conducted for all patients with a general blood test (excluding thrombocytopenia), a study of the coagulogram (APTT, PT, INR).

Therapeutic tactics is determined by the cause of SAH. Currently, no clear algorithms have been devised for the management of children with SAH. Neurosurgeons, neurologists, and interventional surgery specialists act based on clinical recommendations, devised for the treatment of adult patients, but taking into account the peculiarities of the management of children's patients. For example, if there are signs of the traumatic SAH, a neurosurgeon necessarily conducts a consultation to determine the possibility of surgical treatment and the choice of operative tactics (endovascular intervention or brain surgery). If there is a suspicion or signs of an ICP increase, it is necessary to install an ICP sensor. External ventricular drainage is installed according to the indications. A patient should be observed in an intensive care unit for neurological patients. In the case of non-traumatic subarachnoid hemorrhage, it is necessary to establish and eliminate the etiology of the hemorrhage. Neurosurgical tactics depends on the causes of the hemorrhage, the patient's age, general condition, and anatomical and physiological features of the location of the vessel. It is mandatory to evaluate the risks of the surgical intervention and the possibility of conservative management of children. The risks of repeated hemorrhages and vascular ruptures in children are higher than in adult patients due to the peculiarities of the anatomical structure of the aneurysms (fusiform aneurysms) (Ghali et al. 2018, 294-307). It is also necessary to take into account the high risks of secondary infectious complications of the brain (meningitis) during performing "open" brain surgery.

The open neurosurgical operations with SAH include microsurgical clipping of a cerebral aneurysm; external decompression with the plastic of the dura mater, ventriculostomy, and installation of an ICP sensor.

Methods of aneurysms treatment by the clipping or endovascular occlusion are a priority in indications for surgical intervention. The advantages of these surgical techniques are the possibility of preserving and restoring blood supply and blood flow through the brain vessels, reducing the risks of secondary complications.

Microsurgical clipping is the best option when the morphology and etiology of the aneurysm are a contraindication to endovascular intervention. According to laboratory examinations, it is performed evaluations on the size of the aneurysm, its diameter, the convenience of surgical access, the absence of infectious pathology in the patient, and low risks of bleeding (Xia et al. 2017, 411-420; Liu and Huang 2015).

The endovascular method is embolization of the cerebral aneurysm. Thus, surgical and endovascular intervention is the most effective method of treatment for SAH.

At the same time, surgical methods are often associated with high risks of complications and death. For example, spontaneous thrombosis of a damaged artery often occurs in children and good results can be achieved by using conservative methods of treatment. It is not recommended to use the surgical methods for multiple aneurysms and SAH in the outcome of bacterial infections (endocarditis, sepsis).

The endovascular methods are preferred in children with SAH, given the low invasiveness and traumatism. The endovascular treatment is performed with removable platinum spirals. It is considered a first-line treatment for adult patients with ruptured intracranial aneurysms. Figure 3 shows the data of the patient Sh., 16 years old, who had staged embolization of the affected vessel.

The main complications during the endoscopic interventions are aneurysm rupture, stroke, and aneurysm dissection, but it should always be remembered that there may be recurrences of SAH directly from the maternal aneurysm. The endovascular interventions are often associated with high risks of thromboembolic complications and bleeding at the same time, therefore, antiplatelet and/or anticoagulant therapy is necessary (Vachhani et al. 2016; Vargas et al. 2016, 41-45). General algorithms for the treatment of SAH in children, dosages of antiplatelet agents or anticoagulants are often chosen empirically depending on the patient's condition, concomitant diseases, the risk of thromboembolic complications, the patient age. Some studies have demonstrated that long-term monotherapy with antiplatelet drugs is safe for the patient (Bowry et al. 2008, 960-966).

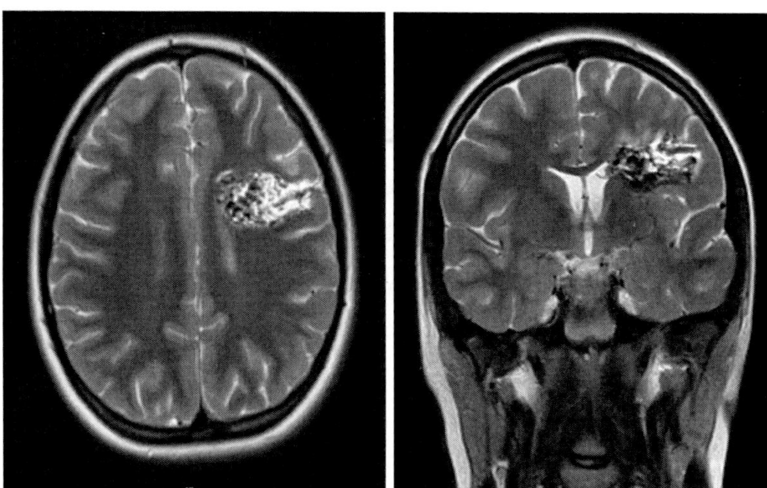

A B

Figure 3. Patient Sh., 16 years old. Condition after intravascular embolization of AVM of the left frontal lobe. On a series of MRI brain T2-VI in axial projection (A) and T2-VI in coronary projection (B) in the left frontal lobe, against the background of a zone of cystic-atrophic changes, AVM with traces of embolizate is detected.

In case of difficulties with the clipping or endovascular interventions, some neurosurgeons consider options for the surgical treatment using bypass blood supply method, shunting of brain vessels. Such aneurysms do not recur in retrospective studies. The necessary conditions for performing these interventions are the presence of the giant (complex) aneurysm, good collateral blood flow through nearby vessels, which can compensate for itself, the operation of a "switched-off" vessel, and the impossibility of performing other surgical interventions (Ganesh Kumar 2017, 250-255).

The main risks with such types of surgery are most often the development of regional hypoperfusion with ischemia of the brain area and an increase in hemodynamic strain on compensatory vessels. It can cause the re-development of the aneurysm in a previously intact vessel due to increased blood flow. It was proposed to use methods of reconstruction of the vessel with a bypass of the site of aneurysmal expansion and bleeding to avoid the progress of such formidable complications. Such methods are used in the treatment of giant aneurysms located in the bifurcation zone of the upper middle cerebral artery (Ganesh Kumar 2017, 250-255).

Such types of surgical aids are associated with general risks of microsurgery, including intraoperative aneurysm rupture, stroke, and graft thrombosis (Ganesh Kumar 2017, 250-255).

An international study of the subarachnoid aneurysm showed that the chances of independent survival for 1 year were significantly higher after the endovascular treatment than after neurosurgical intervention. Modern advances in technology and equipment allow performing the endovascular interventions in infants and newborns (Saraf et al. 2021, 748-750).

Increased intracranial pressure (ICP) is one of the most common causes of secondary brain damage in SAH. It is necessary to constantly monitor the pressure level with the ICP increase to optimize treatment tactics, determine the prognosis of the disease, and monitor the current condition of a patient. The world's leading associations of neurosurgeons have proposed the use of continuous monitoring of ICP to control ICP (Cremer 2005, 2207-2213; Marmarou 1991, 59-66). Monitoring is also actively used for the temporary resolution of hydrocephalus.

It is customary to use "classic" drainage with controlled hydrostatic pressure and drip chambers to control ICP and drainage function, which is the gold standard (Linsler 2013, 1589-1594). However, the disadvantages of this system are the use of droppers restricts the mobility of the patient and may cause unintentional excessive or insufficient drainage during Valsalva maneuvers or patient movements. Therefore, patients are immobilized during drainage (Arts et al. 2021).

Recently, there has been a tendency to use automated ICP control drainage systems. The automated system is a system of cerebrospinal fluid drainage. The system is used for the early mobilization of patients. Its use is destined for patients who require drainage of cerebrospinal fluid due to plastic surgery of the thoracoabdominal aortic aneurysm, and for neurosurgical patients who need ICP regulation. The device is an automated pressure-based cerebrospinal fluid drainage system connected to a catheter. He measures ICP using a pressure sensor, which is fixed by an electrocardiographic sticker on the skin above the temporal bone at the height of the Monroe hole (Kwon et al. 2016, 28-33).

It should be noted that measuring only ICP may not be entirely effective for patients with subarachnoid hemorrhage. Normotensive hydrocephalus is usually diagnosed with this disease, which can cause a high number of premature shutdowns. Perhaps the standard pressure settings in these patients are insufficient. The authors of the study recommend a gradual decrease in pressure parameters or a transition to drainage with a controlled volume to overcome this problem (Arts et al. 2021).

In addition, when patients are in an upright position, the physiological intracranial pressure can become negative, changing with physical exertion or movement (Brimioulle et al. 1997, 1682-1689; Haykowsky et al. 2003, 65-68). This can cause insufficient drainage during mobilization, as the pressure settings remain unchanged during mobilization. The expected pressure adjustment during the prone position was not confirmed. It can be assumed that the regulation of ICP and the dynamics of the cerebrospinal fluid is a complex, multicomponent process that depends on a combination of many factors, and not only on the control of the cerebrospinal fluid.

The conservative methods are the treatment of the underlying disease, which has been complicated by the progress of SAH, for example, generalized infectious diseases, cardiovascular pathology (aortic coarctation), hemolytic disease of newborns, etc. Also, antiepileptic and antihypertensive antibacterial drugs are used as non-surgical methods according to indications.

Cerebral vasospasm is one of the most serious complications after undergoing SAH. The spasm of the cerebral vessels can cause delayed cerebral ischemia, secondary cerebral infarction, and repeated bleeding, which are the main causes of disability, long-term rehabilitation, and death of the patient. Some neurosurgeons and neurologists recommend using drugs that reduce resistance and relax the vessels of the brain to correct the vasospasm. For example, in the literature, you can often find information about the use of the calcium channel blocker nimodipine in children with a clinical picture of SAH. Nimodipine is a blocker of 1,4-dihydropyridine calcium channels. It blocks the calcium channels of the cell membrane in the central nervous system, inhibits the extracellular influx of Ca^{2+} into the smooth muscles of blood vessels, reduces the fragility of red blood cells and blood viscosity, and also effectively prevents and treats ischemic brain damage caused by SAH. In addition, Nimodipine can selectively dilate the vessels of the brain and practically does not affect peripheral vessels (Cho et al. 2016, 718-724; van Gijn and Rinkel 2001, 249-278). Magnesium sulfate is also used to relieve the central vasospasm. Mg^{2+} can suppress the activity of the central nervous system, relax the smooth muscles of the vessels and relieve vascular spasm. Mg^{2+} begins to act immediately with intravenous induction; the effect of the drug is limited to 30 minutes. Since extracellular Mg^{2+} is a natural physiological blocker of Ca^{2+} channels, it competes with bound Ca^{2+}, inhibits the influx of Ca^{2+}, and prevents calcium overload. Mg^{2+} can block ion channels, which reduces the influx of Na+ and Ca2+ and the outflow of K+. Mg^{2+} supports normal sodium–potassium metabolism through the cell membrane prevents cell edema [Muir et al. 2004, 439-445; Kato 2004, 76-80; Macdonald et al. 2004, 106-110), and thereby prevents and treats the central vasospasm. Mg^{2+} acts on glutamate receptors inhibit their activation, reduces the release of glutamate, reduces neuron necrosis (an den Bergh et al. 2005, 1011-1015; Chang et al. 2014, 52), and thereby reduces mortality.

A special role in therapy is played by the early start of rehabilitation (the first 72 hours) in the intensive care unit, and the involvement of neuropsychologists, neurologists, and speech therapists in rehabilitation. The particular importance of this concept is the possibility of preserving the physical condition of the body and the social status of the patient after a stroke (Krings et al. 2008). The selection of rehabilitation methods is performed depending on the age of the child and his cognitive functions. The program necessarily includes physical exercises, and classes with a neuropsychologist and a speech therapist.

The criteria for the effectiveness of therapy are the absence of cerebral blood flow of the aneurysm or vascular malformation, which was the direct cause of SAH, (assessment is performed according to the results of cerebral angiography); stabilization of the patient's condition, absence of the need to maintain vital functions in the intensive care unit (independent breathing, support of hemodynamics, water-electrolyte balance, carbohydrate metabolism); absence of neurological complications and deficiencies (relief of cerebral edema, absence of convulsive syndrome, resolution of acute occlusive hydrocephalus, cerebral vasospasm). All positive results must be confirmed by the results of neuroimaging (CT, MRI, ultrasound). If possible complications are detected, it is necessary to stop somatic complications (pneumonia, infections), normalize laboratory parameters, and correct neurological deficits to a minimum or complete regression.

Conclusion

SAH in children is a fairly rare pathology. Most often, the causes of hemorrhages are the presence of cerebral aneurysms as a result of genetic, traumatic factors, certain diseases; vascular-venous malformations, and spontaneous hemorrhages. Currently, there are no well-developed algorithms for the most effective methods of surgical and conservative treatment for SAH. The commission examination of the patient (neurologist, neurosurgeon, pediatrician or neonatologist, anesthesiologist, rehabilitation specialist) must justify the choice of management tactics. It is necessary to evaluate all the risk factors of the operation and the possibilities of conservative treatment during the surgical intervention. Endovascular techniques and minor invasive neurosurgery are the preferred methods of surgical treatment.

References

Abla A. A, Lekovic G. P, Turner J. D., de Oliveira J. G., Porter R., Spetzler R. F. Advances in the treatment and outcome of brainstem cavernous malformation surgery: A single-center case series of 300 surgically treated patients. *Neurosurgery*. 2011;68:403–15.

Abraham M. K., Chang W. W. Subarachnoid Hemorrhage. *Emerg Med Clin North Am*. 2016 Nov;34(4):901-916. doi: 10.1016/j.emc.2016.06.011. PMID: 27741994.

Amelot, A., Saliou, G., Benichi, S., Alias, Q., Boulouis, G., Zerah, M., Aghakhani, N., Ozanne, A., Blauwblomme, T., & Naggara, O. Long-term outcomes of cerebral aneurysms in children. *Pediatrics*. 2019;143: 20183036.

Araki S., Shirahata A. Vitamin K Deficiency Bleeding in Infancy. *Nutrients*. 2020 Mar 16;12(3):780. doi: 10.3390/nu12030780. PMID: 32187975; PMCID: PMC7146284.

Arts S., van Bilsen M., van Lindert E. J., Bartels R. H., Aquarius R., Boogaarts H. D. Implementation of an Automated Cerebrospinal Fluid Drainage System for Early Mobilization in Neurosurgical Patients. *Brain Sci*. 2021 May 22;11(6):683.

Barrow D. L, Prats A. R. Infectious intracranial aneurysms: comparison of groups with and without endocarditis. *Neurosurgery*. 1990;27:562–572, discussion 572–563.

Bohmfalk G. L, Story J. L., Wissinger J. P., Brown W. E. Jr. Bacterial intracranial aneurysm. *J Neurosurg*. 1978;48:369–382.

Bonadio W. Pediatric lumbar puncture and cerebrospinal fluid analysis. *J Emerg Med*. 2014 Jan;46(1):141-50. doi: 10.1016/j.jemermed.2013.08.056. Epub 2013 Nov 1. PMID: 24188604.

Bowry A. D., Brookhart M. A, Choudhry N. K. Meta-analysis of the efficacy and safety of clopidogrel plus aspirin as compared to antiplatelet monotherapy for the prevention of vascular events. *Am J Cardiol.* 2008;101:960-966.

Brimioulle S., Moraine J. J., Norrenberg D., Kahn R. J. Effects of positioning and exercise on intracranial pressure in a neurosurgical intensive care unit. *Phys Ther.* 1997;77: 1682–1689.

Can A., Gross B. A., Du R. The natural history of cerebral arteriovenous malformations. *Handb Clin Neurol.* 2017;143:15-24. doi: 10.1016/B978-0-444-63640-9.00002-3. PMID: 28552137.

Chakravarthy H., Lin T. K., Chen Y. L., Wu Y. M., Yeh C. H., Wong H. F. De novo formation of cerebral cavernous malformation adjacent to existing developmental venous anomaly - an effect of change in venous pressure associated with management of a complex dural arterio-venous fistula. *Neuroradiol J.* 2016 Dec;29(6):458-464. doi: 10.1177/1971400916666558. Epub 2016 Aug 25. PMID: 27562580; PMCID: PMC5131766.

Chang, J. J., Mack, W. J., Saver, J. L., & Sanossian, N. Magnesium: potential roles in neurovascular disease. *Front Neurol.* 2014 Apr;15(5):52. doi:10.3389/fneur.2014.00052. eCollection 2014.

Cho S., Bales J., Tran T. K., Korab, G., Khandelwal, N., Aaron M. Joffe. Effects of 14 versus 21 days of nimodipine therapy on neurological outcomes in aneurysmal subarachnoid hemorrhage patients. *Ann Pharmacother.* 2016;50(9):718–724.

Choux M., Lena G., Genitori L. 1992. "Intracranial aneurysms in children." In *Cerebrovascular Disease in Children,* edited by Raimoni A., Choux M., Di Rocco C., 123-130. Vienna: Springer.

Clare C. E, Barrow D. L. Infectious intracranial aneurysms. *NeurosurgClin N* Am. 1992;3:551–566.

Clatterbuck R. E., Elmaci I., Rigamonti D. The juxtaposition of capillary telangiectasia, cavernous malformation, and developmental venous anomaly in the brainstem of a single patient: case report. *Neurosurgery.* 2001;49:1246–1250.

Cremer O. L., van Dijk G. W., Brekelmans G. J. Effect of intracranial pressure monitoring and targeted intensive care on functional outcome after severe head injury. *Crit Care Med.* 2005; 33:2207-2213.

Dalyai, R. T., Ghobrial, G., Awad, I., Tjoumakaris, S., Gonzalez, L. F., Dumont, A. S., Chalouhi, N., Randazzo, C., Rosenwasser, R., & Jabbour, P. Management of incidental cavernous malformations: A review. *Neurosurg Focus.* 2011;31:E5.

da Cunha C. E. G., da Cunha Correia C. Dilation of the middle cerebral artery and the risk of developing the aneurysmal disease. *J Neurol Sci.* 2018 Jul 15;390:219-221. doi: 10.1016/j.jns.2018.04.040. Epub 2018 Apr 26. PMID: 29801892.

Fernando P. M., Munasinghe B. M., Jayamanne M. D. C. J. P., Jayasundara K. A., Arambepola W. S. N. W. B. M. A. G., Pranavan S., Ranathunge N. D. Cerebral cavernous malformation in a child leading to a fatal subarachnoid hemorrhage - "silent but sinister:" A case report and literature review. *Surg Neurol Int.* 2021 Jun 7;12:253. doi: 10.25259/SNI_248_2021. PMID: 34221584; PMCID: PMC8247693.

Fung C., Mavrakis E., Filis A., Fischer I., Suresh M., Tortora A., Cornelius J. F., Bostelmann R., Gralla J., Beck J., Raabe A., Khan M. O., Steiger H. J., Petridis A. K. Anatomical evaluation of intracranial aneurysm rupture risk in patients with multiple aneurysms. *Neurosurg Rev*. 2019.

Ganesh Kumar, N., Ladner, T. R., Kahn, I. S., Zuckerman, S. L., Baker, C. B., Skaletsky, M., Cushing, D., Sanborn, M. R., Mocco, J., & Ecker, R. D. Parent vessel occlusion for treatment of cerebral aneurysms: is there still an indication? A series of 17 patients. *J Neurol Sci*. 2017;372:250-255.

Ghali M. G. Z., Srinivasan V. M., Cherian J., Wagner K. M., Chen S. R., Johnson J., Lam S. K., Kan P. Multimodal Treatment of Intracranial Aneurysms in Children: Clinical Case Series and Review of the Literature. *World Neurosurg*. 2018 Mar;111:294-307. doi: 10.1016/j.wneu.2017.12.057. Epub 2017 Dec 18. PMID: 29269068.

Hahn Y. S., Welling B., Reichman O. H., Azar-Kia B. Traumatic intracavernous aneurysm in children: massive epistaxis without ophthalmic signs. *Childs Nerv Syst*. 1990;6:360–364.

HaykowskyM. J., Eves N. D., DE R. W., Findlay M. J. Resistance exercise, the Valsalva maneuver, and cerebrovascular transmural pressure. *Med Sci Sports Exerc*. 2003; 35: 65–68.

Hegde A. N., Mohan S., Lim C. C. CNS cavernous haemangioma: "popcorn" in the brain and spinal cord. *Clin Radiol*. 2012;67:380–8.

Huang S., Guo Z. N., Shi M., Yang Y., Rao M. Etiology and pathogenesis of Moyamoya Disease: An update on disease prevalence. *Int J Stroke*. 2017 Apr;12(3):246-253. doi: 10.1177/1747493017694393. Epub 2017 Jan 1. PMID: 28381201.

Josephson C. B., Bhattacharya J. J., Counsell C. E., Papanastassiou V., Ritchie V., Roberts R., Sellar R., Warlow C. P., Al-Shahi Salman R. Scottish Audit of Intracranial Vascular Malformations (SAIVMs) steering committee and collaborators. Seizure risk with AVM treatment or conservative management: a prospective, population-based study. *Neurology*. 2012 Aug 7;79(6):500-7. doi: 10.1212/WNL.0b013e3182635696. Epub 2012 Jul 3. PMID: 22764257; PMCID: PMC3413766.

Kato T. Role of magnesium ions on the regulation of NMDA receptor–a pharmacopathology of memantine. *Clin Calcium*. 2004;14(8):76–80.

Kikuchi K., Kowada M., Sasajima H. Vascular malformations of the brain in hereditary hemorrhagic telangiectasia (Rendu-Osler-Weber disease). *Surg Neurol*. 1994 May;41(5):374-80. doi: 10.1016/0090-3019(94)90030-2. PMID: 8009411.

Krings T., Geibprasert S., terBrugge K. G. Pathomechanisms and treatment of pediatric aneurysms. *Childs Nerv Syst*. 2010;26:1309-18.

Krings T., Lasjaunias P., Geibprasert S., Pereira V., Hans F. J. The aneurysmal wall. The key to a subclassification of intracranial arterial aneurysm vasculopathies? *Interv Neuroradiol*. 2008;14:315–329.

Krystkiewicz K., Ciszek B., Szylberg L., Tosik M., Harat M. Morphological analysis of cerebral artery fenestration and their correlation with intracranial aneurysms. *World Neurosurg*. 2021 Dec;156: 85-92. doi: 10.1016/j.wneu.2021.08.137. Epub 2021 Sep 7. PMID: 34506985.

Kwon Y. S., Lee Y. H., Cho J. M. Early Experience of Automated Intraventricular Type Intracranial Pressure Monitoring (LiquoGuard^{R}) for Severe Traumatic Brain Injury Patients. *Korean J Neurotrauma.* 2016;12:28–33.

Lasjaunias P. From aneurysm to aneurysmal vasculopathies. *Operative Techniques in Neurosurgery.* 2000;3:160–165.

Lasjaunias P., Wuppalapati S., Alvarez H., Rodesch G., Ozanne A. Intracranial aneurysms in children aged under 15 years: a review of 59 consecutive children with 75 aneurysms. *Childs Nerv Syst.* 2005;21:437–450.

Levy M. L., Levy D. M., Manna B. Pediatric Cerebral Aneurysm. 2021 Aug 12. In: StatPearls [Internet]. Treasure Island (FL): *StatPearls Publishing*; 2022 Jan. PMID: 30725770.

Linsler S., Schmidtke M., Steudel W. I., Kiefer M., Oertel J. Automated intracranial pressure-controlled cerebrospinal fluid external drainage with LiquoGuard. *Acta Neurochir.* 2013; 155: 1589–1594.

Liu A., Huang J. Treatment of intracranial aneurysms: clipping versus coiling. *Curr Cardiol Rep.* 2015;17:628.

Lawton M. T., Jacobowitz R., Spetzler R. F. Redefined role of angiogenesis in the pathogenesis of dural arteriovenous malformations. *J Neurosurg.* 1997 Aug;87(2):267-74. doi: 10.3171/jns.1997.87.2.0267. PMID: 9254092.

Macdonald, R. L., Curry, D. J., Aihara, Y., Zhang, Z.-D., Jahromi, B. S., & Yassari, R. Magnesium and experimental vasospasm. *J Neurosurg.* 2004;100(1):106–110.

Marsot-Dupuch K., Riachi S., Berthet K., Azizi L. Infectious aneurysms of the cavernous carotid artery. *J Radiol.* 2000;81:891–898.

Marmarou A., Anderson J. D., Ward R. L. Impact of ICP instability and hypotension on outcome in patients with severe head trauma. *J Neurosurgery.* 1991;75:59-66.

Mizutani T., Kojima H. Clinicopathological features of nonatherosclerotic cerebral arterial trunk aneurysms. *Neuropathology.* 2000; 1:91–97.

Muir K. W., Lees K. R., Ford I., Davis, S. Intravenous magnesium efficacy in stroke (IMAGES) study investigators. Magnesium for acute stroke (Intravenous Magnesium Efficacy in Stroke trial): a randomized controlled trial. *Lancet.* 2004;363(9407):439–445.

Nabavizadeh S. A., Mamourian A. C., Vossough A., Loevner L. A., Hurst R. The Many Faces of Cerebral Developmental Venous Anomaly and Its Mimicks: Spectrum of Imaging Findings. *J Neuroimaging.*2016 Sep;26(5):463-72. doi: 10.1111/jon.12373. Epub 2016 Jun 28. PMID: 27350284.

Rigamonti D., Drayer B. P., Johnson P. C., Hadley M. N., Zabramski J., Spetzler R. F. The MRI appearance of cavernous malformations (angiomas*). J Neurosurg.* 1987;67:518–24.

Ross M. E., Waldron P. E., Cashore W. J., de Alarcón P. A. 2013. "Hemolytic disease of the fetus and newborn." In *Neonatal Hematology: Pathogenesis, Diagnosis, and Management of Hematologic Problems,* 2nd ed., edited by de Alarcón P. A., Werner E. J, Christensen R. D., 65. Cambridge: Cambridge University Press.

Ruiz D. S., Yelmaz H., Gailloud P. Cerebral developmental venous ´anomalies: current concepts. *Ann Neurol.* 2009;66:271-83.

Saraf R., Garg T., Parvathi S. Endovascular Therapy in Paediatric Dissecting Intracranial Aneurysm: A Case Report. *Neurol India*. 2021 May-Jun;69(3):748-750. doi: 10.4103/0028-3886.317236. PMID: 34169882.

Shinkawa T., Ramakrishnaiah R. H., Eble B. K. Subarachnoid haemorrhage from an undiagnosed mycotic aortic aneurysm in a child. *Cardiol Young*. 2018 Mar;28(3):461-463. [PubMed].

Shipman K. E., Ramalingam S. K., Dawson C. H., Yasear Z. A. Subarachnoid haemorrhage. *Clin Med (Lond)*. 2019 Jan;19(1):88-89.

Shope C., Alshareef M., Larrew T., Bolling C., Reagan J., Yazdani M., Spampinato M., Eskandari R. Utility of a pediatric fast magnetic resonance imaging protocol as surveillance scanning for traumatic brain injury. *J Neurosurg Pediatr*. 2021 Feb 5;27(4):475-481. doi: 10.3171/2020.8.PEDS20496. PMID: 33545669.

Skoch J., Tahir R., Abruzzo T., Taylor J. M., Zuccarello M., Vadivelu S. Predicting symptomatic cerebral vasospasm after aneurysmal subarachnoid hemorrhage with an artificial neural network in a pediatric population. *Childs Nerv Syst*. 2017 Dec;33(12):2153-2157. [PubMed].

Ventureyra E. C., Higgins M. J. Traumatic intracranial aneurysms in childhood and adolescence. Case reports and review of the literature. *Childs Nerv Syst* 1994;10:361–379.

Yazbak P. A., McComb J. G., Raffel C. Pediatric traumatic intracranial aneurysms. *Pediatr Neurosurg*. 1995;22:15–19.

Vachhani J. A., Nickele C. M., Elijovich L., Klimo P., Arthur A. S. Flow diversion for treatment of growing A2 aneurysm in a child: case report and review of flow diversion for intracranial aneurysms in pediatric patients. *World Neurosurg*. 2016;96:607.

van den Bergh W. M., Algra A., van Kooten F. MASH study group. Magnesium sulfate in aneurysmal subarachnoid hemorrhage: a randomized controlled trial. *Stroke*. 2005;1011–1015.

van Gijn J., Rinkel G. J. Subarachnoid haemorrhage: diagnosis, causes, and management. *Brain*. 2001;124(Pt 2):249–278.

Vargas S. A., Diaz C., Herrera D. A., Dublin A. B. Intracranial aneurysms in children: the role of stenting and flow-diversion. *J Neuroimaging*. 2016; 26:41-45.

Xia, Z. W., Liu, X. M., Wang, J. Y., Cao, H., Chen, F. H., Huang, J., Li, Q. Z., Fan, S. S., Jiang, B., Chen, Z. G., & Cheng, Q. Coiling is not superior to clipping in patients with high-grade aneurysmal subarachnoid hemorrhage: systematic review and meta-analysis. *World Neurosurg*. 2017;98:411-420. https://www.neurosklif.ru/Diseases/Avm date 30.03.22 (Google 2022).

Chapter 8

Concerns, Developments, and Future Direction of Aneurysmal Subarachnoid Hemorrhage Management

Yusuf Mehkri[1], William Dodd[1], Abeer Dagra[1], Alec Clark[2] and Brandon Lucke-Wold[1,*], MD, PhD, MCTS

[1]Department of Neurosurgery, University of Florida, Gainesville, FL, USA

[2]College of Medicine, University of Central Florida, Orlando, FL, USA

Abstract

Subarachnoid hemorrhage can have debilitating outcomes for patients following aneurysm rupture. Recent evidence has emerged showing new treatments and guiding recommendations. These treatments will be highlighted soon in the new American Heart Association Guidelines. We discuss some of the key findings from recent studies and highlight avenues for further investigation. These knowledge gaps will be the focus of renewed interest over the coming decades. This expert commentary discusses some of the primary concerns regarding subarachnoid hemorrhage. We delve into future directions such as headache management. Finally, we present several avenues that warrant clear and focused pre-clinical and clinical study. By addressing these unanswered questions, true breakthroughs can be made for patients.

Keywords: subarachnoid hemorrhage, updates, headache, management, clinical concerns

[*]Corresponding Author's Email: Brandon.lucke-wold@neurosurgery.ufl.edu.

In: Aneurysmal Subarachnoid Hemorrhage
Editor: Irina Savvina
ISBN: 979-8-88697-251-1

Introduction

Subarachnoid hemorrhage has potential devastating outcomes for patients. With a 50% mortality and 30% of remaining survivors developing symptomatic vasospasm, the need for improved treatment is apparent. This expert commentary section highlights the current management strategies with emphasis on endovascular treatment of the aneurysm. Furthermore, we discuss issues related to rebleeding, treatment of vasospasm, and intensive care unit stay. We then delve into the new clinical trials that are changing the field. In the final section, we highlight future directions and what is needed to take the field to the next level for the care of patients.

Current Management of aSAH

The management of aneurysmal subarachnoid hemorrhage (aSAH) has two general goals: securing the culprit aneurysm and minimizing complications. Once a patient presenting with aSAH is stabilized, CTA or another imaging modality such as MRA, can identify the aneurysm and help guide the treatment strategy. Endovascular treatment is now the first line option for most patients (Molyneux and Kerr 2005, 809), although many anatomic considerations necessitate continued need for surgical clip ligation. Coil embolization, also called coiling, is the primary means of endovascular treatment; however, stents, flow diverters, and flow disrupters may also be deployed via an endovascular route (Pierot and Wakhloo 2013, 2046). These devices are especially useful when treating an aneurysm not suitable to clipping or coiling alone such as a blister aneurysm or wide-neck aneurysms of the of the posterior circulation (Tsianaka et al., 2019; Zhao et al., 2016; Peitz and Sy 2017, 42). The most powerful predictor of death following aSAH is rebleeding of the culprit aneurysm (Stienen et al., 2018). Rebleeding can be minimized by careful execution of the initial aneurysm treatment as well as ensuring satisfactory aneurysm occlusion with follow-up cerebral angiography. Rates of rebleeding may also be lower with surgical clipping compared to endovascular coiling (Molyneux and Kerr 2005, 809; Li et al., 2013). This however is debated and indicates room for improvement of endovascular techniques. Inadequate aneurysm occlusion may warrant repeat treatment to secure the aneurysm. The rise in popularity of endovascular therapies have presented a unique challenge to neurointerventionalists; the use of anti-coagulant and anti-platelet drugs is necessary to reduce device-induced thrombosis yet may also contribute to hemorrhage severity in cases of aneurysm rebleeding (Altenburg and Haage 2012,30; Limaye et al., 2019; Samaniego et al., 2019). The optimal strategies for minimizing these complications are still being rigorously investigated.

Once the aneurysm is secured, the managing physician must proactively identify and treat emerging complications. Many patients develop hydrocephalus after aSAH requiring the placement of external ventricular drains. Hydrocephalus and cerebral edema are associated with poor long-term outcome after SAH (Claassen et al., 2002; Rabinstein et al., 2005; Alotaibi et al., 2017). Similarly, headache, hyponatremia, seizure, and depression are all common complications of aSAH that remain understudied and difficult to effectively treat (Tang et al., 2020; Huckhagel et al., 2020; Connolly et al., 2012). After rebleeding, the next predictor of poor outcome is cerebral infarction due to delayed cerebral ischemia (DCI) (Stienen et al., 2018). DCI is a highly complex process and thus can be difficult to identify and treat. The current standard is to treat all aSAH patients with oral nimodipine as DCI prophylaxis. Nimodipine, a dihydropyridine-class L-type calcium channel blocker is the only drug that improves long-term outcome after aSAH (Dorhout Mees et al., 2007). One of the many factors that contribute to DCI is cerebral vasospasm, characterized by decreased luminal diameter of affected vessels occurring most often 5-10 days post-ictus (Dodd et al., 2021). Moderate-to-severe vasospasm occurs in approximately 30% of aSAH patients (Dorsch and King 1994,19). The gold standard for diagnosing vasospasm is cerebral angiography, although it is regularly observed via CTA as well (Chaudhary et al., 2008; Joo et al., 2006; Arias et al., 2015). Transcranial doppler (TCD) ultrasonography is used as a non-invasive method to monitor for the development of cerebral vasospasm prior to CTA or angiography (Connolly et al., 2012; Bathala and Mehndiratta 2013, 174). TCD findings of increased flow velocities (> 100-120 cm/s) are concerning for vasospasm based on Poiseuille's law of fluid dynamics. The law states that the pressure gradient between two points of a vessel is proportional to the flow rate and inversely proportional to the cross-sectional area, thus the physiologic response to vasospasm is increased pressure (and velocity) to maintain cerebral blood flow. The underlying assumption that cerebral blood flow will remain consistent, however; is not always accurate and one of the weaknesses of TCD monitoring (Barthélémy and Damoisel 2019, e385; Samagh and Bhagat 2019,12). Nevertheless, TCD has sufficiently high sensitivity and negative predictive value to be routinely used for vasospasm screening

(Kumar and Shahripour 2016,1257). First line treatment for cerebral vasospasm is permissive hypertension (systolic BP > 160 mmHg) to increase cerebral perfusion pressure (Connolly et al., 2012). In patients who do not respond to first line therapy, endovascular intervention may be warranted. This includes mechanical angioplasty and intraarterial delivery of anti-spasmodics such as nimodipine, nicardipine, verapamil, and milrinone (Pandey et al., 2013; Higashida et al., 1989; Kassell et al., 1992). Mechanical manipulation of the cerebrovasculature has several potential complications, the most drastic of which is intraoperative arterial rupture (Hoh and Ogilvy 2005, 501; Haque et al., 2009). These modalities may be of some benefit to specific patient population. Despite decades of investigation, there remains an urgent need for better medical and interventional therapies to improve outcomes following aSAH.

Novel Treatments in Clinical Trials

Delayed cerebral ischemia (DCI) following aneurysmal subarachnoid hemorrhage (SAH) is a major source of additional morbidity and mortality in an already vulnerable situation. One of the most important therapies for cerebral infarction secondary to SAH has been the cornerstone pharmacologic therapy nimodipine, a dihydropyridine calcium channel antagonist. It is preferable to other calcium channel antagonists because of its relative selectivity for the cerebral vasculature, lipophilic nature, and ability to traverse the blood brain barrier (Castanares-Zapatero and Hantson 2011,12). Although nimodipine's capacity to block calcium influx through L-type calcium channels may not dramatically cure angiographic vasospasm, it may resist calcium-mediated excitotoxicity (Feigin et al., 1998). It has also been proposed that, as compared to other calcium channel antagonists, nimodipine's capacity to improve endogenous fibrinolytic activity may limit the production of microthromboses, which have become a key consideration in the establishment of DCI (Vergouwen et al., 2007). A randomized controlled trial investigating the administration of intraventricular nimodipine microparticles found no significant increase in favorable outcome in the study population when compared to standard of care (Carlson et al., 2020). Chemical angioplasty with intra-arterial infusion of vasodilators and mechanical dilatation with a percutaneous transluminal balloon angioplasty (PTCA) are two more common treatments that are included in the current AHA/ASA guidelines for SAH treatment as a Class IIb, Level of Evidence B. In large capacitance arteries, PTCA has been demonstrated to be efficient in mechanically reversing vasospasm (Zubkov andNikiforov 1984, 65). It is extremely effective in proximal arteries with thick muscle walls, such as the internal carotid artery or the vertebral arteries. It loses effectiveness beyond second order segments (Eskridge and Song 1997, 1653). With the development of micro-catheter technology, it is now possible to treat vasospasm in vessels beyond second order segments with vasodilators. Intra-aortic balloon counter pulsation pumps (IABP) have been described for the management of concomitant symptomatic cerebral vasospasm and neurogenic stress cardiomyopathy after SAH (Al-Mufti et al., 2016). It reduces left ventricular stress and myocyte oxygen demand by enhancing coronary perfusion during diastole and lowering afterload (Naidech et al., 2005). IABP can also lead to the gradual withdrawal of vasopressors, which can aggravate low cardiac output (Ducruet et al., 2013). Furthermore, studies have shown that sympatholytic therapy can help with SAH management, with increased CBF and fewer neurological impairments. One way could be to temporarily block sympathetic ganglion cells to enhance patient outcomes while avoiding the long-term implications of permanent sympathetic blockade. A potential target is the stellate ganglion, which is made up of the inferior cervical and first thoracic ganglions. After stellate ganglion block, one group found that flow velocities improved on the contralateral side (Jain et al., 2011). In comparison to a superior cervical ganglion block, which needs fluoroscopy, a stellate ganglion block can be performed at the patient's bedside (Prabhakar et al., 2007). Finally, the FDA has approved the CoAxiaNeuroFloTM device under the Humanitarian Device Exemption (HDE) pathway for the treatment of cerebral ischemia caused by symptomatic vasospasm after aneurysmal subarachnoid hemorrhage in patients who have failed to respond to medical treatment (COAXIA NEUROFLO CATHETER 2022). While the specific mechanism of action is unknown and likely multifactorial (Liebeskind 2008, 31-36), it has been demonstrated to improve cerebral blood flow even after the device has been removed (Lylyk et al., 2005). Increased collateral blood flow through leptomeningeal arteries is thought to be responsible for a large part of the effect (Ramakrishnan et al., 2016). There have been instances of considerable clinical improvement in aSAH patients after its use (Alnaami and Saqqur 2009, 417). The manufacturer funded SENTIS trial provides the most robust evidence for its safety profile. The study found that about 50% of treated patients experienced a 3-point or greater reduction in NIH Stroke Scale ratings in the experimental group, with the benefit lasting at least 24 hours (COAXIA NEUROFLO CATHETER 2022). It was demonstrated to increase middle cerebral artery mean velocities in 20 of 24 participants in another investigation (Lylyk et al., 2005). It has also been explored for usage in ischemic stroke patients who aren't candidates for tPA or who don't respond to tPA (Emery et al., 2011). Thesc treatments and those under investigation provide a promising future for effective management of these cerebral events aiming at minimizing the long-term impairments.

Future Directions

A few aSAH treatment modalities are being investigated in preclinical studies, with many more options being hypothesized based on more recent exploration into the pathophysiology behind aSAH. Several current preclinical studies are aimed at more efficient attenuation of cerebral vasospasm, a main mechanism by which aSAH causes severe complications, such as DCI (Ikram et al., 2021; Carr and Zuckerman 2013, 506584). In 2022, an in vivo study showed significant increase in vessel diameter to near pre-vasospasm baseline levels in vessels exposed to ultrasound-induced release of nimodipine in cerebral vasospasm models using chicken chorioallantoic membranes (Döring et al., 2022). Authors noted that these results justify further investigation using rat SAH models and may prove to be a promising method for on-demand direct release of nimodipine to vasospastic vessels. This could potentially bypass the issue of poor bioavailability of nimodipine in aSAH models (Luo et al., 2016). On a similar note, it has been recently postulated that prevention of endothelial glycocalyx shedding of cerebral vessels may help reduce the negative impact of delayed cerebral ischemia following aSAH (Schenck et al., 2021). As shedding of the glycocalyx has been demonstrated in response to several intrinsic mechanisms, such as mechanical stress and ischemia-reperfusion injury, a deeper understanding and strategic targeting of this shedding could assist in improving both timing and method of treatment modalities used in response to aSAH (Schenck et al., 2021; Pillinger and Kam 2017, 295). In addition, other preclinical studies are being performed on the use of new models of self-expanding stents aimed at diminishing delayed cerebral vasospasm, with early results demonstrating an ability for these stents to increase vessel diameter by up to 300% (Bhogal et al., 2021).

There now exists a plethora of hypothetical aSAH treatment options involving the targeting of inflammatory mediators, which have been widely demonstrated to contribute to the pathogenesis of aSAH and its sequelae (Dienel et al., 2021; Muhammad and Hänggi 2021, 22). Since toll-like receptors (TLRs) are well-known propagators of inflammation, they are becoming one of the more commonly described targets in this context (Vijay 2018, 391-412). Furthermore, attenuation of essentially all the well-known pro-inflammatory mediators have now been hypothesized as therapeutic targets for aSAH treatment. These include various cytokines, such as tumor necrosis factor-α (TNF-α) and interleukin (IL-6), and chemokines, such as CCL5 (Weiland et al., 2021). Furthermore, the neutrophil-to-lymphocyte ratio (NLR), an increasingly well-known biomarker of inflammation, may have efficacy as an indicator of aSAH severity and risk for complications. This may serve as an eventual target for the reduction of inflammation-induced damage in aSAH (Cai et al., 2021). C-reactive protein has also been shown to serve as an independent predictor of poor outcomes following aSAH and may similarly serve as a potential target (Gaastra et al., 2021). Another potential mechanism that may merit further investigation is the role of platelets in aSAH-induced inflammation and subsequent vasospasm and microthrombi development (Dienel et al., 2021). In this context, there may be several potential targets. For example, von Willebrand factor (vWF) promotes platelet binding to both other platelets and to endothelium. As such, targeting either the production or binding of vWF would thus reduce the downstream effects of inflammation, microthrombi formation, and vasospasm, thereby attenuating the propagation of cerebral vasospasm and resultant DCI as a complication of aSAH (Dienel et al., 2021; Hassan and Saxena 2012,11). Specifically, targeting a disintegrin and metalloproteinase with a thrombospondin type 1 motif member 13 (ADAMTS13), which frees individual vWF molecules from multimers, has already shown promise by reducing brain damage in preclinical aSAH animal models (Wan et al., 2018).

Conclusion

In sum, both current preclinical studies and hypothesized targets are showing significant promise in the way of developing more effective treatment modalities for aSAH and its sequelae. Targets aimed at reducing inflammatory mediators and subsequent cerebral vasospasm appear to have the most relative focus in the literature and, as such, show the most promise as it currently stands. These new treatments have the potential to modify disease course and improve outcomes. Great work is still needed, but the field is changing with emphasis on approved outcomes for patients. The coming decades will continue to bring novel and innovative changes.

References

Al-Mufti, F., Morris, N., Lahiri, S., Roth, W., Witsch, J., Machado, I., Agarwal, S., Park, S., Meyers, P. M., Connolly, E. S., Claassen, J. Use of Intra-aortic- Balloon Pump Counterpulsation in Patients with Symptomatic Vasospasm Following Subarachnoid Hemorrhage and Neurogenic Stress Cardiomyopathy. *J. Vasc. Interv. Neurol.* Jun 2016;9(1):28-34.

Alnaami, I., Saqqur, M., & Chow, M. A novel treatment of distal cerebral vasospasm. A case report. *Interv. Neuroradiol.* Dec 2009;15(4):417-420.

Alotaibi, N. M., Wang, J. Z., Pasarikovski, C. R., Guha, D., Al-Mufti, F., Mamdani, M., Saposnik, G., Schweizer, T. A., Macdonald, R. L. Management of raised intracranial pressure in aneurysmal subarachnoid hemorrhage: Time for a consensus? *Neurosurgical Focus.* 2017;43(5).

Altenburg, A., Haage, P. Antiplatelet and anticoagulant drugs in interventional radiology. Vol 35: *Cardiovasc. Intervent. Radiol.*; 2012:30-42.

Arias, E. J., Vajapey, S., Reynolds, M. R., Chicoine, M. R., Rich, K. M., Dacey, R. G., Jr, Dorward, I. G., Derdeyn, C. P., Moran, C. J., Cross, D. T., 3rd, Zipfel, G. J., & Dhar, R. Utility of Screening for Cerebral Vasospasm Using Digital Subtraction Angiography. *Stroke.* 2015;46(11):3137-3141.

Barthélémy, R., Damoisel, C., Chousterman, B. G. Transcranial Doppler and Cerebral Vasospasm: It Is Time to Move On. *Critical care medicine.* 2019;47(4):e385-e385.

Bathala, L., Mehndiratta, M., Sharma, V. Transcranial doppler: Technique and common findings (Part 1). *Annals of Indian Academy of Neurology.* 2013;16(2):174-174.

Bhogal, P., Simpanen, T., Wong, K., Bushi, D., Sirakov, M. A., Sirakov, S., Aggour, M., & Makalanda, L. Use of the Cascade expandable net to treat cerebral vasospasm - initial clinical experience from a single centre with in vitro benchside tests. *CVIR Endovasc.* Dec 8 2021;4(1):82.

Cai, L., Zeng, H., Tan, X., Wu, X., Qian, C., Chen, G. The Role of the Blood Neutrophil-to-Lymphocyte Ratio in Aneurysmal Subarachnoid Hemorrhage. *Front. Neurol.* 2021;12:671098.

Carlson, A. P., Hänggi, D., Wong, G. K., Etminan, N., Mayer, S. A., Aldrich, F., Diringer, M. N., Schmutzhard, E., Faleck, H. J., Ng, D., Saville, B. R., Bleck, T., Grubb, R., Jr, Miller, M., Suarez, J. I., Proskin, H. M., Macdonald, R. L., NEWTON Investigators. Single-Dose Intraventricular Nimodipine Microparticles Versus Oral Nimodipine for Aneurysmal Subarachnoid Hemorrhage. *Stroke.* 04 2020;51(4):1142-1149.

Carr, K. R., Zuckerman, S. L., Mocco, J. Inflammation, cerebral vasospasm, and evolving theories of delayed cerebral ischemia. *Neurol. Res. Int.* 2013;2013:506584.

Castanares-Zapatero, D., Hantson, P. Pharmacological treatment of delayed cerebral ischemia and vasospasm in subarachnoid hemorrhage. *Ann. Intensive Care.* May 24 2011;1(1):12.

Chaudhary, S. R., Ko, N., Dillon, W. P., Yu, M. B., Liu, S., Criqui, G. I., Higashida, R. T., Smith, W. S., Wintermark, M. Prospective evaluation of multidetector-row CT angiography for the diagnosis of vasospasm following subarachnoid hemorrhage: A comparison with digital subtraction angiography. *Cerebrovascular Diseases.* 2008;25(1-2):144-150.

Claassen, J., Carhuapoma, J. R., Kreiter, K. T., Du, E. Y., Connolly, E. S., Mayer, S. A. Global cerebral edema after subarachnoid hemorrhage: frequency, predictors, and impact on outcome. *Stroke.* May 2002;33(5):1225-1232.

COAXIA NEUROFLO CATHETER Humanitarian Device Exemption (HDE). 2022. Accessed 04/09, 2022.

Connolly, E. S., Jr, Rabinstein, A. A., Carhuapoma, J. R., Derdeyn, C. P., Dion, J., Higashida, R. T., Hoh, B. L., Kirkness, C. J., Naidech, A. M., Ogilvy, C. S., Patel, A. B., Thompson, B. G., Vespa, P., American Heart Association Stroke Council, Council on Cardiovascular Radiology and Intervention, Council on Cardiovascular Nursing, Council on Cardiovascular Surgery and Anesthesia, Council on Clinical Cardiology. Guidelines for the management of aneurysmal subarachnoid hemorrhage: a guideline for healthcare professionals from the American Heart Association/american Stroke Association. *Stroke.* 2012;43(6):1711-1737.

Dienel, A., Kumar, T. P., Blackburn, S. L., McBride, D. W. Role of platelets in the pathogenesis of delayed injury after subarachnoid hemorrhage. *J. Cereb. Blood Flow Metab.* Nov 2021;41(11):2820-2830.

Dodd, W. S., Laurent, D., Dumont, A. S., Hasan, D. M., Jabbour, P. M., Starke, R. M., Hosaka, K., Polifka, A. J., Hoh, B. L., & Chalouhi, N. Pathophysiology of Delayed Cerebral Ischemia After Subarachnoid Hemorrhage: A Review. *J. Am. Heart Assoc.* Aug 3 2021;10(15):e021845.

Dorhout Mees, S. M., Rinkel, G. J., Feigin, V. L., Algra, A., van den Bergh, W. M., Vermeulen, M., van Gijn, J. Calcium antagonists for aneurysmal subarachnoid haemorrhage. *The Cochrane database of systematic reviews.* 2007(3):CD000277-CD000277.

Döring, K., Sperling, S., Ninkovic, M., Schroeder, H., Fischer, A., Stadelmann, C., Streit, F., Binder, L., Mielke, D., Rohde, V., & Malinova, V. Ultrasound-Induced Release of Nimodipine from Drug-Loaded Block Copolymer Micelles: In Vivo Analysis. *Transl. Stroke Res.* Jan 5 2022.

Dorsch, N. W., King, M. T. A review of cerebral vasospasm in aneurysmal subarachnoid haemorrhage Part I: Incidence and effects. *Journal of Clinical Neuroscience.* 1994;1(1):19-26.

Ducruet, A. F., Albuquerque, F. C., Crowley, R. W., Williamson, R., Forseth, J., McDougall, C. G. Balloon-pump counterpulsation for management of severe cardiac dysfunction after aneurysmal subarachnoid hemorrhage. *World Neurosurg.* Dec 2013;80(6):e347-352.

Emery, D. J., Schellinger, P. D., Selchen, D., Douen, A. G., Chan, R., Shuaib, A., & Butcher, K. S. Safety and feasibility of collateral blood flow augmentation after intravenous thrombolysis. *Stroke.* Apr 2011;42(4):1135-1137.

Eskridge, J. M., Song, J. K. A practical approach to the treatment of vasospasm. *AJNR Am. J. Neuroradiol.* Oct 1997;18(9):1653-1660.

Feigin, V. L., Rinke, G. J. E., Algra, A., Vermeulen, M., van Gijn, J. Calcium antagonists in patients with aneurysmal subarachnoid hemorrhage: a systematic review. *Neurology.* Apr 1998;50(4):876-883.

Gaastra, B., Barron, P., Newitt, L., Chhugani, S., Turner, C., Kirkpatrick, P., MacArthur, B., Galea, I., & Bulters, D. CRP (C-Reactive Protein) in Outcome Prediction After Subarachnoid Hemorrhage and the Role of Machine Learning. *Stroke.* Oct 2021;52(10):3276-3285.

Haque, R., Kellner, C. P., Komotar, R. J., Connolly, E. S., Lavine, S. D., Solomon, R. A., & Meyers, P. M. Mechanical treatment of vasospasm. *Neurological research.* 2009;31(6):638-643.

Hassan, M. I., Saxena, A., Ahmad, F. Structure and function of von Willebrand factor. *Blood Coagul Fibrinolysis.* Jan 2012;23(1):11-22.

Higashida, R. T., Halbach, V. V., Cahan, L. D., Brant-Zawadzki, M., Barnwell, S., Dowd, C., & Hieshima, G. B. Transluminal angioplasty for treatment of intracranial arterial vasospasm. *Journal of Neurosurgery.* 1989;71(5 I):648-653.

Hoh, B. L., Ogilvy, C. S. Endovascular treatment of cerebral vasospasm: transluminal balloon angioplasty, intra-arterial papaverine, and intra-arterial nicardipine. *Neurosurgery clinics of North America.* 2005;16(3):501-516.

Huckhagel, T., Klinger, R., Schmidt, N. O., Regelsberger, J., Westphal, M., Czorlich, P. The burden of headache following aneurysmal subarachnoid hemorrhage: a prospective single-center cross-sectional analysis. *Acta Neurochirurgica.* 2020; 162(4):893-903.

Ikram, A., Javaid, M. A., Ortega-Gutierrez, S., Selim, M., Kelangi, S., Anwar, S., Torbey, M. T., & Divani, A. A. Delayed Cerebral Ischemia after Subarachnoid Hemorrhage. *J. Stroke Cerebrovasc. Dis.* Nov 2021;30(11):106064.

Jain, V., Rath, G. P., Dash, H. H., Bithal, P. K., Chouhan, R. S., Suri, A. Stellate ganglion block for treatment of cerebral vasospasm in patients with aneurysmal subarachnoid hemorrhage - A preliminary study. *J. Anaesthesiol. Clin. Pharmacol.* Oct 2011;27(4): 516-521.

Joo, S. P., Kim, T. S, Moon, K. S., Lee, J. K., Kim, J. H., Kim, S. H. Clinical utility of multislice computed tomographic angiography for detection of cerebral vasospasm in acute subarachnoid hemorrhage. *Minimally Invasive Neurosurgery.* 2006;49(5):286-290.

Kassell, N. F., Helm, G., Simmons, N., Phillips, C. D., Cail, W. S. Treatment of cerebral vasospasm with intra-arterial papaverine. *Journal of Neurosurgery.* 1992;77(6):848-852.

Kumar, G., Shahripour, R. B., Harrigan, M. R. Vasospasm on transcranial Doppler is predictive of delayed cerebral ischemia in aneurysmal subarachnoid hemorrhage: a systematic review and meta-analysis. *J. Neurosurg.* May 2016;124(5):1257-1264.

Li, H., Pan, R., Wang, H., Rong, X., Yin, Z., Milgrom, D. P., Shi, X., Tang, Y., & Peng, Y. Clipping versus coiling for ruptured intracranial aneurysms: a systematic review and meta-analysis. *Stroke.* 2013;44(1):29-37.

Liebeskind, D. S. Aortic occlusion for cerebral ischemia: from theory to practice. *Curr. Cardiol. Rep.* Feb 2008;10(1):31-36.

Limaye, K., Zanaty, M., Hudson, J., Nakagawa, D., Al Kasab, S., Alvarez, C., Dandapat, S., Kung, D. K., Ortega-Gutierrez, S., Jabbour, P., Samaniego, E. A., & Hasan, D. The Safety and Efficacy of Continuous Tirofiban as a Monoantiplatelet Therapy in the Management of Ruptured Aneurysms Treated Using Stent-Assisted Coiling or Flow Diversion and Requiring Ventricular Drainage. *Neurosurgery.* 2019;85(6):E1037-E1042.

Luo, J. W., Zhang, Z. R, Gong, T., Fu, Y. One-step self-assembled nanomicelles for improving the oral bioavailability of nimodipine. *Int. J. Nanomedicine.* 2016;11:1051-1065.

Lylyk, P., Vila, J. F., Miranda, C., Ferrario, A., Romero, R., Cohen, J. E. Partial aortic obstruction improves cerebral perfusion and clinical symptoms in patients with symptomatic vasospasm. *Neurol. Res.* 2005;27 Suppl 1:S129-135.

Molyneux, A. J., Kerr, R. S., Yu, L. M., Clarke, M., Sneade, M., Yarnold, J. A., Sandercock, P., International Subarachnoid Aneurysm Trial (ISAT) Collaborative Group. International Subarachnoid Aneurysm Trial (ISAT) of neurosurgical clipping versus endovascular coiling in 2143 patients with ruptured intracranial aneurysms: A randomised comparison of effects on survival, dependency, seizures, rebleeding, subgroups, and aneurysm occlusion. *Lancet.* 2005;366(9488):809-817.

Muhammad, S., Hänggi, D. Inflammation and Anti-Inflammatory Targets after Aneurysmal Subarachnoid Hemorrhage. *Int. J. Mol. Sci.* Jul 8 2021;22(14).

Naidech, A. M., Kreiter, K. T., Janjua, N., Ostapkovich, N. D., Parra, A., Commichau, C., Fitzsimmons, B. F., Connolly, E. S., & Mayer, S. A. Cardiac troponin elevation, cardiovascular morbidity, and outcome after subarachnoid hemorrhage. *Circulation.* Nov 01 2005;112(18):2851-2856.

Pandey, A. S., Elias, A. E., Chaudhary, N., Thompson, B. G., Gemmete, J. J. Endovascular treatment of cerebral vasospasm: vasodilators and angioplasty. *Neuroimaging clinics of North America.* 2013;23(4):593-604.

Peitz, G. W., Sy, C. A., Grandhi, R. Endovascular treatment of blister aneurysms. *Neurosurgical focus.* 2017;42(6).

Pierot, L., Wakhloo, A. K. Endovascular treatment of intracranial aneurysms: Current status. *Stroke.* 2013;44(7):2046-2054.

Pillinger, N. L., Kam, P. Endothelial glycocalyx: basic science and clinical implications. *Anaesth. Intensive Care.* May 2017;45(3):295-307.

Prabhakar, H., Jain, V., Rath, G. P., Bithal, P. K., Dash, H. H. Stellate ganglion block as alternative to intrathecal papaverine in relieving vasospasm due to subarachnoid hemorrhage. *Anesth. Analg.* May 2007;104(5):1311-1312.

Rabinstein, A. A., Weigand, S., Atkinson, J. L., Wijdicks, E. F. Patterns of cerebral infarction in aneurysmal subarachnoid hemorrhage. *Stroke.* 2005;36(5):992-997.

Ramakrishnan, G., Dong, B., Todd, K. G., Shuaib, A., Winship, I. R. Transient Aortic Occlusion Augments Collateral Blood Flow and Reduces Mortality During Severe Ischemia due to Proximal Middle Cerebral Artery Occlusion. *Transl. Stroke Res.* Apr 2016;7(2):149-155.

Samagh, N., Bhagat, H., Jangra, K. Monitoring cerebral vasospasm: How much can we rely on transcranial Doppler. *Journal of Anaesthesiology, Clinical Pharmacology.* 2019;35(1):12-12.

Samaniego, E. A., Gibson, E., Nakagawa, D., Ortega-Gutierrez, S., Zanaty, M., Roa, J. A., Jabbour, P., Hasan, D. M. Safety of tirofiban and dual antiplatelet therapy in treating intracranial aneurysms. *Stroke and Vascular Neurology*. 2019;4(1):36-42.

Schenck, H., Netti, E., Teernstra, O., De Ridder, I., Dings, J., Niemelä, M., Temel, Y., Hoogland, G., Haeren, R. The Role of the Glycocalyx in the Pathophysiology of Subarachnoid Hemorrhage-Induced Delayed Cerebral Ischemia. *Front. Cell Dev. Biol.* 2021;9:731641.

Shuaib, A., Bornstein, N. M., Diener, H. C., Dillon, W., Fisher, M., Hammer, M. D., Molina, C. A., Rutledge, J. N., Saver, J. L., Schellinger, P. D., Shownkeen, H., SENTIS Trial Investigators. Partial aortic occlusion for cerebral perfusion augmentation: safety and efficacy of NeuroFlo in Acute Ischemic Stroke trial. *Stroke*. Jun 2011;42(6):1680-1690.

Stienen, M. N., Germans, M., Burkhardt, J. K., Neidert, M. C., Fung, C., Bervini, D., Zumofen, D., Röthlisberger, M., Marbacher, S., Maduri, R., Robert, T., Seule, M. A., Bijlenga, P., Schaller, K., Fandino, J., Smoll, N. R., Maldaner, N., Finkenstädt, S., Esposito, G., Schatlo, B., Keller, E., Bozinov, O., Regli, L., Swiss SOS Study Group. Predictors of in-hospital death after aneurysmal subarachnoid hemorrhage: Analysis of a nationwide database (Swiss SOS [Swiss Study on Aneurysmal Subarachnoid Hemorrhage]). *Stroke*. 2018;49(2):333-340.

Tang, W. K., Wang, L., Kwok Chu Wong, G., Ungvari, G. S., Yasuno, F., Tsoi, K., & Kim, J. S. Depression after Subarachnoid Hemorrhage: A Systematic Review. *Journal of Stroke*. 2020;22(1):11-11.

Tsianaka, E., Al-Shawish, A., Potapov, A., Fountas, K., Spyrou, M., Konovalov, N. Clipping versus coiling in posterior circulation intracranial aneurysms: A meta-analysis. *Chinese Neurosurgical Journal*. 2019;5(1):1-12.

Vergouwen, M. D., Vermeulen, M., de Haan, R. J., Levi, M., Roos, Y. B. Dihydropyridine calcium antagonists increase fibrinolytic activity: a systematic review. *J. Cereb. Blood Flow Metab.* Jul 2007;27(7):1293-1308.

Vijay, K. Toll-like receptors in immunity and inflammatory diseases: Past, present, and future. *Int. Immunopharmacol.* Jun 2018;59:391-412.

Wan, H., Wang, Y., Ai, J., Brathwaite, S., Ni, H., Macdonald, R. L., Hol, E. M., Meijers, J., & Vergouwen, M. Role of von Willebrand factor and ADAMTS-13 in early brain injury after experimental subarachnoid hemorrhage. *J. Thromb. Haemost.* Jul 2018;16(7):1413-1422.

Weiland, J., Beez, A., Westermaier, T., Kunze, E., Sirén, A. L., Lilla, N. Neuroprotective Strategies in Aneurysmal Subarachnoid Hemorrhage (aSAH). *Int. J. Mol. Sci.* May 21 2021;22(11).

Zhao, B., Yin, R., Lanzino, G., Kallmes, D. F., Cloft, H. J., Brinjikji, W. Endovascular Coiling of Wide-Neck and Wide-Neck Bifurcation Aneurysms: A Systematic Review and Meta-Analysis. *American Journal of Neuroradiology*. 2016;37(9):1700-1705.

Zubkov, Y. N., Nikiforov, B. M., Shustin, V. A. Balloon catheter technique for dilatation of constricted cerebral arteries after aneurysmal SAH. *Acta Neurochir. (Wien)*. 1984;70(1-2):65-79.

About the Editor

Dr. Irina Alexandrovna Savvina, D. Sc. Med.
Chief Researcher
Russian Polenov Scientific Research Neurosurgical Institute
Branch of the National Almazov Medical Research Centre of Ministry
of Health Care of Russian Federation
Professor of the Vladimir L. Vanevskii Department
of Anaesthesiology and Reanimatology
North-Western State Medical University named after Ilya I. Mechnikov
of Ministry of Health Care of Russian Federation
St. Petersburg, Russian Federation

Biographical Sketches

Andreas Theofanopoulos

Affiliation: University Hospital of Patras
Education: University of Patras School of Medicine
Business Address: University Hospital of Patras, Department of Neurosurgery, Rion 26504, Patras, Greece

Research and Professional Experience and Professional Appointments:

- Feb 2019 – Today: University Hospital of Patras, Neurosurgical Department – Resident Doctor
- Dec 2018 - Feb 2019: University Hospital of Patras, Surgical Department – Resident Doctor
- Sep 2017 - Sep 2018: Hellenic Air Force – Conscript Sergeant Doctor
    - 116 Combat Wing (Mar 2018 - Sep 2018)
    - 251 Hellenic Air Force General Hospital – Neurosurgical Department (Nov 2017 - Feb 2018)
    - 124 Basic Training Wing (Sep 2017 - Oct 2017)

Honours:

- Oct 2011: Fondation Santé award – scholarship for 1st place entry in University of Patras Medical School
- Oct 2011: National Scholarships Foundation - scholarship for 1st place entry in University of Patras Medical School
- Nov 2011: Holy Diocese of Patras award - scholarship for 1st place entry in University of Patras Medical School
- Nov 2011: Eurobank award – scholarship for highest National Level Entrance Examination Grade

Publications from the Last 3 Years:

Papadakos D, Zampakis P, Theofanopoulos A, Constantoyannis C, Panagiotopoulos V. Torcular Dural Arteriovenous Fistula (DAVF) Completely Obliterated by Surgical Clipping: Operational Video. *Clin Surg*. 2021; 6: 3326.

Theofanopoulos A, Zampakis P, Antoniadou E, Papadakos D, Fermeli D, Constantoyannis C, Messinis L, Panagiotopoulos V. Spontaneous thoracolumbar epidural hematoma in an apixaban anticoagulated patient. *Surg Neurol Int*. 2021 Jun 07; 12: 256.

Fermeli DD, Theofanopoulos A, Papadakos D, Boulieris S, Constantoyannis C. Hemorrhage of a Cavernous Hemangioma of the Brainstem Presenting with Fever of Unknown Origin: A Case Report. *Am J Case Rep*. 2021 May 25; 22: e930437. doi: 10.12659/AJCR.930437.

Panagiotopoulos V, Theofanopoulos A, Kourakli A, Symeonidis A, Krisela V, Mastronikolis NS, Zampakis P. Ruptured infectious ICA pseudoaneurysm into the sphenoid sinus after maxillofacial infection, successfully treated by selective embolization. *SurgNeurol Int*. 2021 Apr 26; 12: 191. doi: 10.25259/SNI_52_2021.

Theofanopoulos A, Fermeli D, Boulieris S, Kalantzis G, Kefalopoulou Z, Panagiotopoulos V, Papadakos D, Constantoyannis C. Effects of COVID-19 on the admissions of aneurysmal subarachnoid hemorrhage: the West Greece experience. *Neurol Sci.* 2021 Jun; 42(6): 2167-2172. doi: 10.1007/s10072-021-05190-6.

Papadakos D, Boulieris S, Theofanopoulos A, Fermeli D, Constantoyannis C. Tubular laminectomy and percutaneous vertebroplasty for aggressive vertebral hemangioma. *Surg Neurol Int.* 2021 Jan 20; 12: 27. doi: 10.25259/SNI_888_2020.

Constantine Constantoyannis

Affiliation: University Hospital of Patras, Department of Neurosurgery

Education:

- 1990: Graduate of University of Athens School of Medicine
- 1991 – 1992: General Surgery Resident – General Hospital of Korinthos

- 01/1994 – 07/1994: General Surgery Resident – Evgenideio Hospital, Athens
- 11/1994 – 5/1999: Neurosurgery Resident, University Hosptial of Patras
- 6/10/1998: Successful completion of the Written Examination of the European Association of Neurosurgical Societies (EANS), Madera, Portugal
- 6/1999: Successful completion of Neurosurgery Residency
- 1/2001: PhD Graduate of University of Patras School of Mecicine

Business Address: University Hospital of Patras, Department of Neurosurgery, Rion 26504, Patras, Greece

Research - Professional Experience and Professional Appointments:

8/1999 – 1/2000: Private practice at Hygeia General Hospital, Athens (Director Professor N. Papadakis)
1/02/2001 – 1/8/2001: Fellowship at the Department of Neurosurgery, University of Umea, Sweden
10/10/2001: Attending Physician, Department of Neurosurgery, University Hospital of Patras
1/07/2002 – 1/7/2003: Clinical Fellowship "Stereotactic and Functional Neurosurgery", Surgical Centre of Movement Disorders, Department of Neurosurgery, University of British Columbia Canada
19/12/2005: Assistant Professor of Neurosurgery, University of Patras
14/1/2013-18/1/2013: Visiting Professor in Spine Center, Hospital zum Heiligen Geist, Kempen, Germany
4/2013- 4/2018: Associate Professor of Neurosurgery, University of Patras
8/2018- today: Professor of Neurosurgery, University of Patras
12/2018- today: Director of the Department of Neurosurgery, University of Patras

Honours:

- Curriculum vitae included in 'Who is who in the world' database for the year 2009.

- Election as member in 'top 100 Health Professionals 2009' by the International Biographical Centre, Cambridge, England.
- Our presented work 'SPECT neuroimaging and neuropsychological function' was awarded as best presented work in the 24th National Neurological Congress, Kos 20-23/5/2010.
- Publications in the journal Stereotactic and Functional Neurosurgery are suggested by the editor in the top-10 articles list in the journal's on-line edition.

Publications from the Last 3 Years:

Panagiotopoulos V, Tsitsopoulos PP, Zampakis P, Zolota V, Messinis L, Constantoyannis C. Multimodality Treatment of Low-Grade Ruptured Brain Arteriovenous Malformations Presenting with Life-Threatening Intracranial Hematoma. *Maedica (Bucur).* 2021 Mar; 16(1): 117-124. doi: 10.26574/maedica.2020.16.1.112. PMID: 34221166; PMCID: PMC8224719.

Theofanopoulos A, Zampakis P, Antoniadou E, Papadakos D, Fermeli D, Constantoyannis C, Messinis L, Panagiotopoulos V. Spontaneous thoracolumbar epidural hematoma in an apixaban anticoagulated patient. *Surg Neurol Int.* 2021 Jun 7; 12: 256. doi: 10.25259/SNI_434_2021. PMID: 34221587; PMCID: PMC8247671.

Papadakos D, Boulieris S, Theofanopoulos A, Fermeli D, Constantoyannis C. Tubular laminectomy and percutaneous vertebroplasty for aggressive vertebral hemangioma. *Surg Neurol Int.* 2021 Jan 20; 12: 27. doi: 10.25259/SNI_888_2020. PMID: 33598343; PMCID: PMC7881512.

Theofanopoulos A, Fermeli D, Boulieris S, Kalantzis G, Kefalopoulou Z, Panagiotopoulos V, Papadakos D, Constantoyannis C. Effects of COVID-19 on the admissions of aneurysmal subarachnoid hemorrhage: the West Greece experience. *Neurol Sci.* 2021 Jun; 42(6): 2167-2172. doi: 10.1007/s10072-021-05190-6. Epub 2021 Mar 21. PMID: 33745041; PMCID: PMC7981384.

Panagiotopoulos VE, Messinis L, Constantoyannis C, Zampakis P. Ultrasound-guided transjugular embolization of ruptured huge venous ectasia of a Cognard IV tentorial dural arteriovenous fistula as a first-stage lifesaving procedure: Review of the literature. *Brain Circ.* 2021 Aug 27; 7(3): 211-216. doi: 10.4103/bc.bc_12_21. PMID: 34667906; PMCID: PMC8459695.

Mousele C, Georgiopoulos M, Constantoyannis C. Syringobulbia: A delayed complication following spinal cord injury - case report. *J Spinal Cord Med.* 2019 Mar; 42(2): 260-264. doi: 10.1080/10790268.2018.1439437. Epub 2018 Feb 27. PMID: 29485364; PMCID: PMC6419677.

Brandon Lucke-Wold

eRA COMMONS USER NAME (credential, e.g., agency login): blwold
Position Title: Neurosurgery Resident PGY4

Education/Training:

- 08/2007 – 05-2011: BS in Neuroscience from Baylor University
- 07/2011 – 05/2018: MD, PhD in Neuroscience from West Virginia University
- 05/2016 – 07/2017: MCTS in Clinical Translational Science from West Virginia University
- 07/2018 – Ongoing: Residency/Endovascular Fellowship in Neurosurgery at University of Florida

A.Personal Statement

My MD/PhD and MCTS training at WVU provided me with the initial foundation to build my career as a clinician scientist. I learned how to ask clinically relevant questions, design carefully thought through experiments, write animal protocols and IRBs, publish manuscripts, compete for grants, and balance my time in the laboratory with clinical responsibilities. The focus of my PhD training was centered upon the investigation of secondary injury pathways following neurotrauma that play a role in neurodegeneration. I specifically sought a neurosurgery program that would expand my training environment to become a successful clinician scientist. Under the guidance of my chairman Dr. Brian Hoh at University of Florida, I have continued to develop my clinical skill set in conjunction with furthering my research opportunities and training. As I transition from neurotrauma to the field of subarachnoid hemorrhage and aneurysm research, I am intrigued by issues that directly impact our patients and can be determinants of overall outcomes. I will utilize prior technical skill sets and develop new ones, to tackle the challenging questions regarding vasospasm following subarachnoid hemorrhage. This topic is especially important for improving patient care and will be a topic I will continue to investigate as a cerebrovascular trained neurosurgeon scientist. The proposed project looks at preventative strategies, improving resource options for patients, and opening further avenues of research inquiry. My continued training and support at University of Florida will be the catalyst to launching me into a successful academic career.

Highlighted Research Support from Past 3 Years

Ongoing

- 07/2022: R25 Neurosurgery Clinician Scientist Training Award: Lucke-Wold (PI)
- 06/2018 – Present: INOVA Angel Investment $225,000: Lucke-Wold (Co-PI); Start up funds for Wright Wold Scientific Animal Tagging
- 07/2019 – Present: AlphaLab Pilot Funding $50,000: Lucke-Wold (Co-PI); Start up funds for Laboratory Animal Biometric Data monitoring
- 08/2019 – Present: Innovation Works $50,000: Lucke-Wold (Co-PI); Startup funds for cage vision tracking technology

B. Positions

- 5/2011 – 5/2013: Regional Vice President at Nu Rho Psi-Honor Society
- 1/2012 – 5/2013: Committee Chair for Surgery Interest Group at West Virginia University
- 8/2014 – 5/2016: President of American Association of Pharmeceutical Sciences at West Virginia University
- 1/2015 – 1/2016: Partnerships Committee Liason at American Physician Scientist Association
- 8/2017 – 6/2018: President of Neurosurgery Interest Group
- 7/2019 – Present: Representative of House Staff Council University of Florida

Honors

- John E. Pescott Award for Academic Excellence (Spring 2012)
- *1st Place* Oral Presentation American College of Physicians Scientific Meeting (Fall 2013)
- *1st Place* Oral Presentation American Association of Pharmaceutical Sciences Regional Meeting (Fall 2013)
- *1st Place* Oral Presentation Neurological Surgery Society of Virginias Meeting. The Crutchfield, Gage, and Thomson Award. (Spring 2014)
- Behavioral and Biomedical Sciences Research Scholarship (Spring 2014)
- American Physician Scientist Association Travel Award (Spring 2014)
- *2nd Place* Van Liere Oral Presentation (Spring 2014)
- Synapse Travel Award (Spring 2014)
- American Association of Clinical Investigation Travel Award (Spring 2014)
- Neurotrauma Travel Award (Summer 2014)
- WVU Innovator Award Finalist (Fall 2014)
- *1st Place* Oral Presentation American College of Physicians Scientific Meeting (Fall 2014)
- *1st Place* Oral Presentation American Association of Pharmaceutical Sciences Regional Meeting (Fall 2014)
- *1st Place* Poster Presentation Appalachian Regional Cell Conference (Fall 2014)
- American Society of Pharmacology and Experimental Therapeutics Travel Award (Spring 2015)
- American Society of Pharmacology and Experimental Therapeutics Best Abstract Competition (Spring 2015)
- Central Society for Clinical and Translational Research Travel Award (Spring 2015)
- Behavioral and Biomedical Sciences Research Scholarship (Spring 2015)
- American Federation of Medical Research Scholar (Spring 2015)
- Burroughs-Wellcome Fund Trainee Travel Award Translational Science Meeting (Spring 2015)

- 1st Place Poster Competition National American College of Physicians Meeting (Spring 2015)
- Alzheimer's Association International Conference Travel Fellowship (Summer 2015)
- Cranial Trauma Research Award American Association of Neurological Surgeons/Congress of Neurological Surgeons Section on Neurotrauma and Critical Care (Summer 2015)
- American Association of Pharmaceutical Science Biotec Graduate Student Research Award (Fall 2015)
- WV Rural Health Conference Travel Award (Fall 2015)
- Society of Toxicology Future Tox Silver Award (Fall 2015)
- American College of Physicians Research Meeting 2nd Place (Fall 2015)
- Washington Fellow's Program American Society of Pharmacology and Experimental Therapeutics (2015/2016)
- American Association of Neurological Surgeons Medical Student Summer Research Fellowship Award (Spring 2016)
- American Society of Pharmacology and Experimental Therapeutics Travel Award and Best Abstract Award (Spring 2016)
- Second Place Young Neurosurgeons Electronic Poster Award American Association of Neurological Surgeons (Spring 2016)
- West Virginia University Student Innovator of the Year Award (Spring 2016)
- American Academy of Neurology Student Travel Award (Spring 2016)
- West Virginia University Injury Control Research Center Outstanding Student Research Award (Spring 2016)
- West Virginia University Injury Control Research Center Travel Award (Spring 2016)
- West Virginia Business Competition Finalist (Fall 2016)
- 1st Place Oral Presentation WV Clinical Translational Science Research Conference (Winter 2016)
- 1st Place Oral Presentation WV Trauma Symposium (Spring 2017)
- WVU Department of Surgery Richard A. Vaughan, MD Scholarship (Spring 2017)
- 3rd Place PitchTX Business Start-up Competition (Spring 2017)

- 1st Place Science Technology and Engineering Section of WV Business Plan Competition (Spring 2017)
- Top Pediatric Poster Congress of Neurological Surgeons Meeting (Fall 2017)
- Carl H. Cather, Jr. Service Award (Spring 2018)
- Bryan Robinson Endowment Honorable Mention (Spring 2021)
- Southern Neurosurgical Society Best Basic Science Award (Spring 2022)

C. Contributions to Science

1. *Endoplasmic reticulum stress is involved in the pathophysiology of chronic traumatic encephalopathy.* Chronic traumatic encephalopathy is a devastating neurodegenerative disease that is the result of repetitive traumatic brain injury. The underlying pathophysiology linking traumatic brain injury to chronic traumatic encephalopathy is poorly understood. Through my dissertation work, I investigated the role that endoplasmic reticulum stress plays in disease progression. Using a novel and validated blast traumatic brain injury model, I showed that endoplasmic reticulum stress worsens cognitive performance following traumatic brain injury and accounts for the long-term progression towards tauopathy. By successfully preventing endoplasmic reticulum stress with docosahexaenoic acid, the rodents had improved cognition, decreased tauopathy, and decreased impulsive-like behavior.Using post-mortem human samples from professional athletes, it was found that endoplasmic reticulum stress was significantly increased in cortical areas adjacent to tauopathy. I also showed that endoplasmic reticulum stress is intimately associated with oxidative stress. Targeting oxidative stress has proved beneficial in reducing long-term deficits.

Turner, R.C., **Lucke-Wold, B.P.**, Robson, M.J., Omalu, B.I., Petraglia, A.L., and Bailes, J.E. (2012) Repetitive Traumatic Brain Injury and Development of Chronic Traumatic Encephalopathy: A Potential Role for Biomarkers in Diagnosis, Prognosis, and Treatment? *Frontiers in Neurology: Frontiers in Neurotrauma.* 3: 186.

Lucke-Wold, B.P., Turner, R.C., Logsdon, A.F., Bailes, J.E., Huber, J.D., Rosen, C.L. (2014) Linking Traumatic Brain Injury to Chronic Traumatic Encephalopathy: Identification of Potential Mechanisms Leading to

Neurofibrillary Tangle Development. *Journal of Neurotrauma.* 31(13): 1129-38.

Logsdon, A.F., **Lucke-Wold, B.P.**, Rosen, C.L., Huber, J.D. (2014) Disparity among Neural Injury Models and the Unfolded Protein Response. *Journal of Neurological Disorders and Stroke.* 2(5): 1083.

Lucke-Wold, B.P., Turner, R.C., Logsdon, A.F., Nguyen, L., Bailes, J.E., Lee, J.M., Robson, M.J., Omalu, B.I., Smith, K.E., Huber, J.D., Rosen, C.L. (2015) Endoplasmic Reticulum Stress Implicated in Chronic Traumatic Encephalopathy. *Journal of Neurosurgery.* 18: 1-16.

2. *Oxidative stress is an important component of secondary injury cascades following neurotrauma.* Concussions can cause acute symptoms that can subsequently progress to neurodegenerative disease over time. I found that NADPH mediated oxidative stress plays a critical role in injury expansion using our pre-clinical blast model. In collaboration with our physics colleagues at Iowa State University, we published how the blast model causes injury. Once characterized, I successfully targeted NADPH oxidative stress with lipoic acid. Lipoic acid decreased impulsive like behavior and improved outcomes. Furthermore NADPH oxidative stress is increased in specimens from patients diagnosed with chronic traumatic encephalopathy. NADPH oxidative stress plays a critical role in injury progression and warrants further investigation.

Lucke-Wold, B.P., Naser, Z., Logsdon, A.F., Turner, R.C., Smith, K.E., Robson, M.J., Bailes, J.E., Lee, J.M. Rosen, C.L., Huber, J.D. (2015) Amelioration of NADPH-Mediated Stress Reduces Cell Death following Blast-induced Traumatic Brain Injury. *Translational Research.* 166:509-528.

Turner, R.C.*, **Lucke-Wold, B.P.***, Logsdon, A.F.*, Robson, M.J., Dashnaw, M.L., Huang, J.H., Smith, K.E., Huber, J.D., Rosen, C.L., Petraglia, A.L. (2015) Modeling Chronic Traumatic Encephalopathy: A Multiple Model & Injury Paradigm Experience. *Frontiers in Neurotrauma.* 6: 223.

Logsdon, A*. **Lucke-Wold, B.P.***, Nguyen, L., Matsumoto, R., Turner, R.C., Rosen, C.L., Huber, J.D. (2015) Salubrinal reduces markers of neuroinflammation and improves outcome in a rodent model of traumatic brain injury. *Brain Research.* [Epub Ahead of Print].

Lucke-Wold, B.P., Phillips, M., Turner, R.C., Logsdon, A.F., Smith, K.E., Huber, J.D., Rosen, C.L., Regele, J. (2015) Elucidating the Role of

Compression Waves and Impact Duration for Generating mild Traumatic Brain Injury in Rats. *Brain Injury*. In Press.

3. *Simulation of vascular injury improves neurosurgery residence performance.*In collaboration with Dr. Ciporen at Oregon Health & Science University, I established a simulated model for vascular injury. Carotid injuries are rare but serious events during endoscopic transphenoidal surgeries. The established cadaveric vascular repair model as well as a surgical clipping model has proven valuable for training. These models provide residents with adequate learning environments to reach benchmark standards without risking patient lives. Importantly, I learned microvascular injection techniques that will be helpful in studying vasospasm.

Ciporen, J.N., **Lucke-Wold, B.P.,** Dogan, A., Cetas, J., Cameron, W. (2016). Endoscopic endonasal transclival approach vs dual transorbital port technique for clip application to the posterior circulation: A cadaveric anatomic and cerebral circulation simulation study. *Skull Base.* In Press.

Ciporen, J., **Lucke-Wold, B.P.,** Dogan, A., Cetas, J., Cameron, W.E. (2016). Dual endoscopic endonasal transphenoidal and precaruncular transorbital approaches for clipping the cavernous carotid artery: A cadaveric simulation. *Skull Base.* In Press.

Lucke-Wold, B.P., Gillham, H.E., Baskerville, M., Cameron, W.E., Dillman, D., Haley, C.A., Noles, M., Spight, D., Ciporen, J.N. (2017). Establishing a Multidisciplinary Cavernous Carotid Injury Simulation to Train Neurosurgical, Otolaryngology, and Anesthesia Residents. *Journal of Visualized Experiments.* In Press.

Ciporen, J., Gillham, H., Turner, R.C., **Lucke-Wold, B.P.**(2016) Crisis Management Simulation: Establishing a Dual Neurosurgery and Anesthesia Training Experience. *Journal of Neurosurgical Anesthesiology.* In Press.

Complete List of Published Work
https://pubmed.ncbi.nlm.nih.gov/?term=lucke-wold%2C+b

Irina Alexandrovna Savvina

Affiliation: Almazov National Medical Research Centre of Ministry of Health Care of Russian Federation

Education:

- The First Saint Petersburg Pavlov Medical State University, Saint Petersburg. Residency in Anesthesiology and Intensive Care.
- Postgraduate course in Anesthesiology and Intensive Care.

Business Address: 197341, 2 Akkuratova str., Saint Petersburg, Russian Federation

Research and Professional Experience:

Highly qualified anesthesiologist with 35 years of experience. Specialist in the field of Neuroanesthesiology and NeuroIntensive Care.

I am also committed to conducting scientific research in this area.

My scientific interest is in the study of septic encephalopathy, molecular genetic aspects of general anesthesia and systemic inflammation response during general anesthesia in neurosurgery including pediatric neurosurgery, personified premedication in neurosurgical patients.

In 1994, I defended my PhD thesis "Opioid anesthesia in pediatric neurosurgery", which describes the peculiarities of opioid anesthesia in pediatric patients with intracranial hypertension, intracranial pressure dynamics during induction of anesthesia in neurosurgical patients with brain tumor, hydrocephalus.

In 2000, I defended my doctoral dissertation on the topic "Anesthesia management system of neurosurgical operations and diagnostic proceeders in pediatric patients", which presents the structure of general anesthesia and choice of anesthetic agents according to the anesthetic influence on the stress-limiting antinociceptive neuroregulatory systems of the brain.

In 2001 I received the degree of Doctor of Medical Sciences.

Alongside with the research I performed duties of a clinical anesthesiologist.

Professional Appointments:

- 1987-1988 - postgraduate study at the First Saint Petersburg Pavlov Medical State University, anesthesiologist by profession.
- In 1988, after my postgraduate study I got the position of a scientific researcher on a competitive basis of the Russian

Polenov Scientific Research Neurosurgical Institute. For 30 years of my professional activity, I have gone from an junior researcher to the Chief Researcher.

- 2008-2010 - Head of the Research Department of Anesthesiology and Intensive Care of the Research Institute of Children's Infections, Saint Petersburg, Russian Federation
- From 2001 to the present time – Professor of the Vladimir L. Vanevskii Department of Anaesthesiology and Reanimatology of the North-Western State Medical University named after Ilya I. Mechnikov of Ministry of Health Care of Russian Federation, Saint Petersburg, Russian Federation

Honors: I am awarded the medal "To the 300th anniversary of St. Petersburg", the medal "For contribution to the development of science named after the nobel laureate Ivan P. Pavlov", the medal "Personality of St. Petersburg".

Publications from the Last 3 Years:

Orekhova E S, Gulyaev D A, Savvina I A. Personalized approach to premedication in neurosurgical patients. *Russian Journal of Anaesthesiology and Reanimatology.* 2019; (3): 79-89. https://doi.org/10. 17116/anaesthesiology201903179.

Rasputina D.A., Rutkovsky R.V., Mertsalov S.A., Krupko T.A., Gulyaev M.E., Salogub E.D., Savello A.V., Yakovlev A.N., Zverev D.A., Kozlenok A.V., Savvina I.A. Neurogenic stressor cardiomyopathy caused by aneurysmal subarachnoid hemorrhage. *Russian Journal of Cardiology*. 2019; (2): 81-85. (In Russ.) https://doi.org/10.15829/1560-4071-2019-2-81-85.

Kondratov K A, Fedorov A V, Rasputina D A, Krupko T A, Rutkovskiy R V, Dryagina N V, Petrov A A, Gulyaev D A, Kostareva A A, Savvina I A. Influence of neurosurgical intervention and sevoflurane general anesthesia combined with fentanyl on the concentration of nucleic acids, biomarkers of inflammation and cerebral damage in cerebrospinal fluid of patients with intracranial meningioma: pilot study. *Russian Journal of Anaesthesiology and Reanimatology.* 2019; (3): 71-78. https://doi.org/ 10.17116/anaesthesiology201903171.

Panshin D D, Rasputina D A, Krupko T A, Rutkovskiy R V, Dryagina N V, Petrov A A, Gulyaev D A, Kondratov K A, Fedorov A V, Kostareva A

A, Savvina I A. Effects of neurosurgical intervention and general sevoflurane anesthesia combined with fentanyl on the plasma concentrations of nucleic acids and proinflammatory cytokines in patients with intracranial meningioma: a pilot study. *Russian Journal of Anaesthesiology and Reanimatology.* 2019; (4): 55-60. https://doi.org/ 10.17116/anaesthesiology201904155.

Savvina I A, Cherebillo V Yu, Zabrodskaya Yu M, Petrova A O, Sergeev A V, Paltsev A A, Rutkovskiy R V, Malkhozova A M. The intraoperative prophylaxis of local ischemical brain damage in neurosurgical patients with cerebral aneurysm (in Russian only). *Khirurgiya.* 2019; (5): 57-63. https://doi.org/10.17116/hirurgia 201905157.

Gurskaia V. I., Dryagina N. V., Ivanov V. P., Savvina I.A. General inhalation sevoflurane anesthesia effect on the inflammatory and brain damage biomarkers blood serum levels in the paediatric patients with craniosynostosis during MRI invetigation: a cohort study. *Science.* Education. Practice: materials of the International University Science Forum (Canada, Toronto), April 22, 2020. - Infinity Publishing. - P. 119-124. DOI 10.34660/INF.2020.1.61638 URL http://naupers.ru/wp-content/uploads/ 2020/04/Canada-April-22- Part-2.pdf#page=119.

Savvina I., Orechova E., Gulyaev D. Personify premedication in the structure of general anaesthesia in neurosurgical patients with intracranial neoplasm. *European Journal of Anaesthesiology.* - 2020.-Vol.37, suppl.58. - P. 182-183. www.ejanaesthesiology.com.

Savvina I.A.,. Lavrinenko N.V,. Zabrodskaya Yu. M, Sebelev K. I., Dolmatov.V. Hippocampus role in predictive assessment of sepsis development in patients with severe traumatic brain injury. *European Journal of Anaesthesiology.* - 2020. - Vol.37, suppl.58. - P. 302-303. www.ejanaesthesiology.com.

Savvina I., Anna Petrova, Roman Rutkovskiy, Ekaterina Orechova, Sergey Mertsalov, Anna Novikova. Selective decontamination of the intestine in neurosurgical patients with subarachnoid haemorrhage in the acute period of cerebral aneurysm rupture. *European Journal of Anaesthesiology.* June 2020. - Vol.37, e-Suppl.58. - P. 274-275. www.ejanaesthesiology.com.

Savvina I.A, Alexandrovich Yu S, Lekmanov A.U, Semenova Zh. B, Khachatryan V.A. Management of Pediatric Severe Traumatic Brain Injury: What are News? *EC Anaesthesia.* – 2020. – Vol.6, №10. – P. 1-14. https://www.ecronicon.com/ anaesthesia.php.

Atiskov Yu A., Akshulakov S.K., Belkin A.A., Kondratiev A.N., Larionov S.N., Nazaralieva E.T., Riznich V.P., Savvina I.A., Safin I.Sh., Khachatryan V.A. Craniospinal compliance — new principles for intracranial pressure monitoring. *Russian Journal of Anaesthesiology and Reanimatology.* 2020; (6): 37-43. https://doi.org/10.17116/ anaesthesiology202006137.

Savvina I.A., Kondratieva E.A., Grekhov E.V., Morozov K.A., Biktasheva L.Z., Gurskaya V.I., Stepanova K.V., Novikov V. Yu., Kim A.V., Lebedev K.E., Sereda E.O., Ryzhkov A.V., Efimtsev A. Yu., Trufanov G.E., Ryzhkova D.V., Pervunina T.M., Khachatryan V.A., Shlyakhto E.V. Consciousness recovery in a child with hypoxic brain damage after surgical treatment of congenital heart disease. *Russian Journal of Anaesthesiology and Reanimatology.* 2021;(1):81-90. https://doi.org/10. 17116/anaesthesiology202101181.

Gurskaya V.I., Dryagina N.V., Ivanov V.P., Aleksandrovich Yu. S., Khachatryan V.A., Savvina I.A. Effect of general anesthesia on systemic inflammatory response and neuronal damage in children with craniosynostosis in perioperative period. *Russian Journal of Anaesthesiology and Reanimatology.* 2021;(1):39-45. https://doi.org/10.17116/ anaesthesiology202101139.

Gurskaya V.I., Ivanov V.P., Novikov V.Yu., Dryagina N.V., Savvina IA. Systemic inflammatory response in infants with craniostenosis sedated with propofol. *Russian Journal of Pediatric Surgery, Anesthesia and Intensive Care.* 2021:;11(3): 297-306. DOI: https://doi.org/10.17816/ psaic961.

Irina Alexandrovna Savvina, Anna Olegovna Petrova. The Treatment of Acute Stroke. In: *Ischemic Stroke.* Edited by Pratap Sanchetee. Intech Open, London.-2021. - 117 P. DOI: 10.5772/intechopen.86623 ISBN: 978-1-83962-395-0.

Irina Alexandrovna Savvina, Yulia Mihailovna Zabrodskaya, Anna Olegovna Petrova, Konstantin Alexandrovich Samochernykh. Cerebral vasospasm: Mechanisms, Pathomorphology, Diagnostics, Treatment. In: *Cerebrovascular Diseases.* Edited by Patricia Bozzetto Ambrosi/ IntechOpen, London. - 2021. - 138 P. DOI: http://dx.doi.org/10.5772/ intechopen.101229 ISBN: 978-1-83962-701-9.

Yulia Mikhailovna Zabrodskaya

Affiliation: Russian Polenov Scientific Research Neurosurgical Institute – branch of the Almazov National Medical Research Centre of Ministry of Health Care of Russian Federation, Russian Federation
Education: Leningrad Sanitary and Hygienic Medical Institute, qualification of a general practitioner. Residency in pathological anatomy. Postgraduate course in pathological anatomy.
Business Address: 191014, 12 Mayakovskogo Str., Saint Petersburg, Russian Federation

Research and Professional Experience:

Highly qualified pathologist with more than 25 years of experience. Specialist in the field of pathomorphological diagnostics of diseases of the nervous system and neurooncology.

I am also committed to conducting scientific research in this area.

My scientific interest is in the etiology of brain aneurysm, wound process, pathomorphology and proteomics of epilepsy, apoptosis, structural and metabolic changes of skeletal muscles in intensive care patients, morphological evaluation of the effectiveness of fluorescence navigation with chlorin e6 in surgery for gliomas.

In 1997, I defended my PhD thesis "Pathomorphological characteristics of changes in the articulations of the arteries of the base of the brain (to the problem of the origin of aneurysms)", which describes the previously unknown phenomenon of segmental (metameric) structure of the arterial circle of the brain and morphogenesis of brain aneurysms - stretching of the articulations of the arterial circle of the human brain, studied the structural changes of the arteries in vasospasm after rupture of aneurysms.

In 2012, I defended my doctoral dissertation on the topic "Pathological anatomy of a surgical wound of the brain with modern methods of surgical treatment", which presents the structure of the perifocal zone of brain tumors as an area of the surgical wound, the morphogenesis of the wound process, new data on the peritumorous zone were obtained.

Alongside with the research I performed duties of a clinical pathologist.

Professional Appointments:

- 1992-1995 - postgraduate studies at the Russian Polenov Scientific Research Neurosurgical Institute, pathologist by profession.
- In 1995, after my postgraduate study I got the position of a scientific research on a competitive basis. For 30 years of my professional activity, I have gone from an ordinary researcher to the head of a laboratory.
- Since 2008, Head of the Research Laboratory of Pathomorphology of the Nervous system of the Polenov Russian Neurosurgical Research Institute.
- I am a Professor at the Department of Pathology of the Institute of Medical Education of the Almazov National Medical Research Center.

Honours: I am awarded three medals named after P. L. Kapitsa "To the author of a scientific discovery", the medal "For contribution to the development of medical genomics named after Yu. B. Yurov".

Publications from the Last 3 Years:

Rynda, A. Yu., Zabrodskaya, Yu. M., Olyushin, V.E., Sokolova, T.V., Papayan, G.V. Morphological evaluation of the effectiveness of fluorescence navigation with chlorin e6 in surgery for malignant gliomas. *Arkhiv Patologii.* 2021, 83(5), стр. 13–20.

Rynda, A. Yu., Olyushin, V.E., Rostovtsev, D.M., Tastanbekov, M.M., Papayan, G.V. Intraoperative fluorescence control with chlorin e6 in resection of glial brain tumors. *Zhurnal Voprosy Nejrokhirurgii Imeni N.N. Burdenko.* 2021, 85(4), стр. 20–26.

Sitovskaya, D.A., Zabrodskaya, Y., Sokolova, T.V., Nezdorovina, V.G., Dobrogorskaya, L.N. Structural heterogeneity of epileptic foci in local drug-resistant epilepsy. *Arkhiv Patologii.* 2020, 82(6), стр. 5–15.

Sazhina, T.A., Sitovskaya, D.A., Zabrodskaya, Y.M., Bazhanova, E.D. Functional Imbalance of Glutamate- and GABAergic Neuronal Systems in the Pathogenesis of Focal Drug-Resistant Epilepsy in Humans. *Bulletin of Experimental Biology and Medicine.* 2020, 168(4), стр. 529–532.

Rynda, A. Yu., Rostovtsev, D.M., Olyushin, V.E., Zabrodskaya, Yu. M. Therapeutic pathomorphosis in malignant glioma tissues after photodynamic therapy with chlorin e6 (Reports of two clinical cases). *Biomedical Photonics.* 2020, 9(2), стр. 45–54.

Rynda, A., Olyushin, V.E., Rostovtsev, D.M., Zabrodskaya, Y. Complex treatment of a patient with neurofibromatosis type 2. *Zhurnal Nevrologiii Psihiatriiimeni S.S. Korsakova.* 2020, 120(8), стр. 98–104.

Sidorin, V.S., Zabrodskaya, Y.M., Dobrogorskaya, L.N. Tanatogenetic role of type 2 diabetes in neurosurgical patients. *Arkhiv Patologii.* 2020, 82(1), стр. 38–46.

Emelyanov, A., Shtam, T., Kamyshinsky, R., Pchelina, S., Konevega, A. Cryo-electron microscopy of extracellular vesicles from cerebrospinal fluid. *PLoSONE.* 2020, 15(1), e0227949.

Rynda, A.U., Olyushin, V.E., Zabrodskaya, U.M., Rostovtsev, D.M. Metastasis primary myxofibrosarcoma from the heart of in brain. Case report. *Voprosy Onkologii.* 2019, 65(3), стр. 467–474.

Savvina, I.A., Cherebillo, V.Y., Zabrodskaya, Y.M., Rutkovskiy, R.V., Malkhozova, A.M. The intraoperative prophylaxis of local ischemical brain damage in neurosurgical patients with cerebral aneurysm. *Khirurgiia.* 2019, (5), стр. 57–63.

Bersnev V., Kravtsova S., Stepanova T., Zabrodskaya Yu. M. STRUCTURAL FINDINGS IN PATIENTS WITH PHARMACORESISTANT TEMPORAL EPILEPSY AFTER ANTERIOR TEMPORAL LOBECTOMY WITH A HISTORY OF STATUS EPILEPTICUS *Epilepsy & Behavior.* 2019. T. 101. № Part B. C. 106750.

Rozhchenko Larisa Vitalievna

Affiliation: Russian Polenov Scienific Research Neurosurgical Institute – branch of the Almazov National Medical Research Centre of Ministry of Health Care of Russian Federation

Education: The First Pavlov Saint Petersburg Medical State University

Business Address: 191014, 12 Mayakovskogo Str., Saint Petersburg, Russian Federation.

Research and Professional Experience: surgery and endovascular therapy of cerebral vascular pathology

Professional Appointments: neurosurgeon

Honors: PhD

Publications from the Last 3 Years:

1. Rozhchenko L.V. [Molecular mechanisms of growth and relapse of cerebral arteriovenous malformations]. *Zh Vopr Neirokhir Im N N Burdenko.* 2020; 84(1): 94-100. doi: 10.17116/neiro20208401194. PMID: 32207748 Russian.
2. Rozhchenko L.V., Dryagina N.V., Petrov A.E., Goroshchenko S.A. Molecular mechanisms of growth and recurrence of cerebral arteriovenous malformations: part 2 (our own research). *Zh Vopr Neirokhir Im N N Burdenko.* 2020; 84(2): 35-41. Russian. doi: 10.17116/neiro20208402135.
3. Goroshchenko S.A., Petrov A.E., Rozhchenko L.V., Samochernykh K.A. Endovascular embolization of high-flow arteriovenous fistulae with non-adhesive agents in the structure of cerebral arteriovenous malformations on the background of adenosine-induced cardioplegia. *Zh Vopr Neirokhir Im N N Burdenko.* 2020; 84(3): 21-27. Russian. doi: 10.17116/neiro20208403121.
4. Goroshchenko S.A., Sitovskaya D.A., Petrov A.E., Rozhchenko L.V., Khristoforova M.I., Samochernykh K.A. Unfavorable outcome of giant vertebral artery aneurysm. Clinical case and literature review. *Arkh Patol.* 2021; 83(4): 45-51. Russian. doi: 10.17116/patol20218304145.
5. Goroshchenko S.A., Petrov A.E., Rozhchenko L.V., Blagorazumova G.P., Vyazgina E.M., Ivanov A.Y. [Surgical treatment of large and giant vertebrobasilar aneurysms manifested by brainstem compression symptoms]. *Zh Vopr Neirokhir Im N N Burdenko.* 2018; 82(4): 32-37. Russian. doi: 10.17116/neiro201882432.
6. Goroshchenko, S.A., Rozhchenko, L.V., Petrov, A.E., Ivanova, N.E., Ivanov, A.Yu. Rupture of dissection aneurysm of the vertebral artery followed by formation of epidural hematoma of the cervical spine: *Case report Patologiya Krovoobrashcheniya i Kardiokhirurgiya,* 2018, 22(2), стр. 58–62.
7. Petrov A.E., Goroshchenko S.A., Rozhchenko L.V., Samochernykh K.A. Results of endovascular treatment for high-flow direct carotid-cavernous fistulas. *Journal of Radiology and Nuclear Medicine.* 2020;

101(5): 283–7 (in Russian). https://doi.org/10.20862/0042-4676-2020-101-5-283-287.

8. Petrov A.E., Rozhchenko L.V., Ivanov A.A., Bobinov V.V., Henkes H. [The first experience of endovascular treatment of chronic subdural hematomas with non-adhesive embolization materials of various viscosities: Squid 12 and 18]. *Zh Vopr Neirokhir Im N N Burdenko.* 2021; 85(5): 80-87. doi: 10.17116/neiro2021850 5180.PMID: 34714007 Russian.
9. Petrov A., Ivanov A., Rozhchenko L., Petrova A., Bhogal P., Cimpoca A., Henkes H.J. Endovascular Treatment of Chronic Subdural Hematomas through Embolization: A Pilot Study with a Non-Adhesive Liquid Embolic Agent of Minimal Viscosity (Squid). *Clin Med.* 2021 Sep 27; 10(19): 4436. doi: 10.3390/jcm10194436.PMID: 34640453 Free PMC article.

Goroshchenko Sergey Anatolyevich

Affiliation: Russian Polenov Scienific Research Neurosurgical Institute – branch of the Almazov National Medical Research Centre of Ministry of Health Care of Russian Federation

Education: Petrozavodsk State University

Business Address: 191014, 12 Mayakovskogo Str., Saint Petersburg, Russian Federation.

Research and Professional Experience: surgery and endovascular therapy of cerebral vascular pathology

Professional Appointments: neurosurgeon

Honors: PhD

Publications from the Last 3 Years:

1. Rozhchenko L.V., Dryagina N.V., Petrov A.E., Goroshchenko S.A. Molecular mechanisms of growth and recurrence of cerebral arteriovenous malformations: part 2 (our own research). *Zh Vopr*

Neirokhir Im N N Burdenko. 2020; 84(2): 35-41. Russian. doi: 10.17116/neiro20208402135.

2. Goroshchenko S.A., Petrov A.E., Rozhchenko L.V., Samochernykh K.A. Endovascular embolization of high-flow arteriovenous fistulae with non-adhesive agents in the structure of cerebral arteriovenous malformations on the background of adenosine-induced cardioplegia. *Zh Vopr Neirokhir Im N N Burdenko.* 2020; 84(3): 21-27. Russian. doi: 10.17116/neiro20208403121.
3. Goroshchenko S.A., Sitovskaya D.A., Petrov A.E., Rozhchenko L.V., Khristoforova M.I., Samochernykh K.A. Unfavorable outcome of giant vertebral artery aneurysm. Clinical case and literature review. *Arkh Patol.* 2021; 83(4): 45-51. Russian. doi: 10.17116/patol20218304145.
4. Goroshchenko S.A., Petrov A.E., Rozhchenko L.V., Blagorazumova G.P., Vyazgina E.M., Ivanov A.Y. Khirurgicheskoe lechenie krupnykh i gigantskikh anevrizm vertebrobaziliarnogo basseĭna, proiavliaiushchikhsia simptomatikoĭ kompressii stvola golovnogo mozga [Surgical treatment of large and giant vertebrobasilar aneurysms manifested by brainstem compression symptoms]. *Zh Vopr Neirokhir Im N N Burdenko.* 2018; 82(4): 32-37. Russian. doi: 10.17116/neiro 201882432.
5. Khachatryan V.A., Samochernykh K.A., Mamatkhanov M.R., Potemkina E.G., Goroshchenko S.A., Tadevosyan A.R., Litvinenko P.V. Metody otsenki sostoiatel'nosti nepriamoĭ revaskuliarizatsii golovnogo mozga u deteĭ [Methods to assess competence of indirect cerebral revascularization in children]. *Zh Vopr Neirokhir Im N N Burdenko.* 2018; 82(2): 30-38. Russian. doi: 10.17116/oftalma 201882230-38.
6. Oleynik, A.A., Ivanova, N.E., Goroshchenko, S.A. et al. The quality of life in patients with ruptured multiple cerebral aneurysms after endovascular treatment *Medical News of North Caucasus.* 2020, 15(3), стр. 400–404.
7. Oleinik, A.A., Ivanova, N.E., Goroshchenko, S.A., Oleinik, E.A. Late results and health-related quality of life in patients after endovascular treatment for multiple intracranial aneurysms *Bulletin of Siberian Medicine.* 2020, 19(3), стр. 60–66
8. Goroshchenko, S.A., Rozhchenko, L.V., Petrov, A.E., Ivanova, N.E., Ivanov, A. Yu. Rupture of dissection aneurysm of the vertebral artery followed by formation of epidural hematoma of the cervical spine: Case

report. *Patologiya Krovoobrashcheniya i Kardiokhirurgiya*. 2018, 22(2), стр. 58–62

9. Petrov A.E., Goroshchenko S.A., Rozhchenko L.V., Samochernykh K.A. Results of endovascular treatment for high-flow direct carotid-cavernous fistulas. *Journal of Radiology and Nuclear Medicine.* 2020; 101(5): 283–7 (in Russian). https://doi.org/10.20862/0042-4676-2020-101-5-283-287

Potemkina Elena Gennadevna

Affiliation: Russian Polenov Scienific Research Neurosurgical Institute – branch of the Almazov National Medical Research Centre of Ministry of Health Care of Russian Federation

Education: St. Petersburg State Pediatric Medical University

Business Address: 191014, 12 Mayakovskogo Str., Saint Petersburg, Russian Federation.

Research and Professional Experience: radiation diagnostics of cerebral vascular pathology

Professional Appointments: neurorentgenology

Honors: PhD

Publications from the Last 3 Years:

1. Kondratyeva E.A., Ivanova A.O., Yarmolinskaya M.I., Potemkina E.G. et al. Evaluation of structural variations in the pituitary gland, hormonal status and laboratory markers of the central nervous system functioning in patients with chronic disorders of consciousness. *Journal of obstetrics and women's diseases.* - 2021. - Vol. 70. - N. 5. - P. 23-36. doi: 10.17816/JOWD77930.
2. Potemkina E.G., N.K. Samochernykh, K.B. Abramov, M.S. Nikolaenko [et al.]. Treatment of patients with posthemorrhagic hydrocephalus. *Russian Bulletin of Perinatology and Pediatrics.* - 2021. - Vol. 66. - No. 5. - pp. 97-104. - DOI 10.21508/1027-4065-2021-66-5-97-104.
3. Potemkina E.G., Yu. V. Belyakov, A.M. Meredzhi, A.Y. Orlov [et al.]. Comparative analysis of percutaneous endoscopic intralaminar

discectomy and microdiscectomy in overweight patients. *The Russian Neurosurgical Journal named after Professor A.L. Polenov*. - 2020. - Vol. 12. - No. 1. - pp. 12-15.

4. Potemkina E.G., N.E. Warriors, A.Y. Ulitin, P.V. Lavrovsky [et al.]. Primary multiple cerebral tumors of various histological structures (description of clinical cases). *The Russian Neurosurgical Journal named after Professor A.L. Polenov*. - 2020. - Vol. 12. - No. 1. - pp. 55-63.
5. Potemkina E.G., K.K. Kukanov, A.A. Matrelov, K.A. Samochernykh [et al.]. Comparative analysis of stereotactic and endoscopic methods of brain tumor biopsy (literature review). *The Russian Neurosurgical Journal named after Professor A.L. Polenov*. - 2020. - Vol. 12. - No. 1. - pp. 64-70.
6. Potemkina E.G., N.V. Dryagina, E.A. Kondratieva, S.A. Kondratiev [et al.]. The frequency of infectious complications and features of the systemic inflammatory response in patients with prolonged impaired consciousness. *Journal of Infectology*. - 2020. - Vol. 12. - pp. 21-28. - DOI 10.22625/2072-6732-2020-12-5-21-28.
7. Potemkina E.G., Yu. M. Zabrodskaya, T.V. Zhukova, A.F. Smeyanovich [et al.]. Pathomorphological manifestations of peritumorous inflammation in brain tumors. *Neurology and neurosurgery*. Eastern Europe. - 2020. - Vol. 10. - No. 3. - pp. 392-399. - DOI 10.34883/PI.2020.10.3.034.
8. Potemkina E.G., E.V. Iskhakova, A.S. Lepekhina, Ya. B. Batozhargalova [et al.]. Features of the atrophic process in progressive supranuclear paralysis according to magnetic resonance morphometry. *Russian Electronic Journal of Radiation Diagnostics*. - 2020. - Vol. 10. - No. 1. - pp. 43-49. - DOI 10.21569/2222-7415-2020-10-1-43-49.
9. Potemkina E.G., Y.M. Zabrodskaya, E.V. Sivtsova, S.Y. Pyanzin [et al.]. Clinical and pathomorphological features of atypical teratoid-rhabdoid brain tumor in children on the example of three observations. *Neurosurgery and neurology of childhood*. – 2019. – № 4(62). – Pp. 26-37.
10. Potemkina E.G., V.G. Voronov, S.D. Radzhabov, A.A. Ivanov [et al.]. Clinic, diagnostics, surgical treatment of Chiari malformation type I in adults and adolescents. *Neurosurgery and neurology of childhood*. – 2019. – № 4(62). – Pp. 78-97.
11. Potemkina E.G., V.A. Khachatryan, K.A. Samochernykh, M.R. Mamatkhanov [et al.]. Methods of assessing the viability of indirect

revascularization of the brain in children. *Zh Vopr Neirokhir Im N N Burdenko.* - 2018. - Vol. 82. - No. 2. - pp. 30-38. - DOI 10.17116/oftalma201882230-38.

Petrova Anna Olegovna

Affiliation: Almazov National Medical Research Centre of Ministry of Health Care of Russian Federation
Education: The First Saint Petersburg Pavlov Medical State University
Business Address: 197341, 2 Accuratova Str., Saint Petersburg, Russian Federation.

Research and Professional Experience:

- Anesthesiologic maintenance of neurosurgical interventions
- In 2011, I defended my PhD thesis "Multimodal analgesia in pediatric neurosurgery", which describes the peculiarities of stress reactions in neurosurgery in paediatric patients and multimodal approach to maintenance of analgesia perioperatively in pediatric patients with intracranial hypertension, brain tumor, hydrocephalus.

Professional Appointments: anesthesiologist

Publications from the Last 3 Years:

1. Savvina I.A., Cherebillo V. Yu., Zabrodskaya Yu M., Petrova A.O., Sergeev A.V., Paltsev A.A., Rutkovskiy R.V., Malkhozova A.M. The intraoperative prophylaxis of local ischemical brain damage in neurosurgical patients with cerebral aneurysm (in Russian only). *Khirurgiya.* 2019; (5): 57-63. https://doi.org/10.17116/hirurgia 201905157.
2. Petrov A., Ivanov A., Rozhchenko L., Petrova A., Bhogal P., Cimpoca A., Henkes H.J. Endovascular Treatment of Chronic Subdural Hematomas through Embolization: A Pilot Study with a Non-Adhesive Liquid Embolic Agent of Minimal Viscosity (Squid). *Clin Med.* 2021 Sep 27; 10(19): 4436. doi: 10.3390/jcm10194436.

3. Savvina I., Anna Petrova, Roman Rutkovskiy, Ekaterina Orechova, Sergey Mertsalov, Anna Novikova. Selective decontamination of the intestine in neurosurgical patients with subarachnoid haemorrhage in the acute period of cerebral aneurysm rupture. *European Journal of Anaesthesiology*. June 2020. - Vol.37, e-Suppl.58. - P. 274-275. www.ejanaesthesiology.com.
4. Irina Alexandrovna Savvina, Anna Olegovna Petrova. The Treatment of Acute Stroke. In: *Ischemic Stroke*. Edited by Pratap Sanchetee. IntechOpen, London. - 2021. - 117 P. DOI: 10.5772/intechopen. 86623 ISBN: 978-1-83962-395-0.
5. Irina Alexandrovna Savvina, Yulia Mihailovna Zabrodskaya, Anna Olegovna Petrova, Konstantin Alexandrovich Samochernykh. Cerebral vasospasm: Mechanisms, Pathomorphology, Diagnostics, Treatment. In: *Cerebrovascular Diseases*. Edited by Patricia Bozzetto Ambrosi. IntechOpen, London. - 2021. - 138 P. DOI: http://dx.doi.org/10.5772/intechopen.101229 ISBN: 978-1-83962-701-9.

Samochernykh Konstantin Alexandrovich

Affiliation: Russian Polenov Scienific Research Neurosurgical Institute – branch of the Almazov National Medical Research Centre of Ministry of Health of Russian Federation, St. Petersburg, Russian Federation

Education: The Orenburg State Medical University

Business Address: 191014, 12 Mayakovskogo Str., Saint Petersburg, Russian Federation.

Research and Professional Experience: surgery and endovascular therapy of cerebral vascular pathology, oncology, hydrocephalus

Professional Appointments: neurosurgeon

Honors: PhD

Publications from the Last 3 Years:

Goroshchenko S.A., Petrov A.E., Rozhchenko L.V., Samochernykh K.A. Endovascular embolization of high-flow arteriovenous fistulae with non-adhesive agents in the structure of cerebral arteriovenous malformations on the background of adenosine-induced cardioplegia. *Zh Vopr Neirokhir Im N N Burdenko.* 2020; 84(3): 21-27. Russian. doi: 10.17116/neiro 20208403121.

Petrov A.E., Goroshchenko S.A., Rozhchenko L.V., Samochernykh K.A. Results of endovascular treatment for high-flow direct carotid-cavernous fistulas. *Journal of Radiology and Nuclear Medicine.* 2020; 101(5): 283–7 (in Russian). https://doi.org/10.20862/0042-4676-2020-101-5-283-287.

G. Odintsovaa, K. Samochernykhb, N. Samochernykhb, M. Nikolaenko Arachnoid cyst management in children. *Journal of the Neurological Sciences.* 405S (2019). p.51-52. doi:10.1016/j.jns.2019.10.312.

Samochernykh N., Sysoev K., Kim A., Samochernykh K., Ulitin A. C2 spinal nerve tumors in young adults: report of two cases and review of the literature. *Child's Nervous System.* (2020). https://doi.org/10.1007/s0038 1-020-04777-2.

Семенютин В.Б., Никифорова А., Самочерных К.А. Changes in default mode network connectivity in patients with postmastectomy syndrome. *Journal of the Neurological Sciences.* Vol. 429 Supplement. WCN 2021. XXV World Congress of Neurology. Virtual, 3-7.10.2021 DOI: https://doi.org/10.1016/j.jns.2021.118307.

I.K. Ternovykh, T.A. Bukkieva, M.L. Pospelova, A.Yu. Efimtsev, O.V. Fionik, T.M. Alekseeva, G.E. Trufanov, K.A. Samochernykh, N.E. Ivanova, V.V. Krasnikova, E.A. Gorbunova, A.G. Levchuk, A.A. Kasumova. Changes in default mode network connectivity in patients with postmastectomy syndrome. *Journal of the Neurological Sciences.* Vol. 429 Supplement. WCN 2021. XXV World Congress of Neurology. Virtual, 3-7.10.2021. DOI: https://doi.org/10.1016/j.jns.2021.118307

Dryagina Natalia

Affiliation: RNSI n.a. A.L. Polenov at Almazov National Medical Research Centre, Saint Petersburg, Russia

Education: St. Petersburg State Medical Academy, Russia

Business Address: 12, Mayakovskaya str., 191014, St.Petersburg

Research and Professional Experience: I am a participant of the following scientific programs:

1. state assignment «Development of new technologies for the diagnosis and management of patients with prolonged unconsciousness». 2018-2020.
2. state assignment «Development of a personalized approach to endovascular treatment of cerebral arteriovenous malformations based on the study of molecular mechanisms of neoangiogenesis" GRNTI 76.29.42 neurosurgery EGISU registration number 121031100282-3. 2021-2023
3. RFBR grant № 19-29-01066 «Methods of analyzing large unstructured data for developing a system for assessing the prognosis of restoring integrative brain function and creating treatment methods in conditions of disordered consciousness – a combination of loss and a new pathological integration of the body». 2019-2021.
4. RFBR grant № 20-015-00127 «The role of autoimmune neuroinflammation and apoptosis in the pathogenesis of pharmacoresistant epilepsy». 2020-2022.

Professional Appointments: clinical laboratory diagnostics

Publications from the Last 3 Years:

Gurskaia V.I., Ivanov V.P., Novikov V.Yu., Dryagina N.V., Savvina I.A. Systemic inflammatory response in infants with craniostenosis sedated with propofol. *Russian Journal of Pediatric Surgery, Anesthesia and Intensive Care.* 2021; 11(3): 297–306. (In Russ.). DOI: https://doi.org/10.17816/psaic961.

Kondratyeva E.A., Aybazova M.I., Lesteva N.A., Kondratyev S.A., Dryagina N.V., Kondratyev A.N. Assessment of nociception in patients with chronic disorders of consciousness using the analgesia nociception index. *Russian Journal of Anaesthesiology and Reanimatology =Anesteziologiya I Reanimatologiya.* 2021; 5: 34–39. (In Russ.). https://doi.org/10.17116/anaesthesiology20210513.

Gurskaya V.I., Dryagina N.V., Ivanov V.P., Aleksandrovich Yu. S., Khachatryan V.A., Savvina I.A. Effect of general anesthesia on systemic inflammatory response and neuronal damage in children with craniosynostosis in perioperative period. *Russian Journal of Anesthesiology and Reanimatology = Anesteziologiya i*

Reanimatologiya. 2021 (1): 39–45. (In Russ.) DOI: 10.17116/anaesthesiology202101139.

Dryagina N.V., Kondratyeva E.A., Kondratyev S.A., Potemkina E.G., Kondratyev A.N. Frequency of infectious complications and features of systemic inflammatory response in patients with prolonged disorders of consciousness. *Jurnal Infektologiithis.* 2021; 12(5): 21–28. (In Russ.) DOI: 10.22625/2072-6732-2020-12-5-21-28.

Dryagina N.V., Kondratyeva E.A., Dubrovskii Ya. A., Kondratyev A.N. Metabolome of the brain. *Russian Neurological Journal.* 2020; 25(1): 4–12. (In Russ.) DOI: 10.30629/2658-7947-2020-25-1-4-12.

Rozhchenko L.V., Dryagina N.V., Petrov A.E., Goroshchenko S.A. Molecular mechanisms of growth and recurrence of cerebral arteriovenous malformations: Part 2 (our own research). *Zhurnal Voprosy Nejrokhirurgii Imeni N.N. Burdenko.* 2020; 84(2): 35–41. (In Russ.) DOI: 10.17116/neiro20208402135.

Kondratev S., Dubrovskiy Y., Kondratyeva E., Dryagina N., Verbitskaya E. Metabolomic profiles of patients with unresponsive wakefullness syndrome. WEB OF SCIENCE. Published: Jun 2021 in *European Journal of Neurology.*

Rozhchenko L.V., Dryagina N.V. Modern approaches to treatment of complex cerebral arteriovenous malformations. *Translyatsionnaya meditsina = Translational Medicine.* 2020; 7 (5): 43-52. (In Russ.) DOI: 10.18705/2311-4495-2020-7-5-43-52.

Kondratyeva E., Aybazova M., Korostovtseva L., Ternovykh I., Dryagina N., Kondrayev S. Polysomnography (PSG), melatonin and hormones levels in disorders of consciousness patients. WEB OF SCIENCE. Published: Oct 2019 in *Journal of the Neurological Sciences.* 405:92-93. DOI: 10.1016/J.JNS. 2019.10.1737.

Metsker O., Aybazova M., Kondratyeva E., Dryagina N., Kondratyev A., Efimov E. Sepsis prediction using machine-learning methods: prolonged disorders of consciousness patients. WEB OF SCIENCE. Published: Oct 2019 in *Journal of the Neurological Sciences.* 405: 83. DOI: 10.1016/J.JNS.2019.10.1719.

Kondratyeva E., Aybazova M., Lesteva N., Kondratyev S., Kondratyev A., Dryagina N., Unresponsive wakefulness syndrome (UWS) and minimally conscious state (MCS) patients with myoclonus - Pathological variant organization of brain's function. WEB OF SCIENCE. Published: Oct 2019 in *Journal of the Neurological Sciences.* 405: 98. DOI: 10.1016/J.JNS. 2019.10.1748.

Kondratyeva E., Aybazova M., Dryagina N., Kondratyev A., Kondratev S. Results of the study of hormones and cytokines in patients in unresponsive wakefullness syndrome after TBI. WEB OF SCIENCE. Published: Oct 2019 in *Journal of the Neurological Sciences.* 405: 154-155. DOI: 10.1016/J.JNS.2019.10.735.

Ternovykh I., Kondratyeva E., Korostovtseva L., Dryagina N., Aybazova M., Kondratyev S. Long-term polysomnography (PSG) and melatonin levels in DOC patients as predicting the recovery of consciousness. WEB OF SCIENCE. Published: 2019 in *European Journal of Neurology.* 405:92-93. DOI: 10.1016/j.jns.2019.10.1737.

Baylieva Ainagul Zholdoshevna

Affiliation: Kazan State Medical University, head of the department of anesthesiology and IC, PhD, professor

Education: Kyrgyz State Medical Academy named after. I.K. Akhunbayeva, pediatrics

Business Address: Kazan State Medical University, Health Ministry of Russian Federation; 49 Butlerova Str., Kazan 420015, Russia;

Research and Professional Experience: Anesthesiology and intensive care in obstetrics, cardio and neurosurgery, pain management

Professional Appointments: Head of the clinic in the direction of "anaesthesiology and intensive care" of the Republican Clinical Hospital, Kazan, Republic of Tatarstan, Russia

Honors: Honored Doctor of the Republic of Tatarstan

Publications from the Last 3 Years:

Khasanov A.F., Burmistorov M.V., Bayalieva A. Zh., Shpaner R. Ya., Khasanova N.A., Bebezov S.I. Historical interweaving of surgery of the esophagus and its anesthetic management. Early stage of development. *Povolzhskii oncological bulletin*. No. 2, volume No. 10, pp. 39-51. ISSN: 2078-1466 http://oncovestnik.ru.

Bayalieva A. Zh., Ziganshin I.M., Babintseva A.A. Analysis of respiratory therapy of newborns with extremely low birth weight. *Russian bulletin of perinatology and pediatrics.* 2019 volume 64. P 171-176. Moscow DOI:10.21508.

Ziganshin I.M., Bayalieva A. Zh., Babintseva A.A., Shaimardanova G.R. Study of the effectiveness of artificial lung ventilation with the option of a guaranteed volume in newborns. *Bulletin of Intensive Care.* A.I. Saltanova. 2019 No. 4 Moscow. http://intensive-care.ru/archiv/.

Bayalieva A. Zh., Shpaner R. Ya., Ganeeva I.R., Volodyukhin M. Yu. Comparative evaluation of the methods of treatment of headache with radio-vascular occlusion of aneurysm. *Russian neurological journal named after pr. A.L. Polenova.* No. 3, Volume 11 p. 9-14 St. Petersburg. https://elibrary.ru/title_about.asp?id=30975.

Bayalieva A. Zh., Shpaner R. Ya. Infusion therapy as a correction of hemodynamics in patients with subarachnoid hemorrhage in the acute period. *Practical medicine.* No. 6 (part 1), volume 17.

Bayalieva A. Zh., Shpaner R. Ya., Nabiullina A.D., Davydova V.R. The results of 50 years of work of the Department of Anesthesiology-Resuscitation and Transfusiology of the Kazan State Medical Academy. *Kazan medical journal.* No. 5 Volume 100, p. 860-864 Kazan.

Bayalieva A. Zh., Zefirov R.A., Yankovich Yu. N. Peculiarities of managing patients with gastrointestinal bleeding in intensive care units. *Kazan medical journal.* No. 6 Volume 100, p. 930-934.

Bayalieva A. Zh., Shpaner R. Ya. "Organization of care for patients with non-traumatic subarachnoid hemorrhages in the Republic of Tatarstan" *Bulletin of Modern Clinical Medicine.* Kazan, 2019, Volume 12, issue 1, p. 18-24, DOI: 10.20969/ VSKM.2019. 12(1). 1.

Bayalieva A. Zh., Davydova V.R., Shpaner R. Ya. Adverse effects of intensive care: it is possible to avoid? *Russian neurological journal named after pr. A.L. Polenovap.* 64-73.

S.A. Makoveev, A. Khussein, N.V. Perembetov, A.V. Khlopushin, A.V. Eremeev, D.N. Protsenko, N.V. Tselykh, K.G. Shapovalov, and R. Emelyanov S., Bayalieva A. Zh., Zabolotskikh I.B., Schegolev A.V., Potapov A.F., Matveev A.S., Kirov M. Yu. "The frequency, structure and outcomes of hypothermia in adult patients upon admission to the intensive care unit and intensive care unit: a multicenter retrospective study."*Anesteshiology and IC.* №4 (2019). p.31-38.

R.F. Shavaliyev, M.M. Minnullin, R.A. Zefirov, R.N. Akhundov, A. Zh. Bayalieva, Sh. pancreatitis." *Creative surgery and oncology.* Vol 9, No 4 (2019) https://doi.org/10.24060/2076-3093-2019-9-4-254-260

Bayalieva A. Zh., Shpaner R. Ya. "Effect of inhalation anesthetic (sevoflurane) and propofol on awakening and postoperative complications in neurosurgical interventions." *Russian neurosurgical journal by prof A.L. Polenov.* 2020. Vol. 2. p. 389-390.

L.I. Maltseva, E. Yu. Yupatov, R.S. Zamaleeva, I.F. Fatkullin, A. Zh. Bayalieva, M.E. Zhelezova, T.P. Zefirova, R.I. Gabidullina, I.S. Raginov, L.S. Fatkullina, I.R. Galimova, N.R. Akhmadeev, S.V. Gubaidullina, A.A. Evstratov. Clinical observation of a severe course of a new coronavirus infection COVID-19, which complicated the postpartum period in a puerperal woman who underwent a caesarean section. *Obstetrics, gynecology and reproduction.* 2021. Volume 15, No. 3 Moscow. https://doi.org/10.17749/2313-7347/ob.gyn.rep.2021.19

A. Zh. Bayalieva, S.D. Gardanov, A.A. Surikov. Mediastinitis due to Cervical Osteophytes in a Patient after Hemithyroidectomy. *Turkish journal of anesthesiology and reanimatology.* 2021; 49(3): 250-253 Turkey. https://turkjanaesthesiolreanim.org/ EN/june-2021-0073

Munir Mohsin

Affiliation: Kazan State Medical University, Resident anesthesiology and intensive care. Department of anesthesiology and intensive care.

Education: Semey State Medical University, Kazakhstan

Business Address: Kazan State Medical University, Health Ministry of Russian Federation; 49 Butlerova Str., Kazan 420015, Russia;

Research and Professional Experience: Anesthesiology and intensive care

Professional Appointments: Anesthesiologist and Intensivist. Municipal City Hospital No. 4. City Ust-Kamenogorsk. Kazakhstan.

Davydova Veronika Rustemovna

Affiliation: Kazan State Medical University, department of anesthesiology and IC, PhD, assistant professor

Education: Kazan State Medical University

Business Address: Kazan State Medical University, Health Ministry of Russian Federation; 49 Butlerova Str., Kazan 420015, Russia;

Research and Professional Experience: Anesthesiology and intensive care in obstetrics, oncogynecology, pain management, intensive care of post IC syndrome.

Professional Appointments: anesthesiologist and IC doctor of Clinical city hospital №7, Kazan

Publications from the Last 3 Years:

Bayalieva A. Zh., Shpaner R. Ya., Nabiullina A.D., Davydova V.R. The results of 50 years of work of the Department of Anesthesiology-Resuscitation and Transfusiology of the Kazan State Medical Academy. *Kazan medical journal.* No. 5 Volume 100, p. 860-864. Kazan.

Bayalieva A. Zh., Davydova V. R., Shpaner R. Ya. Adverse effects of intensive care: it is possible to avoid? *Russian neurological journal named after pr. A.L. Polenova.* 2019. p.64-73.

T.A. Fedorova, N.A. Barskovskaya, V.A. Vdovin, O.V. Rogachevskiy, N. Yu. Katkova, V.R. Davydova. Experience in the use of recombinant activated coagulation factor 7 in the treatment of massive obstetric bleeding. *Issues of gynecology, obstetrics and perinatology.* 2021, volume 20, № 6, p. 30-42.

Shpaner Roman Yakovlevich

Affiliation: Kazan State Medical University, head of the department of anesthesiology and IC, PhD, assistant professor

Education: Kazan State Medical University

Business Address: Kazan State Medical University, Health Ministry of Russian Federation; 49 Butlerova Str., Kazan 420015, Russia;

Research and Professional Experience: Anesthesiology and intensive care in neurosurgery surgery, pain management

Professional Appointments: Head of the department of anesthesiology and intensive care of the Republican Clinical Hospital, Kazan, Republic of Tatarstan, Russia

Honors: Certificate of Honor of the Ministry of Health of the Republic of Tatarstan, Certificate of Honor of the Committee for Labor Protection of the State Duma of the Russian Federation

Publications from the Last 3 Years:

Khasanov A.F., Burmistorov M.V., Bayalieva A. Zh., Shpaner R. Ya., Khasanova N.A., Bebezov S.I. Historical interweaving of surgery of the esophagus and its anesthetic management. Early stage of development. *Povolzhskii oncological bulletin*. No. 2, volume No. 10, pp. 39-51. ISSN: 2078-1466. http://oncovestnik.ru.

Bayalieva A. Zh., Shpaner R. Ya., Ganeeva I.R., Volodyukhin M. Yu. Comparative evaluation of the methods of treatment of headache with radio-vascular occlusion of aneurysm. *Russian neurological journal named after pr. A.L. Polenova*. No. 3, Volume 11 p. 9-14 St. Petersburg. https://elibrary.ru/title_about.asp?id=30975.

Bayalieva A. Zh., Shpaner R. Ya. Infusion therapy as a correction of hemodynamics in patients with subarachnoid hemorrhage in the acute period. *Practical medicine*. No. 6 (part 1), volume 17.

Bayalieva A. Zh., Shpaner R. Ya., Nabiullina A.D., Davydova V.R. The results of 50 years of work of the Department of Anesthesiology-Resuscitation and Transfusiology of the Kazan State Medical Academy. *Kazan medical journal.* No. 5 Volume 100, p. 860-864 Kazan.

Bayalieva A. Zh., Shpaner R. Ya. "Organization of care for patients with non-traumatic subarachnoid hemorrhages in the Republic of Tatarstan" *Bulletin of Modern Clinical Medicine.* Kazan, 2019, Volume 12, issue 1, p. 18-24, DOI: 10.20969/VSKM.2019.12(1).1.

Bayalieva A. Zh., Davydova V.R., Shpaner R. Ya. Adverse effects of intensive care: it is possible to avoid? *Russian neurological journal named after pr. A.L. Polenova.* p.64-73.

Bayalieva A. Zh. Shpaner R. Ya. "Effect of inhalation anesthetic (sevoflurane) and propofol on awakening and postoperative complications in neurosurgical interventions." *Russian neurosurgical journal by prof A.L. Polenov.* 2020. Vol. 2.p. 389-390.

Eleonora T. Nazaralieva

Affiliation:

- Department of Paediatric Neurosurgery, Almazov National Medical Research Centre of Ministry of Health Care of Russian Federation, Saint Petersburg, Russian Federation;
- National Hospital of Ministry of Health of Kyrgyzstan Republik, Bishkek, Kyrgyzstan

Education: Kyrgyz State Medical Academy, Bishkek, Kyrgyzstan
Business Address: Department of Paediatric Neurosurgery, Almazov National Medical Research Centre of Ministry of Health Care of Russian Federation Akkuratova str. 197341, Saint Petersburg, Russian Federation

Research and Professional Experience and Professional Appointments:

- May 2021 – Today: Department of Paediatric Neurosurgery, Almazov National Medical Research Centre of Ministry of Health Care of Russian Federation – Researcher, Neurosurgeon
- Dec 2009 - Sep 2018: National Hospital of Ministry of Health of Kyrgyz Republic, Bishkek, Kyrgyzstan - Neurosurgeon

Honours:

- Sep 2014: ASNS – scholarship for or the best achievements in the field of neurooncology among young scientists

Publications from the Last 3 Years:

Yu. A. Atiskov., S.K. Akshulakov., A.A. Belkin., E.T. Nazaralieva., V.P. Riznich., Sh. M. Safin., I. Sh. Safin., B.V. Gaydar., W.A. Khachatryan. Brain biomechanics: monitoring the biomechanical properties of the human craniospinal system. *Russian Journal of Biomechanics.* 2020. Vol.24, No 2: pp.111-124.

Yu. A. Atiskov., W.A. Khachatryan., E.T. Nazaralieva., A. Ya. Malikov., V.P. Riznich. A Craniospinal Compliance Monitor. *Biomedical Engineering.* Vol.54, No.6, March, 2021, pp.380-383.

Nazaralieva E.T., Riznich V.P., Khachatryan W.A. New approaches to the diagnosis of intracranial hypertension. *Russian Neurosurgical Journal.* Professor A.L. Polenov. 2021. Vol. 13. No. S1. pp. 156-157.

Nazaralieva E.T., Gerasimov A.P., Zabrodskaya Yu. M., Ivanova N.E., Shevtsov M.A., Khachatryan W.A. Some genetic markers of low-grade cerebral gliomas in children and their potential importance in the development of therapy. *Russian Neurosurgical Journal.* Professor A.L. Polenov. 2021. V. 13. No. 4. S. 103-110.

Nazaralieva E.T., Cherebillo V. Yu., Khachatryan W.A. Modern aspects of the study of pituitary adenomas and issues of epidemiology. *Modern problems of science and education.* 2021. No. 4. P. 103.

Atiskov Yu. A., Akshulakov S.K., Belkin A.A., Kondratyev A.N., Larionov S.N., Nazaralieva E.T., Riznich V.P., Savvina I.A., Safin I. Sh., Khachatryan W.A. Craniospinal compliance - new principles for monitoring intracranial pressure. *Anesthesiology and resuscitation.* (Media Sphere). 2020. No. 6. S. 37-43.

Akshulakov S.K., Bazarhandaeva T.B., Gaidar B.V., Dallakyan N.O., Don O.A., Kim A.V., Nazaralieva E.T., Olenbay G.I., Safin Sh. M., Khachatryan W.A. Surgery for brainstem tumors. *Neurosurgery and neurology of Kazakhstan.* No. 3 (56), 2019, pp. 3-22.

Khachatryan William A.

Affiliation: Department of Paediatric Neurosurgery, Almazov National Medical Research Centre of Ministry of Health Care of Russian Federation, Saint Petersburg, Russian Federation;

Education: Yerevan Medical Institute, Yerevan, Armenia

Business Address: Department of Paediatric Neurosurgery, Almazov National Medical Research Centre of Ministry of Health Care of Russian Federation Akkuratova str. 197341, Saint Petersburg, Russian Federation

Research and Professional Experience and Professional Appointments:

- May 1980 – Today: Department of Paediatric Neurosurgery, Almazov National Medical Research Centre of Ministry of Health Care of Russian Federation – Head of the Research Laboratory of Pediatric Neurosurgery

Honours:

- 2014: Honorary Professor of the Center for Neurosurgery, Nur-Sultan, Kazakhstan
- 2007: Awarded the title of Academician of the Academy of Medical and Technical Sciences of the Russian Federation.
- 2002: Editor-in-chief of the scientific and practical journal "Neurosurgery and neurology of childhood"
- 1998: Awarded the title of professor.

Publications from the Last 3 Years:

Nizolin D.V., Fedorov E.V., Kim A.V., Mitrofanova L.B., Khachatryan W.A. Combination of tumors of different histogenesis in pediatric neurosurgery. *Questions of neurosurgery.* N.N. Burdenko. 2021. V. 85. No. 2. S. 80-90.

Volkodav O.V., Khachatryan W.A. Methods for improving the effectiveness of hydrocephalus treatment in neonatal practice. *Russian Bulletin of Perinatology and Pediatrics.* 2021. V. 66. No. 4. S. 141-147.

Mamatkhanov M.R., Khachatryan W.A., Lebedev K.E. Analysis of the results of surgical treatment of epilepsy. *Russian Neurosurgical Journal.* Professor A.L. Polenov. 2021. Vol. 13. No. S1. pp. 124-125.

Kim A.V., Fedorov E.V., Khachatryan W.A. Recurrence of neuroepithelial brain tumors in children. *Russian Neurosurgical Journal.* Professor A.L. Polenov. 2021. Vol. 13. No. S1. S. 123.

Yu. A. Atiskov., S.K. Akshulakov., A.A. Belkin., E.T. Nazaralieva., V.P. Riznich., Sh. M. Safin, I. Sh. Safin, B.V. Gaydar., W.A. Khachatryan. Brain biomechanics: monitoring the biomechanical properties of the human craniospinal system. *Russian Journal of Biomechanics.* 2020. Vol.24, No 2: pp.111-124.

Yu. A. Atiskov., W.A. Khachatryan., E.T. Nazaralieva., A. Ya. Malikov., V.P. Riznich. A Craniospinal Compliance Monitor. *Biomedical Engineering.* Vol.54, No.6, March, 2021, pp.380-383.

Nazaralieva E.T., Riznich V.P., Khachatryan W.A. New approaches to the diagnosis of intracranial hypertension. *Russian Neurosurgical Journal.* Professor A.L. Polenov. 2021. Vol. 13. No. S1. pp. 156-157.

Nazaralieva E.T., Gerasimov A.P., Zabrodskaya Yu. M., Ivanova N.E., Shevtsov M.A., Khachatryan W.A. Some genetic markers of low-grade cerebral gliomas in children and their potential importance in the development of therapy. *Russian Neurosurgical Journal.* Professor A.L. Polenov. 2021. V. 13. No. 4. S. 103-110.

Nazaralieva E.T., Cherebillo V. Yu., Khachatryan W.A. Modern aspects of the study of pituitary adenomas and issues of epidemiology. *Modern problems of science and education.* 2021. No. 4.P. 103.

Atiskov Yu. A., Akshulakov S.K., Belkin A.A., Kondratyev A.N., Larionov S.N., Nazaralieva E.T., Riznich V.P., Savvina I.A., Safin I. Sh., Khachatryan W.A. Craniospinal compliance - new principles for monitoring intracranial pressure. *Anesthesiology and resuscitation.* (Media Sphere).2020. No. 6. S. 37-43.

Akshulakov S.K., Bazarhandaeva T.B., Gaidar B.V., Dallakyan N.O., Don O.A., Kim A.V., Nazaralieva E.T., Olenbay G.I., Safin Sh.M., Khachatryan W.A. Surgery for brain stem tumors. *Neurosurgery and neurology of Kazakhstan*. No. 3 (56), 2019, pp. 3-22.

Index